INTRODUCTION TO BACTERIOLOGY

Edited by
Kristy June

ArclerPress

Introduction to Bacteriology

Edited by Kristy June

Edition 2018

ArclerPress

Published by
Arcler Press LLC
708 3rd Avenue, 6th Floor
New York
NY 10017
United States of America
www.arclerpress.com

ISBN: 978-1-68094-527-0 (Hardback)

Printed in United States of America

Library of Congress Control Number: 2017933172

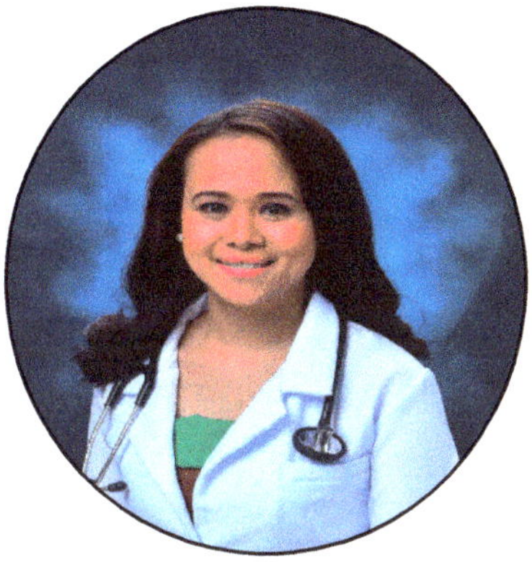

About the Editor

Kristy June

Kristy June is a Doctor of Medicine who also masters copyediting and proofreading scientific and academic research papers. She finished Bachelor of Science in Biology Major in Ecology and Entomology in the University of the Philippines Mindanao as her undergraduate degree where she started engaging herself into writing, editing and proofreading articles and books for publications. She is currently working as both a Medical Doctor and an Editor

Table of Contents

2 BACTERIAL CELL MORPHOLOGY

3 BACTERIAL TAXONOMY

4 BACTERIAL CELL STRUCTURE

5 BACTERIAL GENETICS

6 THEORY OF BACTERIOPHAGE

7 PATHOGENIC BACTERIA

8 HUMAN MICROBIOTA

9 HUMAN VIROME

List of Abbreviations

ANUG	Acute Necrotizing Ulcerative Gingivitis
ACV	Aeropyrum Coil-Shaped Virus
ARMAN	Archaeal Richmond Mine Acidophilic Nanoorganisms
BER	Base Excision Repair
CRP	cAMP Receptor Protein
CAP	Catabolite Activator Protein
Cra	Catabolite Repressor Activator
COPD	Chronic Obstructive Pulmonary Disease
CFU	Colony Forming Units
CDT	Cytolethal Distending Toxin
EPS	Extracellular Polymeric Substances
FDA	Food and Drug Administration
GRAS	Generally Recognized As Safe
HPLC	High Precision Chromatography
HMP	Human Microbiome Project
HPV	Human Papillomaviruses
IARC	International Agency for Research on Cancer
ICSB	International Committee on Systematic Bacteriology
ICTV	International Committee on Taxonomy of Viruses
LPS	Lipopolysaccharide
MAMPs	Microbe-Associated Molecular Patterns
MIC	Minimal Inhibitory Concentration
MDR	Multidrug Resistant

NAG	N-Acetylglucosamine
NAM	N-Acetylmuramic Acid
ORF	Open Reading Frame
OMP	Outer Membrane Protein
PBPs	Penicillin-Binding Proteins
PS	Photosystem
PPLO	Pleuropneumonia-like Organism
PCR	Polymerase Chain Reaction
PAP	Primary Atypical Pneumonia
PLoS	Public Library of Science
ROS	Reactive Oxygen Species
RTE	Ready-to-Eat
RNAP	RNA Polymerase
TLRs	Toll like Receptors
TME	Tumor Microenvironment
USDA	United States Department of Agriculture

Preface

Bacteriology is the study of bacteria. Bacteria are microscopic organisms composed of a single cell. In bacteriology, the structure, functions, and growth of various bacteria have been discovered. Bacteriology has also explored the positive and negative impact of bacteria in the environment and in human beings. Another important function is the identification of bacteria that often cause disease in man and animals, and the mechanisms of how they bring about infection. This is an important aspect of bacteriology, which leads to the development of antibiotics or antibacterial drugs known to treat diseases caused by bacteria. Bacteria are single-celled microorganisms that lack a nuclear membrane, are metabolically active and divide by binary fission. Medically they are a major cause of disease. Superficially, bacteria appear to be relatively simple forms of life; in fact, they are sophisticated and highly adaptable. Many bacteria multiply at rapid rates, and different species can utilize an enormous variety of hydrocarbon substrates, including phenol, rubber, and petroleum. These organisms exist widely in both parasitic and free-living forms. Because they are ubiquitous and have a remarkable capacity to adapt to changing environments by selection of spontaneous mutants, the importance of bacteria in every field of medicine cannot be overstated.

The discipline of bacteriology evolved from the need of physicians to test and apply the germ theory of disease and from economic concerns relating to the spoilage of foods and wine. The initial advances in pathogenic bacteriology were derived from the identification and characterization of bacteria associated with specific diseases. During this period, great emphasis was placed on applying Koch's postulates to test proposed cause-and-effect relationships between bacteria and specific diseases. Today, most bacterial diseases of humans and their etiologic agents have been identified, although important variants continue to evolve and sometimes emerge, e.g., Legionnaire's Disease, tuberculosis and toxic shock syndrome.

Content Coverage

Chapter One introduces the basic concepts of bacteria, such as etymology, evolution, growth and reproduction, as well as classification and identification of bacteria.

Chapters Two presents an emphasis on the morphology of bacteria and bacterial taxonomy.

Chapter Four discusses "about the" bacterial cell structure. Bacteria, despite their simplicity, contain a well-developed cell structure which, is responsible for some of their unique biological structures and pathogenicity. Many structural features are unique to bacteria and are not found among archaea or eukaryotes.

Chapter Five presents the study of the mechanisms of heritable information in bacteria, their chromosomes, plasmids, transposons and phages.

Chapter Six offers the theory of bacteriophage; a virus that infects and replicates within a bacterium. Phages are widely distributed in locations populated by bacterial hosts, such as soil or the intestines of animals.

Chapters Seven and *Eight* discuss "about with" human pathogenic bacteria and human microbiota which is the aggregate of microorganisms, "respectively".

Chapter Nine provides the knowledge of human virome. The human virome is far from being completely explored and new viruses are discovered frequently. Viruses evolve rapidly and hence the human virome changes constantly. Every human being has a unique virome with a unique balance of species

CHAPTER 1

Bacteria: An Introduction

Chapter Contents

- Introduction
- Etymology
- Origin and Early Evolution
- Morphology
- Cellular Structure
- Metabolism
- Growth and Reproduction
- Genomes
- Genetics
- Behaviour
- Classification and Identification
- Interactions with Other Organisms

Bacteria are single-celled microbes. The cell structure is simpler than that of other organisms as there is no nucleus or membrane-bound organelles. Instead their control center containing the genetic information is contained in a single loop of DNA. Some bacteria have an extra circle of genetic material called a plasmid.

INTRODUCTION

Bacteria constitute a large domain of prokaryotic microorganisms. Typically a few micrometres in length, bacteria have a number of shapes, ranging from spheres to rods and spirals. Bacteria are among the first life forms to appear on Earth, and are present in most of its habitats. Bacteria inhabit soil, water, acidic hot springs, radioactive waste, and the deep portions of Earth's crust. Bacteria also live in symbiotic and parasitic relationships with plants and animals.

There are typically 40 million bacterial cells in a gram of soil and a million bacterial cells in a millilitre of fresh water. There are approximately 5×1030 bacteria on Earth, forming a biomass which exceeds that of all plants and animals. Bacteria are vital in recycling nutrients, with many of the stages in nutrient cycles dependent on these organisms, such as the fixation of nitrogen from the atmosphere and putrefaction. In the biological communities surrounding hydrothermal vents and cold seeps, bacteria provide the nutrients needed to sustain life by converting dissolved compounds, such as hydrogen sulphide and methane, to energy. On 17 March 2013, researchers reported data that suggested bacterial life forms thrive in the Mariana Trench, which with a depth of up to 11 kilometres is the deepest part of the Earth's oceans.Other researchers reported related studies that microbes thrive inside rocks up to 580 metres below the sea floor under 2.6 kilometres of ocean off the coast of the northwestern United States. According to one of the researchers, You can find microbes everywhere — they're extremely adaptable to conditions, and survive wherever they are.

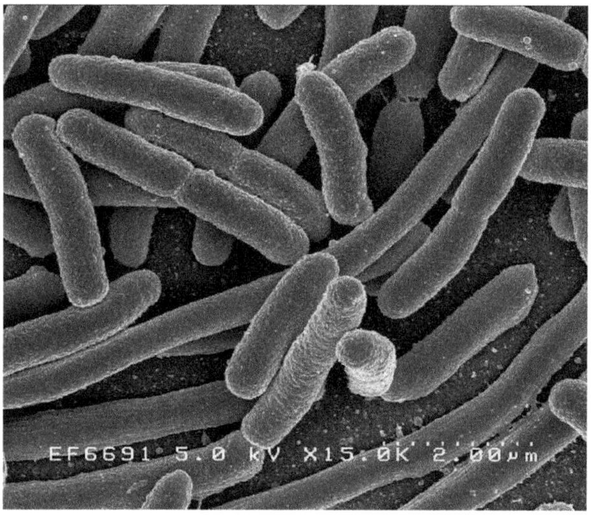

Most bacteria have not been characterised, and only about half of the bacterial phyla have species that can be grown in the laboratory. The study of bacteria is known as bacteriology, a branch of microbiology.

There are approximately ten times as many bacterial cells in the human flora as there are human cells in the body, with the largest number of the human flora being in the gut flora, and a large number on the skin. The vast majority of the bacteria in the body are rendered harmless by the protective effects of the immune system, and some are beneficial. However, several species of bacteria are pathogenic and cause infectious diseases, including cholera, syphilis, anthrax, leprosy, and bubonic plague. The most common fatal bacterial diseases are respiratory infections, with tuberculosis alone killing about 2 million people per year, mostly in sub-Saharan Africa. In developed countries, antibiotics are used to treat bacterial infections and are also used in farming, making antibiotic resistance a growing problem. In industry, bacteria are important in sewage treatment and the breakdown of oil spills, the production of cheese and yogurt through fermentation, and the recovery of gold, palladium, copper and other metals in the mining sector, as well as in biotechnology, and the manufacture of antibiotics and other chemicals.

Once regarded as plants constituting the class Schizomycetes, bacteria are now classified as prokaryotes. Unlike cells of animals and other eukaryotes, bacterial cells do not contain a nucleus and rarely harbour membrane-bound organelles. Although the term bacteria traditionally included all prokaryotes, the scientific classification changed after the discovery in the 1990s that prokaryotes consist of two very different groups of organisms that evolved from an ancient common ancestor. These evolutionary domains are called Bacteria and Archaea.

ETYMOLOGY

The word bacteria is the plural of the New Latin bacterium, which is the latinisation of the Greek βακτήριον (bakterion), the diminutive of βακτηρία (bakteria), meaning "staff, cane", because the first ones to be discovered were rod-shaped.

ORIGIN AND EARLY EVOLUTION

The ancestors of modern bacteria were unicellular microorganisms that were the first forms of life to appear on Earth, about 4 billion years ago. For about 3 billion years, most organisms were microscopic, and bacteria and archaea were the dominant forms of life. In 2008, fossils of macroorganisms were discovered and named as the Francevillian biota. Although bacterial fossils exist, such as stromatolites, their lack of distinctive morphology prevents them from being used to examine the history of bacterial evolution, or to date the time of origin of a particular bacterial species. However, gene sequences can be used to reconstruct the bacterial phylogeny, and these studies indicate that bacteria diverged first from the archaeal/eukaryotic lineage. Bacteria were also involved in the second great evolutionary divergence, that of the archaea and eukaryotes. Here, eukaryotes resulted from the entering of ancient bacteria into endosymbiotic associations with the ancestors of eukaryotic cells, which were themselves possibly related to the Archaea. This involved the engulfment by proto-eukaryotic cells of alphaproteobacterial symbionts to form either mitochondria or hydrogenosomes, which are still found in all known Eukarya (sometimes in highly reduced form, e.g. in ancient amitochondrial protozoa). Later on, some eukaryotes that already contained mitochondria also engulfed cyanobacterial-like organisms. This led to the formation of chloroplasts in algae and plants. There are also some algae that originated from even later endosymbiotic events. Here, eukaryotes engulfed a eukaryotic algae that developed into a "second-generation" plastid. This is known as secondary endosymbiosis.

MORPHOLOGY

Bacteria display a wide diversity of shapes and sizes, called morphologies. Bacterial cells are about one-tenth the size of eukaryotic cells and are typically 0.5–5.0 micrometres in length. However, a few species are visible to the unaided eye — for example, Thiomargarita namibiensis is up to half a millimetre long and Epulopiscium fishelsoni reaches 0.7 mm. Among the smallest bacteria are members of the genus Mycoplasma, which measure only 0.3 micrometres, as small as the largest viruses. Some bacteria may be even smaller, but these ultramicrobacteria are not well-studied.

Most bacterial species are either spherical, called cocci (sing. coccus, from Greek kókkos, grain, seed), or rod-shaped, called bacilli (sing. bacillus, from Latin baculus, stick). Elongation is associated with swimming. Some bacteria, called vibrio, are shaped like slightly curved rods or comma-shaped; others can be spiral-shaped, called spirilla, or tightly coiled, called spirochaetes. A small number of species even have tetrahedral or cuboidal shapes. More recently, some bacteria were discovered deep under Earth's crust that grow as branching filamentous types with a star-shaped cross-section. The large surface area to volume ratio of this morphology may give these bacteria an advantage in nutrient-poor environments. This wide variety of shapes is determined by the bacterial cell wall and cytoskeleton, and is important because it can influence the ability of bacteria to acquire nutrients, attach to surfaces, swim through liquids and escape predators.

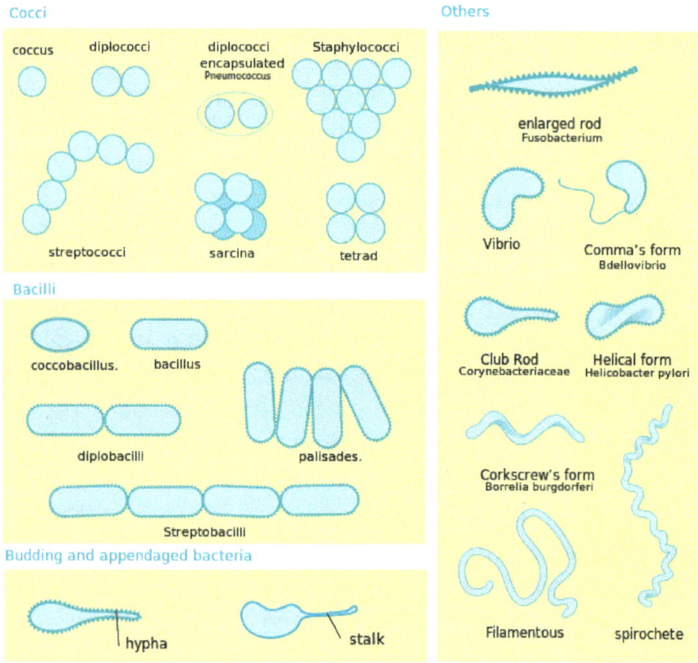

Bacteria display many cell morphologies and arrangements

Many bacterial species exist simply as single cells, others associate in characteristic patterns: Neisseria form diploids (pairs), Streptococcus form chains, and Staphylococcus group together in "bunch of grapes" clusters. Bacteria can also be elongated to form filaments, for example the Actinobacteria. Filamentous bacteria are often surrounded by a sheath that contains many individual cells. Certain types, such as species of the genus Nocardia, even form complex, branched filaments, similar in appearance to fungal mycelia.

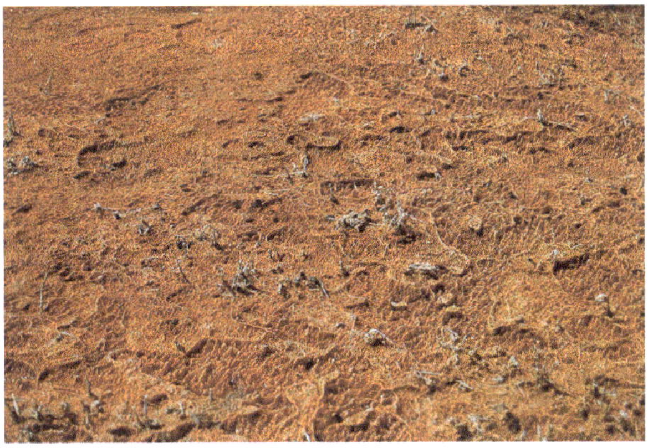

A biofilm of thermophilic bacteria in the outflow of Mickey Hot Springs, Oregon, approximately 20 mm thick.

Bacteria often attach to surfaces and form dense aggregations called biofilms or bacterial mats. These films can range from a few micrometres in thickness to up to half a metre in depth, and may contain multiple species of bacteria, protists and archaea. Bacteria living in biofilms display a complex arrangement of cells and extracellular components, forming secondary structures, such as microcolonies, through which there are networks of channels to enable better diffusion of nutrients. In natural environments, such as soil or the surfaces of plants, the majority of bacteria are bound to surfaces in biofilms. Biofilms are also important in medicine, as these structures are often present during chronic bacterial infections or in infections of implanted medical devices, and bacteria protected within biofilms are much harder to kill than individual isolated bacteria.

Even more complex morphological changes are sometimes possible. For example, when starved of amino acids, Myxobacteria detect surrounding cells in a process known as quorum sensing, migrate towards each other, and aggregate to form fruiting bodies up to 500 micrometres long and containing approximately 100,000 bacterial cells. In these fruiting bodies, the bacteria perform separate tasks; this type of cooperation is a simple type of multicellular organisation. For example, about one in 10 cells migrate to the top of these fruiting bodies and differentiate into a specialised dormant state called myxospores, which are more resistant to drying and other adverse environmental conditions than are ordinary cells.

CELLULAR STRUCTURE

Intracellular Structures

The bacterial cell is surrounded by a cell membrane (also known as a lipid, cytoplasmic or plasma membrane). This membrane encloses the contents of the cell and acts as a barrier to hold nutrients, proteins and other essential components of the cytoplasm within the cell. As they are prokaryotes, bacteria do not usually have membrane-bound organelles in their cytoplasm, and thus contain few large intracellular structures. They lack a true nucleus, mitochondria, chloroplasts and the other organelles present in eukaryotic cells. Bacteria were once seen as simple bags of cytoplasm, but structures such as the prokaryotic cytoskeleton and the localisation of proteins to specific locations within the cytoplasm that give bacteria some complexity have been discovered. These subcellular levels of organisation have been called "bacterial hyperstructures".

Bacterial microcompartments, such as carboxysomes, provide a further level of organisation; they are compartments within bacteria that are surrounded by polyhedral protein shells, rather than by lipid membranes. These "polyhedral organelles" localise and compartmentalise bacterial metabolism, a function performed by the membrane-bound organelles in eukaryotes.

Many important biochemical reactions, such as energy generation, use concentration gradients across membranes. The general lack of internal membranes in bacteria means reactions such as electron transport occur across the cell membrane between the cytoplasm and the periplasmic space. However, in many photosynthetic bacteria the plasma membrane is highly folded and fills most of the cell with layers of light-gathering membrane. These light-gathering complexes may even form lipid-enclosed structures called chlorosomes in green sulfur bacteria. Other proteins import nutrients across the cell membrane, or expel undesired molecules from the cytoplasm.

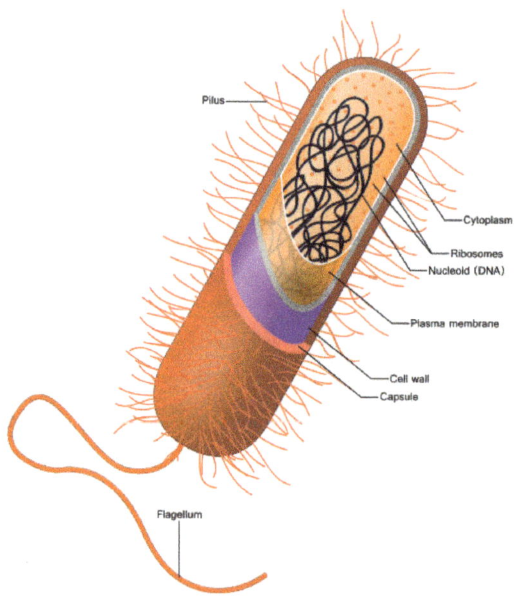

Structure and contents of a typical gram-positive bacterial cell (seen by the fact that only *one* cell membrane is present).

Bacteria do not have a membrane-bound nucleus, and their genetic material is typically a single circular DNA chromosome located in the cytoplasm in an irregularly shaped body called the nucleoid. The nucleoid contains the chromosome with its associated proteins and

RNA. The phylum Planctomycetes and candidate phylum Poribacteria may be exceptions to the general absence of internal membranes in bacteria, because they appear to have a double membrane around their nucleoids and contain other membrane-bound cellular structures. Like all living organisms, bacteria contain ribosomes, often grouped in chains called polyribosomes, for the production of proteins, but the structure of the bacterial ribosome is different from that of eukaryotes and Archaea.

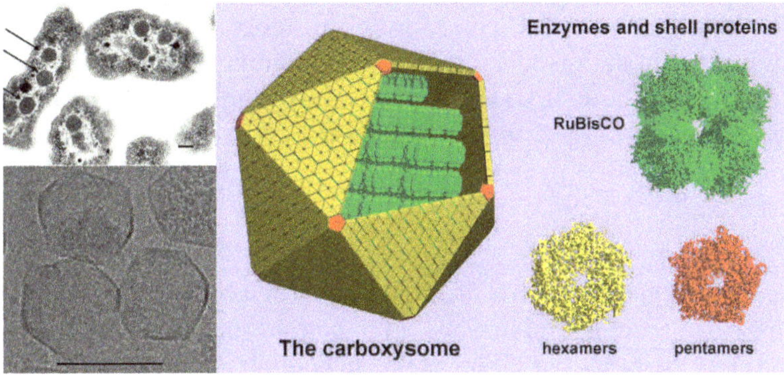

Carboxysomes are protein-enclosed bacterial organelles. Top left is an electron microscope image of carboxysomes in *Halothiobacillus neapolitanus*, below is an image of purified carboxysomes. On the right is a model of their structure. Scale bars are 100 nm.

Bacterial ribosomes have a sedimentation rate of 70S (measured in Svedberg units): their subunits have rates of 30S and 50S. Some antibiotics bind specifically to 70S ribosomes and inhibit bacterial protein synthesis. Those antibiotics kill bacteria without affecting the larger 80S ribosomes of eukaryotic cells and without harming the host.

Some bacteria produce intracellular nutrient storage granules for later use, such as glycogen, polyphosphate, sulfur or polyhydroxyalkanoates. Certain bacterial species, such as the photosynthetic Cyanobacteria, produce internal gas vesicles, which they use to regulate their buoyancy – allowing them to move up or down into water layers with different light intensities and nutrient levels. Intracellular membranes called chromatophores are also found in membranes of phototrophic bacteria. Used primarily for photosynthesis, they contain bacteriochlorophyll pigments and carotenoids. An early idea was that bacteria might contain membrane folds termed mesosomes, but these were later shown to be artefacts produced by the chemicals used to prepare the cells for electron microscopy. Inclusions are considered to be nonliving components of the cell that do not possess metabolic activity and are not bounded by membranes. The most common inclusions are glycogen, lipid droplets, crystals, and pigments. Volutin granules are cytoplasmic inclusions of complexed inorganic polyphosphate. These granules are called metachromatic granules due to their displaying the metachromatic effect; they appear red or blue when stained with the blue dyes methylene blue or toluidine blue. Gas vacuoles, which are freely permeable to gas, are membrane-bound vesicles present in some species of Cyanobacteria. They allow the bacteria to control their buoyancy. Microcompartments are widespread, membrane-bound organelles that are made of a protein shell that surrounds and encloses various enzymes. Carboxysomes are bacterial microcompartments that contain enzymes involved in carbon fixation. Magnetosomes are bacterial microcompartments, present in magnetotactic bacteria, that contain magnetic crystals.

Extracellular Structures

In most bacteria, a cell wall is present on the outside of the cell membrane. The cell membrane and cell wall comprise the cell envelope. A common bacterial cell wall material is peptidoglycan (called "murein" in older sources), which is made from polysaccharide chains cross-linked by peptides containing D-amino acids. Bacterial cell walls are different from the cell walls of plants and fungi, which are made of cellulose and chitin, respectively. The cell wall of bacteria is also distinct from that of Archaea, which do not contain peptidoglycan. The cell wall is essential to the survival of many bacteria, and the antibiotic penicillin is able to kill bacteria by inhibiting a step in the synthesis of peptidoglycan.

There are broadly speaking two different types of cell wall in bacteria, a thick one in the gram-positives and a thinner one in the gram-negatives. The names originate from the reaction of cells to the Gram stain, a long-standing test for the classification of bacterial species.

Gram-positive bacteria possess a thick cell wall containing many layers of peptidoglycan and teichoic acids. In contrast, gram-negative bacteria have a relatively thin cell wall consisting of a few layers of peptidoglycan surrounded by a second lipid membrane containing lipopolysaccharides and lipoproteins. Lipopolysaccharides, also called endotoxins, are composed of polysaccharides and lipid A that is responsible for much of the toxicity of gram-negative bacteria. Most bacteria have the gram-negative cell wall, and only the Firmicutes and Actinobacteria have the alternative gram-positive arrangement. These two groups were previously known as the low G+C and high G+C gram-positive bacteria, respectively. These differences in structure can produce differences in antibiotic susceptibility; for instance, vancomycin can kill only gram-positive bacteria and is ineffective against gram-negative pathogens, such as Haemophilus influenzae or Pseudomonas aeruginosa. If the bacterial cell wall is entirely removed, it is called a protoplast, whereas if it is partially removed, it is called a spheroplast. β-Lactam antibiotics, such as penicillin, inhibit the formation of peptidoglycan cross-links in the bacterial cell wall. The enzyme lysozyme, found in human tears, also digests the cell wall of bacteria and is the body's main defence against eye infections.

Acid-fast bacteria, such as Mycobacteria, are resistant to decolorisation by acids during staining procedures. The high mycolic acid content of Mycobacteria, is responsible for the staining pattern of poor absorption followed by high retention. The most common staining technique used to identify acid-fast bacteria is the Ziehl-Neelsen stain or acid-fast stain, in which the acid-fast bacilli are stained bright-red and stand out clearly against a blue background. L-form bacteria are strains of bacteria that lack cell walls. The main pathogenic bacteria in this class is Mycoplasma (not to be confused with Mycobacteria).

In many bacteria, an S-layer of rigidly arrayed protein molecules covers the outside of the cell. This layer provides chemical and physical protection for the cell surface and can act as a macromolecular diffusion barrier. S-layers have diverse but mostly poorly understood functions, but are known to act as virulence factors in Campylobacter and contain surface enzymes in Bacillus stearothermophilus.

Flagella are rigid protein structures, about 20 nanometres in diameter and up to 20 micrometres in length, that are used for motility. Flagella are driven by the energy released by the transfer of ions down an electrochemical gradient across the cell membrane.

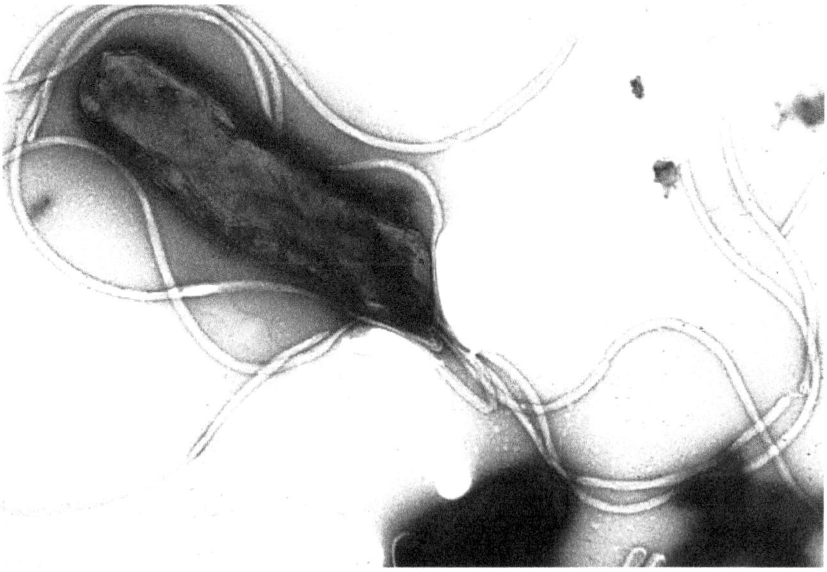

Helicobacter pylori electron micrograph, showing multiple flagella on the cell surface

Fimbriae (sometimes called "attachment pili) are fine filaments of protein, usually 2–10 nanometres in diameter and up to several micrometres in length. They are distributed over the surface of the cell, and resemble fine hairs when seen under the electron microscope. Fimbriae are believed to be involved in attachment to solid surfaces or to other cells, and are essential for the virulence of some bacterial pathogens. Pili (sing. pilus) are cellular appendages, slightly larger than fimbriae, that can transfer genetic material between bacterial cells in a process called conjugation where they are called conjugation pili or "sex pili (see bacterial genetics, below). They can also generate movement where they are called type IV pili (see movement, below).

Glycocalyx are produced by many bacteria to surround their cells, and vary in structural complexity: ranging from a disorganised slime layer of extra-cellular polymer to a highly structured capsule. These structures can protect cells from engulfment by eukaryotic cells such as macrophages (part of the human immune system). They can also act as antigens and be involved in cell recognition, as well as aiding attachment to surfaces and the formation of biofilms.

The assembly of these extracellular structures is dependent on bacterial secretion systems. These transfer proteins from the cytoplasm into the periplasm or into the environment around the cell. Many types of secretion systems are known and these structures are often essential for the virulence of pathogens, so are intensively studied.

Endospores

Certain genera of gram-positive bacteria, such as Bacillus, Clostridium, Sporohalobacter, Anaerobacter, and Heliobacterium, can form highly resistant, dormant structures called endospores. In almost all cases, one endospore is formed and this is not a reproductive process, although Anaerobacter can make up to seven endospores in a single cell. Endospores have a central core of cytoplasm containing DNA and ribosomes surrounded by a cortex layer and protected by an impermeable and rigid coat. Dipicolinic acid is a chemical compound that composes 5% to 15% of the dry weight of bacterial spores. It is implicated as responsible for the heat resistance of the endospore.

Endospores show no detectable metabolism and can survive extreme physical and chemical stresses, such as high levels of UV light, gamma radiation, detergents, disinfectants, heat, freezing, pressure, and desiccation. In this dormant state, these organisms may remain viable for millions of years, and endospores even allow bacteria to survive exposure to the vacuum and radiation in space. According to scientist Dr. Steinn Sigurdsson, "There are viable bacterial spores that have been found that are 40 million years old on Earth — and we know they're very hardened to radiation."Endospore-forming bacteria can also cause disease: for example, anthrax can be contracted by the inhalation of Bacillus anthracis endospores, and contamination of deep puncture wounds with Clostridium tetani endospores causes tetanus.

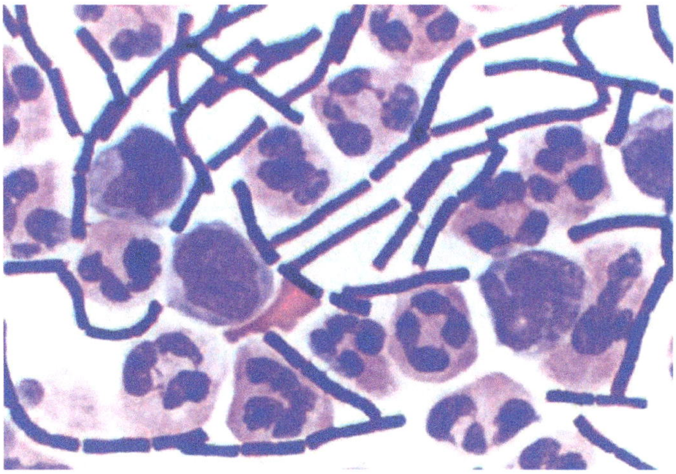

Bacillus anthracis (stained purple) growing in cerebrospinal fluid

METABOLISM

Bacteria exhibit an extremely wide variety of metabolic types. The distribution of metabolic traits within a group of bacteria has traditionally been used to define their taxonomy, but these traits often do not correspond with modern genetic classifications. Bacterial metabolism is classified into nutritional groups on the basis of three major criteria: the kind of energy used for growth, the source of carbon, and the electron donors used for growth. An additional criterion of respiratory microorganisms are the electron acceptors used for aerobic or anaerobic respiration.

Nutritional types in bacterial metabolism

Nutritional type	Source of energy	Source of carbon	Examples
Phototrophs	Sunlight	Organic compounds (photoheterotrophs) or carbon fixation (photoautotrophs)	Cyanobacteria, Green sulfur bacteria, Chloroflexi, or Purple bacteria
Lithotrophs	Inorganic compounds	Organic compounds (lithoheterotrophs) or carbon fixation (lithoautotrophs)	Thermodesulfobacteria, *Hydrogenophilaceae*, or Nitrospirae
Organotrophs	Organic compounds	Organic compounds (chemoheterotrophs) or carbon fixation (chemoautotrophs)	*Bacillus*, *Clostridium* or *Enterobacteriaceae*

Carbon metabolism in bacteria is either heterotrophic, where organic carbon compounds are used as carbon sources, or autotrophic, meaning that cellular carbon is obtained by fixing carbon dioxide. Heterotrophic bacteria include parasitic types. Typical autotrophic bacteria are phototrophic cyanobacteria, green sulfur-bacteria and some purple bacteria, but also many chemolithotrophic species, such as nitrifying or sulfur-oxidising bacteria. Energy metabolism of bacteria is either based on phototrophy, the use of light through photosynthesis, or based on chemotrophy, the use of chemical substances for energy, which are mostly oxidised at the expense of oxygen or alternative electron acceptors (aerobic/anaerobic respiration).

Bacteria are further divided into lithotrophs that use inorganic electron donors and organotrophs that use organic compounds as electron donors. Chemotrophic organisms use the respective electron donors for energy conservation (by aerobic/anaerobic respiration or fermentation) and biosynthetic reactions (e.g., carbon dioxide fixation), whereas phototrophic organisms use them only for biosynthetic purposes. Respiratory organisms use chemical compounds as a source of energy by taking electrons from the reduced substrate and transferring them to a terminal electron acceptor in a redox reaction. This reaction releases energy that can be used to synthesise ATP and drive metabolism. In aerobic organisms, oxygen is used as the electron acceptor. In anaerobic organisms other inorganic compounds, such as nitrate, sulfate or carbon dioxide are used as electron acceptors. This leads to the ecologically important processes of denitrification, sulfate reduction, and acetogenesis, respectively.

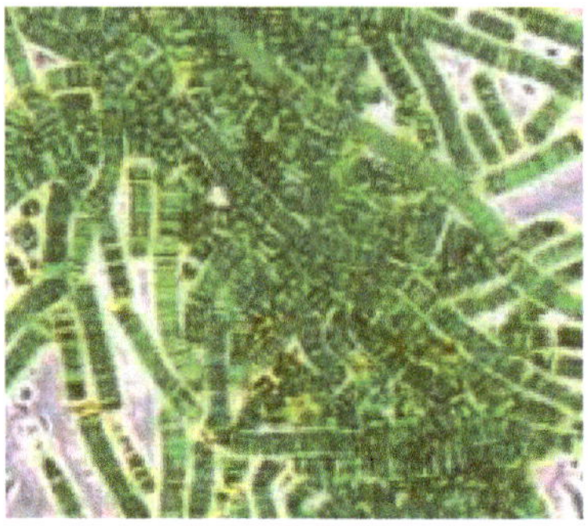

Filaments of photosyntheticcyanobacteria

Another way of life of chemotrophs in the absence of possible electron acceptors is fermentation, wherein the electrons taken from the reduced substrates are transferred to oxidised intermediates to generate reduced fermentation products (e.g., lactate, ethanol, hydrogen, butyric acid). Fermentation is possible, because the energy content of the substrates is higher than that of the products, which allows the organisms to synthesise ATP and drive their metabolism.

These processes are also important in biological responses to pollution; for example, sulfate-reducing bacteria are largely responsible for the production of the highly toxic forms of mercury (methyl- and dimethylmercury) in the environment. Non-respiratory anaerobes use fermentation to generate energy and reducing power, secreting metabolic by-products (such as ethanol in brewing) as waste. Facultative anaerobes can switch between fermentation and different terminal electron acceptors depending on the environmental conditions in which they find themselves.

Lithotrophic bacteria can use inorganic compounds as a source of energy. Common inorganic electron donors are hydrogen, carbon monoxide, ammonia (leading to nitrification), ferrous iron and other reduced metal ions, and several reduced sulfur compounds. In unusual circumstances, the gas methane can be used by methanotrophic bacteria as both a source of electrons and a substrate for carbon anabolism. In both aerobic phototrophy and chemolithotrophy, oxygen is used as a terminal electron acceptor, whereas under anaerobic conditions inorganic compounds are used instead. Most lithotrophic organisms are autotrophic, whereas organotrophic organisms are heterotrophic.

In addition to fixing carbon dioxide in photosynthesis, some bacteria also fix nitrogen gas (nitrogen fixation) using the enzyme nitrogenase. This environmentally important trait can be found in bacteria of nearly all the metabolic types listed above, but is not universal.

Regardless of the type of metabolic process they employ, the majority of bacteria are able to take in raw materials only in the form of relatively small molecules, which enter the cell by diffusion or through molecular channels in cell membranes. The Planctomycetes are the exception (as they are in possessing membranes around their nuclear material). It has recently been shown that Gemmata obscuriglobus is able to take in large molecules via a process that in some ways resembles endocytosis, the process used by eukaryotic cells to engulf external items.

GROWTH AND REPRODUCTION

Unlike in multicellular organisms, increases in cell size (cell growth) and reproduction by cell division are tightly linked in unicellular organisms. Bacteria grow to a fixed size and then reproduce through binary fission, a form of asexual reproduction.

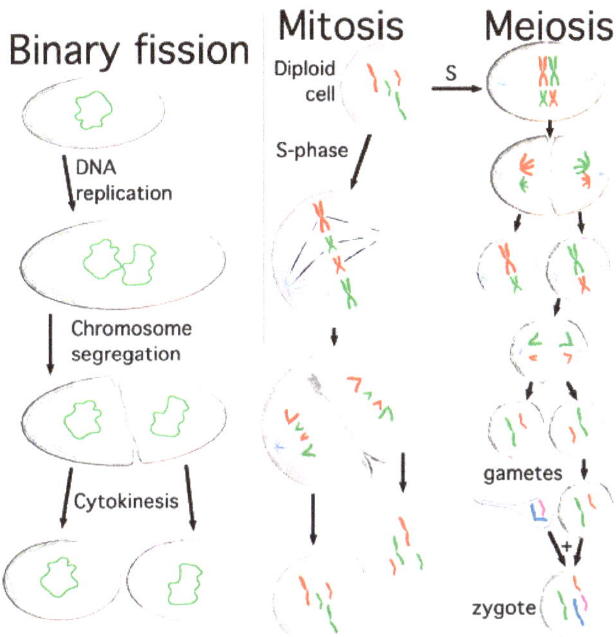

Many bacteria reproduce through binary fission, which is compared to mitosis and meiosis in this image.

Under optimal conditions, bacteria can grow and divide extremely rapidly, and bacterial populations can double as quickly as every 9.8 minutes. In cell division, two identical clone daughter cells are produced. Some bacteria, while still reproducing asexually, form more complex reproductive structures that help disperse the newly formed daughter cells. Examples include fruiting body formation by Myxobacteria and aerial hyphae formation by Streptomyces, or budding. Budding involves a cell forming a protrusion that breaks away and produces a daughter cell.

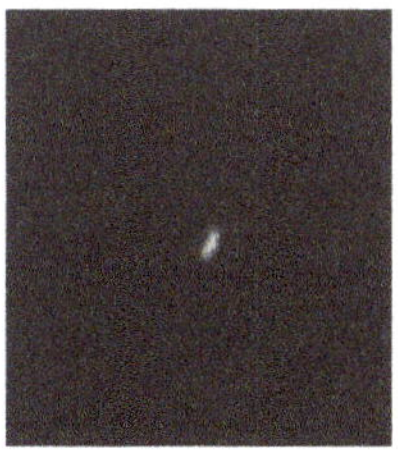

A colony of *Escherichia coli*

In the laboratory, bacteria are usually grown using solid or liquid media. Solid growth media, such as agar plates, are used to isolate pure cultures of a bacterial strain. However, liquid growth media are used when measurement of growth or large volumes of cells are required. Growth in stirred liquid media occurs as an even cell suspension, making the cultures easy to divide and transfer, although isolating single bacteria from liquid media is difficult. The use of selective media (media with specific nutrients added or deficient, or with antibiotics added) can help identify specific organisms.

Most laboratory techniques for growing bacteria use high levels of nutrients to produce large amounts of cells cheaply and quickly. However, in natural environments, nutrients are limited, meaning that bacteria cannot continue to reproduce indefinitely. This nutrient limitation has led the evolution of different growth strategies (see r/K selection theory). Some organisms can grow extremely rapidly when nutrients become available, such as the formation of algal (and cyanobacterial) blooms that often occur in lakes during the summer. Other organisms have adaptations to harsh environments, such as the production of multiple antibiotics by Streptomyces that inhibit the growth of competing microorganisms. In nature, many organisms live in communities (e.g., biofilms) that may allow for increased supply of nutrients and protection from environmental stresses. These relationships can be essential for growth of a particular organism or group of organisms (syntrophy).

Bacterial growth follows four phases. When a population of bacteria first enter a high-nutrient environment that allows growth, the cells need to adapt to their new environment. The first phase of growth is the lag phase, a period of slow growth when the cells are adapting to the high-nutrient environment and preparing for fast growth. The lag phase has high biosynthesis rates, as proteins necessary for rapid growth are produced.The second phase of growth is the log phase, also known as the logarithmic or exponential phase. The log phase is marked by rapid exponential growth. The rate at which cells grow during this phase is known as the growth rate (k), and the time it takes the cells to double is known as the generation time (g). During log phase, nutrients are metabolised at maximum speed until one of the nutrients is depleted and starts limiting growth. The third phase of growth is the stationary phase and is caused by depleted nutrients. The cells reduce their metabolic activity and consume non-essential cellular proteins. The stationary phase is a transition from rapid growth to a stress response state and there is increased expression of genes involved in DNA repair, antioxidant metabolism and nutrient transport. The final phase is the death phase where the bacteria run out of nutrients and die.

GENOMES

The genomes of thousands of bacterial species have been sequenced, with at least 9,000 sequences completed and more than 42,000 left as "permanent" drafts (as of Sep 2016).

Most bacteria have a single circular chromosome that can range in size from only 160,000 base pairs in the endosymbiotic bacteria Candidatus Carsonella ruddii, to 12,200,000 base pairs in the soil-dwelling bacteria Sorangium cellulosum. The genes in bacterial genomes are usually a single continuous stretch of DNA and although several different types of introns do exist in bacteria, these are much rarer than in eukaryotes.Some bacteria, including the Spirochaetes of the genus Borrelia are a notable exception to this arrangement. Borrelia burgdorferi, the cause of Lyme disease, contains a single linear chromosome and several linear and circular plasmids.

Plasmids are small extra-chromosomal DNAs that may contain genes for antibiotic resistance or virulence factors. Plasmids replicate independently of chromosomes, so it is possible that plasmids could be lost in bacterial cell division. Against this possibility is the fact that a single bacterium can contain hundreds of copies of a single plasmid.

GENETICS

Bacteria, as asexual organisms, inherit identical copies of their parent's genes (i.e., they are clonal). However, all bacteria can evolve by selection on changes to their genetic material DNA caused by genetic recombination or mutations. Mutations come from errors made during the replication of DNA or from exposure to mutagens. Mutation rates vary widely among different species of bacteria and even among different clones of a single species of bacteria. Genetic changes in bacterial genomes come from either random mutation during replication or stress-directed mutation, where genes involved in a particular growth-limiting process have an increased mutation rate.

DNA Transfer

Some bacteria also transfer genetic material between cells. This can occur in three main ways. First, bacteria can take up exogenous DNA from their environment, in a process called *transformation*. Genes can also be transferred by the process of *transduction*, when the integration of a bacteriophage introduces foreign DNA into the chromosome. The third method of gene transfer is *conjugation*, whereby DNA is transferred through direct cell contact.

Transduction of bacterial genes by bacteriophage appears to be a consequence of infrequent errors during intracellular assembly of virus particles, rather than a bacterial adaptation. Conjugation, in the much-studied E. coli system is determined by plasmid genes, and is an adaptation for transferring copies of the plasmid from one bacterial host to another. It is seldom that a conjugative plasmid integrates into the host bacterial chromosome, and subsequently transfers part of the host bacterial DNA to another bacterium. Plasmid-mediated transfer of host bacterial DNA also appears to be an accidental process rather than a bacterial adaptation.

Transformation, unlike transduction or conjugation, depends on numerous bacterial gene products that specifically interact to perform this complex process, and thus transformation is clearly a bacterial adaptation for DNA transfer. In order for a bacterium to bind, take up and recombine donor DNA into its own chromosome, it must first enter a special physiological state termed competence (see Natural competence). In Bacillus subtilis, about 40 genes are required for the development of competence. The length of DNA transferred during B. subtilis transformation can be between a third of a chromosome up to the whole chromosome. Transformation appears to be common among bacterial species, and thus far at least 60 species are known to have the natural ability to become competent for transformation. The development of competence in nature is usually associated with stressful environmental conditions, and seems to be an adaptation for facilitating repair of DNA damage in recipient cells.

In ordinary circumstances, transduction, conjugation, and transformation involve transfer of DNA between individual bacteria of the same species, but occasionally transfer may occur between individuals of different bacterial species and this may have significant consequences, such as the transfer of antibiotic resistance. In such cases, gene acquisition from other bacteria or the environment is called horizontal gene transfer and may be common under natural conditions. Gene transfer is particularly important in antibiotic resistance as it allows the rapid transfer of resistance genes between different pathogens.

Bacteriophages

Bacteriophages are viruses that infect bacteria. Many types of bacteriophage exist, some simply infect and lyse their host bacteria, while others insert into the bacterial chromosome. A bacteriophage can contain genes that contribute to its host's phenotype: for example, in the evolution of Escherichia coli O157:H7 and Clostridium botulinum, the toxin genes in an integrated phage converted a harmless ancestral bacterium into a lethal pathogen. Bacteria resist phage infection through restriction modification systems that degrade foreign DNA, and a system that uses CRISPR sequences to retain fragments of the genomes of phage that the bacteria have come into contact with in the past, which allows them to block virus replication through a form of RNA interference. This CRISPR system provides bacteria with acquired immunity to infection.

BEHAVIOUR

Secretion

Bacteria frequently secrete chemicals into their environment in order to modify it favourably. The secretions are often proteins and may act as enzymes that digest some form of food in the environment.

Bioluminescence

A few bacteria have chemical systems that generate light. This bioluminescence often occurs in bacteria that live in association with fish, and the light probably serves to attract fish or other large animals.

Multicellularity

Bacteria often function as multicellular aggregates known as biofilms, exchanging a variety of molecular signals for inter-cell communication, and engaging in coordinated multicellular behaviour. The communal benefits of multicellular cooperation include a cellular division of labour, accessing resources that cannot effectively be used by single cells, collectively defending against antagonists, and optimising population survival by differentiating into distinct cell types. For example, bacteria in biofilms can have more than 500 times increased resistance to antibacterial agents than individual "planktonic" bacteria of the same species. One type of inter-cellular communication by a molecular signal is called quorum sensing, which serves the purpose of determining whether there is a local population density that is sufficiently high that it is productive to invest in processes that are only successful if large numbers of similar organisms behave similarly, as in excreting digestive enzymes or emitting light. Quorum sensing allows bacteria to coordinate gene expression, and enables them to produce, release and detect autoinducers or pheromones which accumulate with the growth in cell population.

Movement

Many bacteria can move using a variety of mechanisms: flagella are used for swimming through fluids; bacterial gliding and twitching motility move bacteria across surfaces; and changes of buoyancy allow vertical motion.

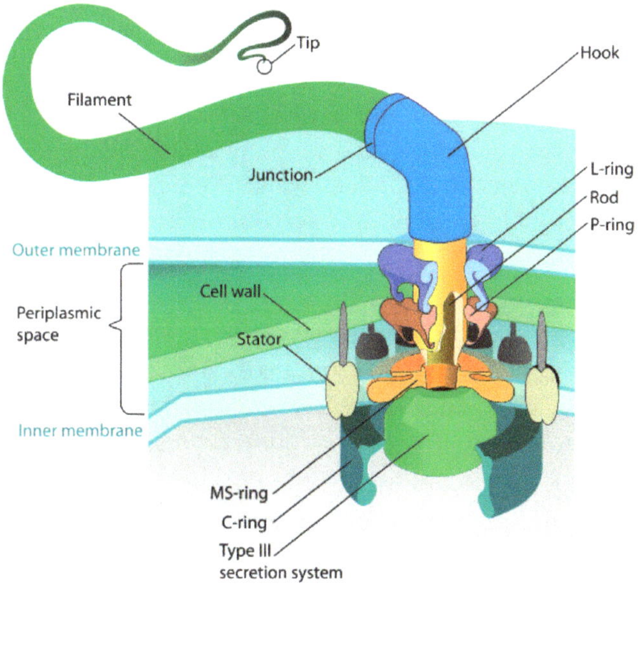

Flagellum of gram-negative bacteria. The base drives the rotation of the hook and filament.

Swimming bacteria frequently move near 10 body lengths per second and a few as fast as 100. This makes them at least as fast as fish, on a relative scale.

In bacterial gliding and twitching motility, bacteria use their type IV pili as a grappling hook, repeatedly extending it, anchoring it and then retracting it with remarkable force (>80 pN).

"Our observations redefine twitching motility as a rapid, highly organized mechanism of bacterial translocation by which Pseudomonas aeruginosa can disperse itself over large areas to colonize new territories. It is also now clear, both morphologically and genetically, that twitching motility and social gliding motility, such as occurs in Myxococcus xanthus, are essentially the same process.

—A re-examination of twitching motility in Pseudomonas aeruginosa – Semmler, Whitchurch & Mattick (1999)

Flagella are semi-rigid cylindrical structures that are rotated and function much like the propeller on a ship. Objects as small as bacteria operate a low Reynolds number and cylindrical forms are more efficient than the flat, paddle-like, forms appropriate at human-size scale.

Bacterial species differ in the number and arrangement of flagella on their surface; some have a single flagellum (monotrichous), a flagellum at each end (amphitrichous), clusters of flagella at the poles of the cell (lophotrichous), while others have flagella distributed over the entire surface of the cell (peritrichous). The bacterial flagella is the best-understood motility structure in any organism and is made of about 20 proteins, with approximately another 30 proteins required for its regulation and assembly. The flagellum is a rotating structure driven by a reversible motor at the base that uses the electrochemical gradient across the membrane for power. This motor drives the motion of the filament, which acts as a propeller.

Many bacteria (such as E. coli) have two distinct modes of movement: forward movement (swimming) and tumbling. The tumbling allows them to reorient and makes their movement a three-dimensional random walk. (See external links below for link to videos.) The flagella of a unique group of bacteria, the spirochaetes, are found between two membranes in the periplasmic space. They have a distinctive helical body that twists about as it moves.

Motile bacteria are attracted or repelled by certain stimuli in behaviours called taxes: these include chemotaxis, phototaxis, energy taxis, and magnetotaxis. In one peculiar group, the myxobacteria, individual bacteria move together to form waves of cells that then differentiate to form fruiting bodies containing spores. The myxobacteria move only when on solid surfaces, unlike E. coli, which is motile in liquid or solid media.

Several Listeria and Shigella species move inside host cells by usurping the cytoskeleton, which is normally used to move organelles inside the cell. By promoting actin polymerisation at one pole of their cells, they can form a kind of tail that pushes them through the host cell's cytoplasm.

CLASSIFICATION AND IDENTIFICATION

Classification seeks to describe the diversity of bacterial species by naming and grouping organisms based on similarities. Bacteria can be classified on the basis of cell structure, cellular metabolism or on differences in cell components, such as DNA, fatty acids, pigments, antigens and quinones. While these schemes allowed the identification and classification of bacterial strains, it was unclear whether these differences represented variation between distinct species or between strains of the same species. This uncertainty was due to the lack of distinctive structures in most bacteria, as well as lateral gene transfer between unrelated species. Due to lateral gene transfer, some closely related bacteria can have very different morphologies and metabolisms. To overcome this uncertainty, modern bacterial classification emphasises molecular systematics, using genetic techniques such as guanine cytosine ratio determination, genome-genome hybridisation, as well as sequencing genes that have not undergone extensive lateral gene transfer, such as the rRNA gene. Classification of bacteria is determined by publication in the International Journal of Systematic Bacteriology, and Bergey's Manual of Systematic Bacteriology. The International Committee on Systematic Bacteriology (ICSB) maintains international rules for the naming of bacteria and taxonomic categories and for the ranking of them in the International Code of Nomenclature of Bacteria.

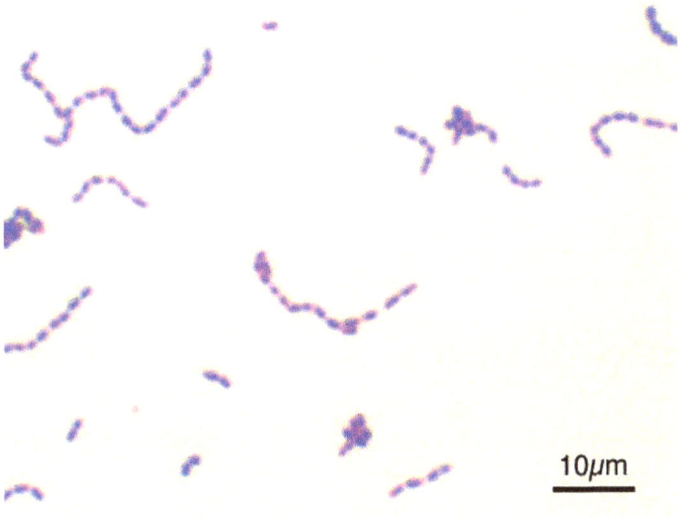

Streptococcus mutans visualised with a Gram stain

The term bacteria was traditionally applied to all microscopic, single-cell prokaryotes. However, molecular systematics showed prokaryotic life to consist of two separate domains, originally called Eubacteria and Archaebacteria, but now called Bacteria and Archaea that evolved independently from an ancient common ancestor. The archaea and eukaryotes are more closely related to each other than either is to the bacteria. These two domains, along with Eukarya, are the basis of the three-domain system, which is currently the most widely used classification system in microbiolology. However, due to the relatively recent introduction of molecular systematics and a rapid increase in the number of genome sequences that are available, bacterial classification remains a changing and expanding field. For example, a few biologists argue that the Archaea and Eukaryotes evolved from gram-positive bacteria.

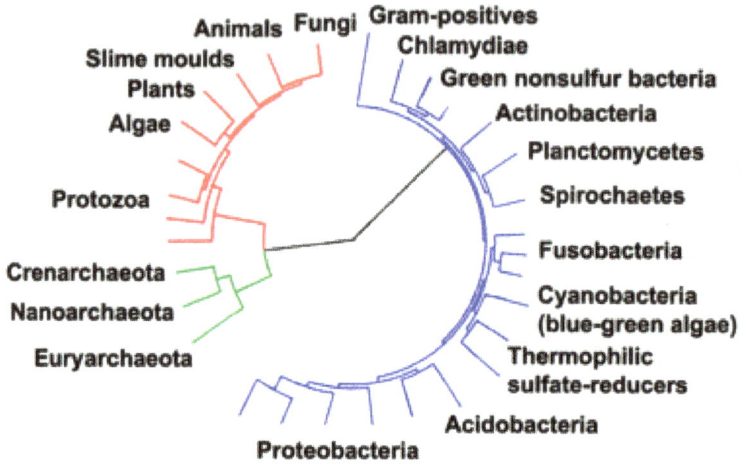

Phylogenetic tree showing the diversity of bacteria, compared to other organisms. Eukaryotes are coloured red, archaea green and bacteria blue.

The identification of bacteria in the laboratory is particularly relevant in medicine, where the correct treatment is determined by the bacterial species causing an infection. Consequently, the need to identify human pathogens was a major impetus for the development of techniques to identify bacteria.

The Gram stain, developed in 1884 by Hans Christian Gram, characterises bacteria based on the structural characteristics of their cell walls. The thick layers of peptidoglycan in the "gram-positive" cell wall stain purple, while the thin "gram-negative" cell wall appears pink. By combining morphology and Gram-staining, most bacteria can be classified as belonging to one of four groups (gram-positive cocci, gram-positive bacilli, gram-negative cocci and gram-negative bacilli). Some organisms are best identified by stains other than the Gram stain, particularly mycobacteria or Nocardia, which show acid-fastness on Ziehl–Neelsen or similar stains. Other organisms may need to be identified by their growth in special media, or by other techniques, such as serology.

Culture techniques are designed to promote the growth and identify particular bacteria, while restricting the growth of the other bacteria in the sample. Often these techniques are designed for specific specimens; for example, a sputum sample will be treated to identify organisms that cause pneumonia, while stool specimens are cultured on selective media to identify organisms that cause diarrhoea, while preventing growth of non-pathogenic bacteria. Specimens that are normally sterile, such as blood, urine or spinal fluid, are cultured under conditions designed to grow all possible organisms. Once a pathogenic organism has been isolated, it can be further characterised by its morphology, growth patterns (such as aerobic or anaerobic growth), patterns of hemolysis, and staining.

As with bacterial classification, identification of bacteria is increasingly using molecular methods. Diagnostics using DNA-based tools, such as polymerase chain reaction, are increasingly popular due to their specificity and speed, compared to culture-based methods.

These methods also allow the detection and identification of viable but nonculturable cells that are metabolically active but non-dividing. However, even using these improved methods, the total number of bacterial species is not known and cannot even be estimated with any certainty. Following present classification, there are a little less than 9,300 known species of prokaryotes, which includes bacteria and archaea; but attempts to estimate the true number of bacterial diversity have ranged from 107 to 109 total species – and even these diverse estimates may be off by many orders of magnitude.

INTERACTIONS WITH OTHER ORGANISMS

Despite their apparent simplicity, bacteria can form complex associations with other organisms. These symbiotic associations can be divided into parasitism, mutualism and commensalism. Due to their small size, commensal bacteria are ubiquitous and grow on animals and plants exactly as they will grow on any other surface. However, their growth can be increased by warmth and sweat, and large populations of these organisms in humans are the cause of body odour.

Predators

Some species of bacteria kill and then consume other microorganisms, these species are called predatory bacteria. These include organisms such as Myxococcus xanthus, which forms swarms of cells that kill and digest any bacteria they encounter. Other bacterial predators either attach to their prey in order to digest them and absorb nutrients, such as Vampirovibrio chlorellavorus, or invade another cell and multiply inside the cytosol, such as Daptobacter. These predatory bacteria are thought to have evolved from saprophages that consumed dead microorganisms, through adaptations that allowed them to entrap and kill other organisms.

Mutualists

Certain bacteria form close spatial associations that are essential for their survival. One such mutualistic association, called interspecies hydrogen transfer, occurs between clusters of anaerobic bacteria that consume organic acids, such as butyric acid or propionic acid, and produce hydrogen, and methanogenic Archaea that consume hydrogen. The bacteria in this association are unable to consume the organic acids as this reaction produces hydrogen that accumulates in their surroundings. Only the intimate association with the hydrogen-consuming Archaea keeps the hydrogen concentration low enough to allow the bacteria to grow.

In soil, microorganisms that reside in the rhizosphere (a zone that includes the root surface and the soil that adheres to the root after gentle shaking) carry out nitrogen fixation, converting nitrogen gas to nitrogenous compounds. This serves to provide an easily absorbable form of nitrogen for many plants, which cannot fix nitrogen themselves. Many other bacteria are found as symbionts in humans and other organisms. For example, the presence of over 1,000 bacterial species in the normal human gut flora of the intestines can contribute to gut immunity, synthesise vitamins, such as folic acid, vitamin K and biotin, convert sugars to lactic acid (see Lactobacillus), as well as fermenting complex undigestible carbohydrates. The presence of this gut flora also inhibits the growth of potentially pathogenic bacteria (usually through competitive exclusion) and these beneficial bacteria are consequently sold as probiotic dietary supplements.

Pathogens

If bacteria form a parasitic association with other organisms, they are classed as pathogens. Pathogenic bacteria are a major cause of human death and disease and cause infections such as tetanus, typhoid fever, diphtheria, syphilis, cholera, foodborne illness, leprosy and tuberculosis. A pathogenic cause for a known medical disease may only be discovered many years after, as was the case with Helicobacter pylori and peptic ulcer disease. Bacterial diseases are also important in agriculture, with bacteria causing leaf spot, fire blight and wilts in plants, as well as Johne's disease, mastitis, salmonella and anthrax in farm animals.

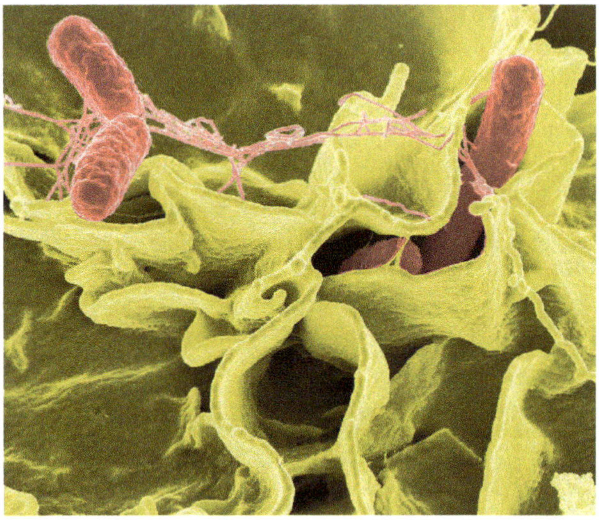

Colour-enhanced scanning electron micrograph showing *Salmonella typhimurium* (red) invading cultured human cells

Each species of pathogen has a characteristic spectrum of interactions with its human hosts. Some organisms, such as Staphylococcus or Streptococcus, can cause skin infections, pneumonia, meningitis and even overwhelming sepsis, a systemic inflammatory response producing shock, massive vasodilation and death. Yet these organisms are also part of the normal human flora and usually exist on the skin or in the nose without causing any disease at all. Other organisms invariably cause disease in humans, such as the Rickettsia, which are obligate intracellular parasites able to grow and reproduce only within the cells of other organisms. One species of Rickettsia causes typhus, while another causes Rocky Mountain spotted fever. Chlamydia, another phylum of obligate intracellular parasites, contains species that can cause pneumonia, or urinary tract infection and may be involved in coronary heart disease. Finally, some species, such as Pseudomonas aeruginosa, Burkholderia cenocepacia, and Mycobacterium avium, are opportunistic pathogens and cause disease mainly in people suffering from immunosuppression or cystic fibrosis.

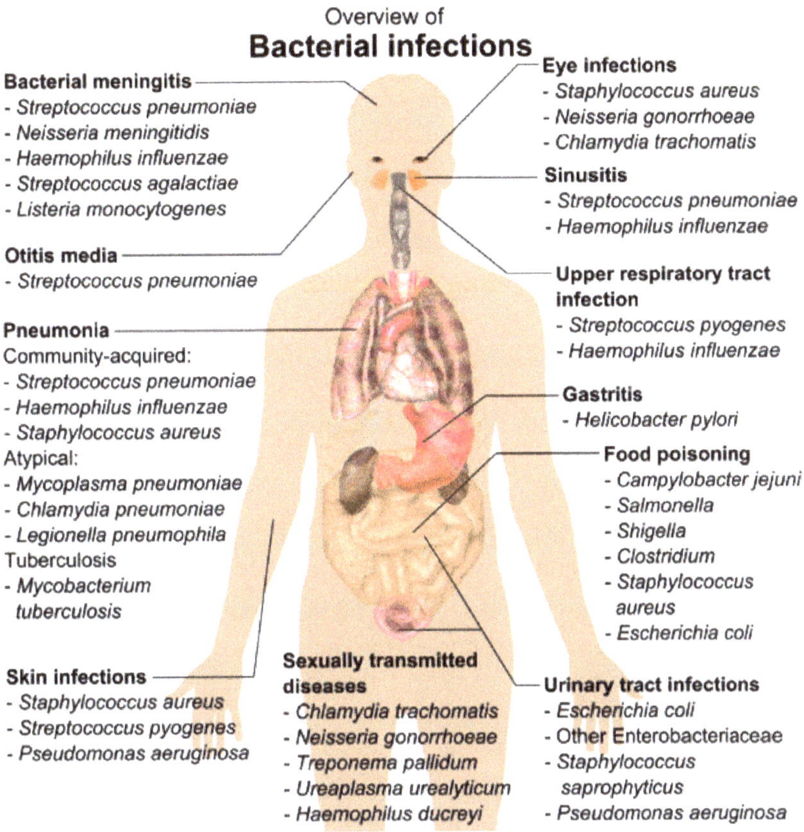

Overview of bacterial infections and main species involved

Bacterial infections may be treated with antibiotics, which are classified as bacteriocidal if they kill bacteria, or bacteriostatic if they just prevent bacterial growth. There are many types of antibiotics and each class inhibits a process that is different in the pathogen from that found in the host. An example of how antibiotics produce selective toxicity are chloramphenicol and puromycin, which inhibit the bacterial ribosome, but not the structurally different eukaryotic ribosome. Antibiotics are used both in treating human disease and in intensive farming to promote animal growth, where they may be contributing to the rapid development of antibiotic resistance in bacterial populations.Infections can be prevented by antiseptic measures such as sterilising the skin prior to piercing it with the needle of a syringe, and by proper care of indwelling catheters. Surgical and dental instruments are also sterilised to prevent contamination by bacteria. Disinfectants such as bleach are used to kill bacteria or other pathogens on surfaces to prevent contamination and further reduce the risk of infection.

Significance in Technology and Industry

Bacteria, often lactic acid bacteria, such as Lactobacillus and Lactococcus, in combination with yeasts and moulds, have been used for thousands of years in the preparation of fermented foods, such as cheese, pickles, soy sauce, sauerkraut, vinegar, wine and yogurt.

The ability of bacteria to degrade a variety of organic compounds is remarkable and has been used in waste processing and bioremediation. Bacteria capable of digesting the hydrocarbons in petroleum are often used to clean up oil spills. Fertiliser was added to some of the beaches in Prince William Sound in an attempt to promote the growth of these naturally occurring bacteria after the 1989 Exxon Valdez oil spill. These efforts were effective on beaches that were not too thickly covered in oil. Bacteria are also used for the bioremediation of industrial toxic wastes. In the chemical industry, bacteria are most important in the production of enantiomerically pure chemicals for use as pharmaceuticals or agrichemicals.

Bacteria can also be used in the place of pesticides in the biological pest control. This commonly involves Bacillus thuringiensis (also called BT), a gram-positive, soil dwelling bacterium. Subspecies of this bacteria are used as a Lepidopteran-specific insecticides under trade names such as Dipel and Thuricide. Because of their specificity, these pesticides are regarded as environmentally friendly, with little or no effect on humans, wildlife, pollinators and most other beneficial insects.

Because of their ability to quickly grow and the relative ease with which they can be manipulated, bacteria are the workhorses for the fields of molecular biology, genetics and biochemistry. By making mutations in bacterial DNA and examining the resulting phenotypes, scientists can determine the function of genes, enzymes and metabolic pathways in bacteria, then apply this knowledge to more complex organisms. This aim of understanding the biochemistry of a cell reaches its most complex expression in the synthesis of huge amounts of enzyme kinetic and gene expression data into mathematical models of entire organisms. This is achievable in some well-studied bacteria, with models of Escherichia coli metabolism now being produced and tested. This understanding of bacterial metabolism and genetics allows the use of biotechnology to bioengineer bacteria for the production of therapeutic proteins, such as insulin, growth factors, or antibodies.

Because of their importance for research in general, samples of bacterial strains are isolated and preserved in Biological Resource Centers. This ensures the availability of the strain to scientists worldwide.

History of Bacteriology

Bacteria were first observed by the Dutch microscopist Antonie van Leeuwenhoek in 1676, using a single-lens microscope of his own design. He then published his observations in a series of letters to the Royal Society of London. Bacteria were Leeuwenhoek's most remarkable microscopic discovery. They were just at the limit of what his simple lenses could make out and, in one of the most striking hiatuses in the history of science, no one else would see them again for over a century. Only then were his by-then-largely-forgotten observations of bacteria — as opposed to his famous animalcules (spermatozoa) — taken seriously.

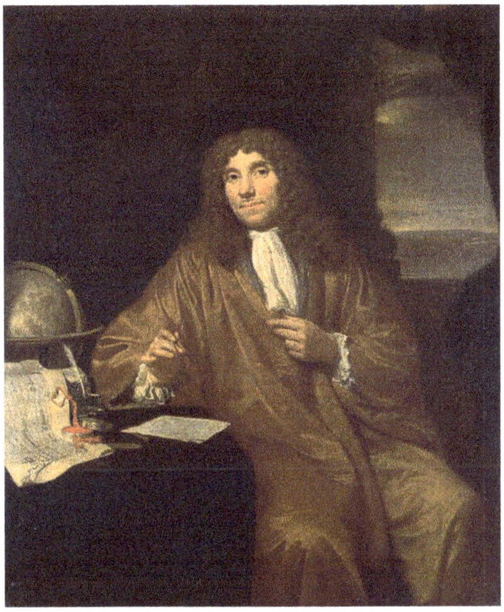

Antonie van Leeuwenhoek, the first microbiologist and the first person to observe bacteria using a microscope.

Christian Gottfried Ehrenberg introduced the word "bacterium" in 1828. In fact, his Bacterium was a genus that contained non-spore-forming rod-shaped bacteria, as opposed to Bacillus, a genus of spore-forming rod-shaped bacteria defined by Ehrenberg in 1835.

Louis Pasteur demonstrated in 1859 that the growth of microorganisms causes the fermentation process, and that this growth is not due to spontaneous generation. (Yeasts and moulds, commonly associated with fermentation, are not bacteria, but rather fungi.) Along with his contemporary Robert Koch, Pasteur was an early advocate of the germ theory of disease.

Robert Koch, a pioneer in medical microbiology, worked on cholera, anthrax and tuberculosis. In his research into tuberculosis Koch finally proved the germ theory, for which he received a Nobel Prize in 1905. In Koch's postulates, he set out criteria to test if an organism is the cause of a disease, and these postulates are still used today.

Though it was known in the nineteenth century that bacteria are the cause of many diseases, no effective antibacterial treatments were available. In 1910, Paul Ehrlich developed the first antibiotic, by changing dyes that selectively stained Treponema pallidum — the spirochaete that causes syphilis — into compounds that selectively killed the pathogen. Ehrlich had been awarded a 1908 Nobel Prize for his work on immunology, and pioneered the use of stains to detect and identify bacteria, with his work being the basis of the Gram stain and the Ziehl–Neelsen stain.

A major step forward in the study of bacteria came in 1977 when Carl Woese recognised that archaea have a separate line of evolutionary descent from bacteria. This new phylogenetic taxonomy depended on the sequencing of 16S ribosomal RNA, and divided prokaryotes into two evolutionary domains, as part of the three-domain system.

REFERENCES

1. "2002 WHO mortality data". Retrieved 20 January 2007.
2. "Bacteria (eubacteria)". Taxonomy Browser, US National Institute of Health. Retrieved 10 September 2008.
3. "Bergey's Manual Trust". Bergeys.org. Retrieved 4 November 2011.
4. "Biography of Paul Ehrlich". Nobelprize.org. Archived from the original on 28 November 2006. Retrieved 26 November 2006.
5. "Genomes Online Database". Genomes Online Database. Joint Genome Institute. Retrieved 14 Sep 2016.
6. "IJSEM Home". Ijs.sgmjournals.org. 28 October 2011. Retrieved 4 November 2011.
7. "Metal-Mining Bacteria Are Green Chemists". Science Daily. 2 September 2010.
8. "Pasteur's Papers on the Germ Theory". LSU Law Center's Medical and Public Health Law Site, Historic Public Health Articles. Archived from the original on 18 December 2006. Retrieved 23 November 2006.
9. "The Nobel Prize in Physiology or Medicine 1905". Nobelprize.org. Archived from the original on 10 December 2006. Retrieved 22 November 2006.
10. Williams C (2011). "Who are you calling simple?". New Scientist. 211 (2821): 38–41. doi:10.1016/S0262-4079(11)61709-0.
11. Akamatsu T, Taguchi H (2001). "Incorporation of the whole chromosomal DNA in protoplast lysates into competent cells of Bacillus subtilis". Biosci. Biotechnol. Biochem. 65 (4): 823–9. doi:10.1271/bbb.65.823. PMID 11388459.
12. Almaas E, Kovács B, Vicsek T, Oltvai ZN, Barabási AL (2004). "Global organization of metabolic fluxes in the bacterium Escherichia coli". Nature. 427 (6977): 839–43. arXiv:q-bio/0403001Freely accessible. Bibcode:2004Natur.427..839A. doi:10.1038/nature02289. PMID 14985762.
13. Aronson AI, Shai Y (2001). "Why Bacillus thuringiensis insecticidal toxins are so effective: unique features of their mode of action". FEMS Microbiol. Lett. 195 (1): 1–8. doi:10.1111/j.1574-6968.2001.tb10489.x. PMID 11166987.
14. Asimov, Isaac (1982), Asimov's Biographical Encyclopedia of Science and Technology, 2nd edition, Garden City, New York: Doubleday and Company, pg 143.
15. bacterium, on Oxford Dictionaries.
16. Bardy S, Ng S, Jarrell K (2003). "Prokaryotic motility structures". Microbiology. 149 (Pt 2): 295–304. doi:10.1099/mic.0.25948-0. PMID 12624192.
17. Barea JM, Pozo MJ, Azcón R, Azcón-Aguilar C (2005). "Microbial co-operation in the rhizosphere". J Exp Bot. 56 (417): 1761–78. doi:10.1093/jxb/eri197. PMID 15911555.
18. Barrangou R, Fremaux C, Deveau H, Richards M, Boyaval P, Moineau S, Romero DA, Horvath P (2007). "CRISPR provides acquired resistance against viruses in prokaryotes". Science. 315 (5819): 1709–12. Bibcode:2007Sci...315.1709B.

doi:10.1126/science.1138140. PMID 17379808.

19. BBC Staff (23 August 2011). "Impacts 'more likely' to have spread life from Earth". BBC. Retrieved 24 August 2011.
20. Beachey EH (1981). "Bacterial adherence: adhesin-receptor interactions mediating the attachment of bacteria to mucosal surface". J Infect Dis. 143 (3): 325–45. doi:10.1093/infdis/143.3.325. PMID 7014727.
21. Belfort M, Reaban ME, Coetzee T, Dalgaard JZ (1 July 1995). "Prokaryotic introns and inteins: a panoply of form and function". J. Bacteriol. 177 (14): 3897–903. PMC 177115Freely accessible. PMID 7608058.
22. Belland RJ, Ouellette SP, Gieffers J, Byrne GI (2004). "Chlamydia pneumoniae and atherosclerosis". Cell Microbiol. 6 (2): 117–27. doi:10.1046/j.1462-5822.2003.00352.x. PMID 14706098.
23. Berg JM, Tymoczko JL, Stryer L (2002). Molecular Cell Biology (5th ed.). WH Freeman. ISBN 0-7167-4955-6.
24. Bernstein H, Bernstein C, Michod RE (2012). "DNA repair as the primary adaptive function of sex in bacteria and eukaryotes". Chapter 1: pp. 1–49 in: DNA Repair: New Research, Sakura Kimura and Sora Shimizu (eds.). Nova Sci. Publ., Hauppauge, N.Y. ISBN 978-1-62100-808-8.
25. Beveridge TJ, Pouwels PH, Sára M, Kotiranta A, Lounatmaa K, Kari K, Kerosuo E, Haapasalo M, Egelseer EM, Schocher I, Sleytr UB, Morelli L, Callegari ML, Nomellini JF, Bingle WH, Smit J, Leibovitz E, Lemaire M, Miras I, Salamitou S, Béguin P, Ohayon H, Gounon P, Matuschek M, Koval SF (1997). "Functions of S-layers". FEMS Microbiol Rev. 20 (1–2): 99–149. doi:10.1016/S0168-6445(97)00043-0. PMID 9276929.
26. Bickle TA, Krüger DH (1993). "Biology of DNA restriction". Microbiol. Rev. 57 (2): 434–50. PMC 372918Freely accessible. PMID 8336674.
27. Bobik TA (2006). "Polyhedral organelles compartmenting bacterial metabolic processes". Applied Microbiology and Biotechnology. 70 (5): 517–25. doi:10.1007/s00253-005-0295-0. PMID 16525780.
28. Bobik TA (2007). "Bacterial Microcompartments" (PDF). Microbe. Am Soc Microbiol. 2: 25–31. doi:10.1128/microbe.2.25.1. Archived from the original (PDF) on 2 August 2008.
29. Boucher Y, Douady CJ, Papke RT, Walsh DA, Boudreau ME, Nesbo CL, Case RJ, Doolittle WF (2003). "Lateral gene transfer and the origins of prokaryotic groups". Annu Rev Genet. 37: 283–328. doi:10.1146/annurev.genet.37.050503.084247. PMID 14616063.
30. Bozsik A (2006). "Susceptibility of adult Coccinella septempunctata (Coleoptera: Coccinellidae) to insecticides with different modes of action". Pest Manag Sci. 62 (7): 651–4. doi:10.1002/ps.1221. PMID 16649191.
31. Branda SS, Vik S, Friedman L, Kolter R (2005). "Biofilms: the matrix revisited". Trends Microbiol. 13 (1): 20–6. doi:10.1016/j.tim.2004.11.006. PMID 15639628.
32. Breed RS, Conn HJ (1936). "The Status of the Generic Term Bacterium Ehrenberg

1828". Journal of Bacteriology. 31 (5): 517–518. PMC 543738Freely accessible. PMID 16559906.

33. Brouns SJ, Jore MM, Lundgren M, Westra ER, Slijkhuis RJ, Snijders AP, Dickman MJ, Makarova KS, Koonin EV, van der Oost J (2008). "Small CRISPR RNAs guide antiviral defense in prokaryotes". Science. 321 (5891): 960–4. Bibcode:2008Sci...321..960B. doi:10.1126/science.1159689. PMID 18703739.
34. Brown JR, Doolittle WF (1997). "Archaea and the prokaryote-to-eukaryote transition". Microbiology and Molecular Biology Reviews. 61 (4): 456–502. PMC 232621Freely accessible. PMID 9409149.
35. Brune DC (1995). "Isolation and characterization of sulfur globule proteins from Chromatium vinosum and Thiocapsa roseopersicina". Archives of Microbiology. 163 (6): 391–9. doi:10.1007/BF00272127. PMID 7575095.
36. Brüssow H, Canchaya C, Hardt WD (2004). "Phages and the evolution of bacterial pathogens: from genomic rearrangements to lysogenic conversion". Microbiology and Molecular Biology Reviews. 68 (3): 560–602. doi:10.1128/MMBR.68.3.560-602.2004. PMC 515249Freely accessible. PMID 15353570.
37. Bryant DA, Frigaard NU (2006). "Prokaryotic photosynthesis and phototrophy illuminated". Trends Microbiol. 14 (11): 488–96. doi:10.1016/j.tim.2006.09.001. PMID 16997562.
38. C.Michael Hogan. 2010. Bacteria. Encyclopedia of Earth. eds. Sidney Draggan and C.J.Cleveland, National Council for Science and the Environment, Washington DC
39. Cabeen MT, Jacobs-Wagner C (2005). "Bacterial cell shape". Nature Reviews Microbiology. 3 (8): 601–10. doi:10.1038/nrmicro1205. PMID 16012516.
40. Cano RJ, Borucki MK (1995). "Revival and identification of bacterial spores in 25- to 40-million-year-old Dominican amber". Science. 268 (5213): 1060–4. Bibcode:1995Sci...268.1060C. doi:10.1126/science.7538699. PMID 7538699.
41. Cavalier-Smith T (2002). "The neomuran origin of archaebacteria, the negibacterial root of the universal tree and bacterial megaclassification". Int J Syst Evol Microbiol. 52 (Pt 1): 7–76. doi:10.1099/00207713-52-1-7. PMID 11837318.
42. Challis GL, Hopwood DA (2003). "Synergy and contingency as driving forces for the evolution of multiple secondary metabolite production by Streptomyces species". Proceedings of the National Academy of Sciences of the United States of America. 100 Suppl 2 (90002): 14555–61. Bibcode:2003PNAS..10014555C. doi:10.1073/pnas.1934677100. PMC 304118Freely accessible. PMID 12970466.
43. Chattopadhyay A, Bhatnagar NB, Bhatnagar R (2004). "Bacterial insecticidal toxins". Crit Rev Microbiol. 30 (1): 33–54. doi:10.1080/10408410490270712. PMID 15116762.
44. Chen I, Dubnau D (2004). "DNA uptake during bacterial transformation". Nature Reviews Microbiology. 2 (3): 241–9. doi:10.1038/nrmicro844. PMID 15083159.
45. Choi CQ (17 March 2013). "Microbes Thrive in Deepest Spot on Earth". LiveScience. Retrieved 17 March 2013.
46. Ciccarelli FD, Doerks T, von Mering C, Creevey CJ, Snel B, Bork P (March

2006). "Toward automatic reconstruction of a highly resolved tree of life". Science. 311 (5765): 1283–7. Bibcode:2006Sci...311.1283C. doi:10.1126/science.1123061. PMID 16513982.

47. Cohen Y (2002). "Bioremediation of oil by marine microbial mats". Int Microbiol. 5 (4): 189–93. doi:10.1007/s10123-002-0089-5. PMID 12497184.
48. Costerton JW, Lewandowski Z, Caldwell DE, Korber DR, Lappin-Scott HM (1995). "Microbial biofilms". Annu. Rev. Microbiol. 49: 711–45. doi:10.1146/annurev.mi.49.100195.003431. PMID 8561477.
49. Curtis TP, Sloan WT, Scannell JW (2002). "Estimating prokaryotic diversity and its limits". Proceedings of the National Academy of Sciences of the United States of America. 99 (16): 10494–9. Bibcode:2002PNAS...9910494C. doi:10.1073/pnas.142680199. PMC 124953Freely accessible. PMID 12097644.
50. Daffé M, Etienne G (1999). "The capsule of Mycobacterium tuberculosis and its implications for pathogenicity". Tuber Lung Dis. 79 (3): 153–69. doi:10.1054/tuld.1998.0200. PMID 10656114.
51. Dalton H (2005). "The Leeuwenhoek Lecture 2000 the natural and unnatural history of methane-oxidizing bacteria". Philosophical Transactions of the Royal Society B. 360 (1458): 1207–22. doi:10.1098/rstb.2005.1657. PMC 1569495Freely accessible. PMID 16147517.
52. Davey ME, O'toole GA (2000). "Microbial biofilms: from ecology to molecular genetics". Microbiol Mol Biol Rev. 64 (4): 847–67. doi:10.1128/MMBR.64.4.847-867.2000. PMC 99016Freely accessible. PMID 11104821.
53. Davison J (1999). "Genetic exchange between bacteria in the environment". Plasmid. 42 (2): 73–91. doi:10.1006/plas.1999.1421. PMID 10489325.
54. DeLong EF, Pace NR (2001). "Environmental diversity of bacteria and archaea". Syst Biol. 50 (4): 470–8. doi:10.1080/106351501750435040. PMID 12116647.
55. Denamur E, Matic I (2006). "Evolution of mutation rates in bacteria". Mol Microbiol. 60 (4): 820–7. doi:10.1111/j.1365-2958.2006.05150.x. PMID 16677295.
56. Donlan RM (2002). "Biofilms: microbial life on surfaces". Emerg Infect Dis. 8 (9): 881–90. doi:10.3201/eid0809.020063. PMC 2732559Freely accessible. PMID 12194761.
57. Donlan RM, Costerton JW (2002). "Biofilms: survival mechanisms of clinically relevant microorganisms". Clin Microbiol Rev. 15 (2): 167–93. doi:10.1128/CMR.15.2.167-193.2002. PMC 118068Freely accessible. PMID 11932229.
58. Doolittle RF (2005). "Evolutionary aspects of whole-genome biology". Current Opinion in Structural Biology. 15 (3): 248–53. doi:10.1016/j.sbi.2005.04.001. PMID 15963888.
59. Douwes KE, Schmalzbauer E, Linde HJ, Reisberger EM, Fleischer K, Lehn N, Landthaler M, Vogt T (2003). "Branched filaments no fungus, ovoid bodies no bacteria: Two unusual cases of mycetoma". J Am Acad Dermatol. 49 (2 Suppl Case Reports): S170–3. doi:10.1067/mjd.2003.302. PMID 12894113.
60. Drake HL, Daniel SL, Küsel K, Matthies C, Kuhner C, Braus-Stromeyer S

(1997). "Acetogenic bacteria: what are the in situ consequences of their diverse metabolic versatilities?". BioFactors. 6 (1): 13–24. doi:10.1002/biof.5520060103. PMID 9233536.

61. Dusenbery, David B. (1996). Life at Small Scale. Scientific American Library. ISBN 0-7167-5060-0.
62. Dusenbery, David B. (2009). Living at Micro Scale, Chapter 13. Harvard University Press, Cambridge, Mass. ISBN 978-0-674-03116-6.
63. Dusenbery, David B. (2009). Living at Micro Scale, p. 136. Harvard University Press, Cambridge, Mass. ISBN 978-0-674-03116-6.
64. Dusenbery, David B. (2009). Living at Micro Scale, pp. 20–25. Harvard University Press, Cambridge, Mass. ISBN 978-0-674-03116-6.
65. Dyall SD, Brown MT, Johnson PJ (2004). "Ancient invasions: from endosymbionts to organelles". Science. 304 (5668): 253–7. Bibcode:2004Sci...304..253D. doi:10.1126/science.1094884. PMID 15073369.
66. Eagon RG (1962). "Pseudomonas natriegens, a marine bacterium with a generation time of less than 10 minutes". Journal of Bacteriology. 83 (4): 736–7. PMC 279347Freely accessible. PMID 13888946.
67. EHRENBERG (C.G.): Dritter Beitrag zur Erkenntniss grosser Organisation in der Richtung des kleinsten Raumes. Physikalische Abhandlungen der Koeniglichen Akademie der Wissenschaften zu Berlin aus den Jahren 1833–1835, 1835, pp. 143–336.
68. Ehrenberg's Symbolae Physioe. Animalia evertebrata. Decas prima. Berlin, 1828.
69. Engelhardt H, Peters J (1998). "Structural research on surface layers: a focus on stability, surface layer homology domains, and surface layer-cell wall interactions". J Struct Biol. 124 (2–3): 276–302. doi:10.1006/jsbi.1998.4070. PMID 10049812.
70. Euzéby JP (8 December 2011). "Number of published names". List of Prokaryotic names with Standing in Nomenclature. Archived from the original on 19 January 2012. Retrieved 10 December 2011.
71. Fieseler L, Horn M, Wagner M, Hentschel U (June 2004). "Discovery of the novel candidate phylum "Poribacteria" in marine sponges". Applied and Environmental Microbiology. 70 (6): 3724–32. doi:10.1128/AEM.70.6.3724-3732.2004. PMC 427773Freely accessible. PMID 15184179.
72. Finlay BB, Falkow S (1997). "Common themes in microbial pathogenicity revisited". Microbiology and Molecular Biology Reviews. 61 (2): 136–69. PMC 232605Freely accessible. PMID 9184008.
73. Fish DN (2002). "Optimal antimicrobial therapy for sepsis". Am J Health Syst Pharm. 59 Suppl 1: S13–9. PMID 11885408.
74. Fisher B, Harvey RP, Champe PC (2007). Lippincott's Illustrated Reviews: Microbiology (Lippincott's Illustrated Reviews Series). Hagerstwon, MD: Lippincott Williams & Wilkins. pp. Chapter 33, pages 367–392. ISBN 0-7817-8215-5.
75. Frankel R, Bazylinski D, Johnson M, Taylor B (1997). "Magneto-aerotaxis in marine

coccoid bacteria". Biophys J. 73 (2): 994–1000. Bibcode:1997BpJ....73..994F. doi:10.1016/S0006-3495(97)78132-3. PMC 1180996Freely accessible. PMID 9251816.

76. Fraser, Claire M.; Casjens, Sherwood; Huang, Wai Mun; Sutton, Granger G.; Clayton, Rebecca; Lathigra, Raju; White, Owen; Ketchum, Karen A.; Dodson, Robert (1997-12-11). "Genomic sequence of a Lyme disease spirochaete, Borrelia burgdorferi". Nature. 390 (6660): 580–586. doi:10.1038/37551. ISSN 0028-0836.

77. Fredrickson JK, Zachara JM, Balkwill DL, Kennedy D, Li SM, Kostandarithes HM, Daly MJ, Romine MF, Brockman FJ (2004). "Geomicrobiology of high-level nuclear waste-contaminated vadose sediments at the Hanford site, Washington state". Applied and Environmental Microbiology. 70 (7): 4230–41. doi:10.1128/AEM.70.7.4230-4241.2004. PMC 444790Freely accessible. PMID 15240306.

78. Fritz I, Strömpl C, Abraham WR (2004). "Phylogenetic relationships of the genera Stella, Labrys and Angulomicrobium within the 'Alphaproteobacteria' and description of Angulomicrobium amanitiforme sp. nov". Int J Syst Evol Microbiol. 54 (Pt 3): 651–7. doi:10.1099/ijs.0.02746-0. PMID 15143003.

79. Fuerst JA (2005). "Intracellular compartmentation in planctomycetes". Annu Rev Microbiol. 59: 299–328. doi:10.1146/annurev.micro.59.030804.121258. PMID 15910279.

80. Gitai Z (2005). "The new bacterial cell biology: moving parts and subcellular architecture". Cell. 120 (5): 577–86. doi:10.1016/j.cell.2005.02.026. PMID 15766522.

81. Glud R, Wenzhöfer F, Middelboe M, Oguri K, Turnewitsch R, Canfield DE, Kitazato H (2013). "High rates of microbial carbon turnover in sediments in the deepest oceanic trench on Earth". Nature Geoscience. 6 (4): 284–288. Bibcode:2013NatGe...6..284G. doi:10.1038/ngeo1773.

82. Goldberg MB (2001). "Actin-based motility of intracellular microbial pathogens". Microbiol Mol Biol Rev. 65 (4): 595–626, table of contents. doi:10.1128/MMBR.65.4.595-626.2001. PMC 99042Freely accessible. PMID 11729265.

83. Gorbach SL (1990). "Lactic acid bacteria and human health". Annals of Medicine. 22 (1): 37–41. doi:10.3109/07853899009147239. PMID 2109988.

84. Gram, HC (1884). "Über die isolierte Färbung der Schizomyceten in Schnitt- und Trockenpräparaten". Fortschr. Med. 2: 185–189.

85. Graumann K, Premstaller A (2006). "Manufacturing of recombinant therapeutic proteins in microbial systems". Biotechnol J. 1 (2): 164–86. doi:10.1002/biot.200500051. PMID 16892246.

86. Gromov, BV. "Electron Microscope Study of Parasitism by Bdellovibrio Chorellavorus Bacteria on Cells of the Green Alga Chorella Vulgaris." Tsitologiya 14.2 (1972): 256-60. Print.

87. Guerrero R, Pedros-Alio C, Esteve I, Mas J, Chase D, Margulis L (April 1986). "Predatory prokaryotes: predation and primary consumption evolved in bacteria". Proceedings of the National Academy of Sciences of the United States of America. 83 (7): 2138–42. Bibcode:1986PNAS...83.2138G. doi:10.1073/pnas.83.7.2138.

PMC 323246Freely accessible. PMID 11542073.

88. Gupta R (2000). "The natural evolutionary relationships among prokaryotes". Crit Rev Microbiol. 26 (2): 111–31. doi:10.1080/10408410091154219. PMID 10890353.
89. Hagedorn S, Kaphammer B (1994). "Microbial biocatalysis in the generation of flavor and fragrance chemicals". Annu. Rev. Microbiol. 48: 773–800. doi:10.1146/annurev.mi.48.100194.004013. PMID 7826026.
90. Harold FM (1972). "Conservation and transformation of energy by bacterial membranes". Bacteriological Reviews. 36 (2): 172–230. PMC 408323Freely accessible. PMID 4261111.
91. Harper, Douglas. "bacteria". Online Etymology Dictionary.
92. Hastings PJ, Rosenberg SM, Slack A (2004). "Antibiotic-induced lateral transfer of antibiotic resistance". Trends Microbiol. 12 (9): 401–4. doi:10.1016/j.tim.2004.07.003. PMID 15337159.
93. Hatheway CL (1990). "Toxigenic clostridia". Clinical Microbiology Reviews. 3 (1): 66–98. PMC 358141Freely accessible. PMID 2404569.
94. Hecker M, Völker U (2001). "General stress response of Bacillus subtilis and other bacteria". Adv Microb Physiol. Advances in Microbial Physiology. 44: 35–91. doi:10.1016/S0065-2911(01)44011-2. ISBN 978-0-12-027744-5. PMID 11407115.
95. Heise ER (1982). "Diseases associated with immunosuppression". Environmental Health Perspectives. 43: 9–19. doi:10.2307/3429162. JSTOR 3429162. PMC 1568899Freely accessible. PMID 7037390.
96. Hellingwerf KJ, Crielaard W, Hoff WD, Matthijs HC, Mur LR, van Rotterdam BJ (1994). "Photobiology of bacteria". Antonie Van Leeuwenhoek. 65 (4): 331–47. doi:10.1007/BF00872217. PMID 7832590.
97. Hinnebusch J, Tilly K (1993). "Linear plasmids and chromosomes in bacteria". Mol Microbiol. 10 (5): 917–22. doi:10.1111/j.1365-2958.1993.tb00963.x. PMID 7934868.
98. Hugenholtz P (2002). "Exploring prokaryotic diversity in the genomic era". Genome Biology. 3 (2): reviews0003.1–reviews0003.8. doi:10.1186/gb-2002-3-2-reviews0003. PMC 139013Freely accessible. PMID 11864374.
99. Ishige T, Honda K, Shimizu S (2005). "Whole organism biocatalysis". Current Opinion in Chemical Biology. 9 (2): 174–80. doi:10.1016/j.cbpa.2005.02.001. PMID 15811802.
100. Johnsborg O, Eldholm V, Håvarstein LS (2007). "Natural genetic transformation: prevalence, mechanisms and function". Res. Microbiol. 158 (10): 767–78. doi:10.1016/j.resmic.2007.09.004. PMID 17997281.
101. Johnson ME, Lucey JA (2006). "Major technological advances and trends in cheese". J Dairy Sci. 89 (4): 1174–8. doi:10.3168/jds.S0022-0302(06)72186-5. PMID 16537950.
102. Kadouri D, Jurkevitch E, Okon Y, Castro-Sowinski S (2005). "Ecological and

agricultural significance of bacterial polyhydroxyalkanoates". Critical Reviews in Microbiology. 31 (2): 55–67. doi:10.1080/10408410590899228. PMID 15986831.

103. Kaiser D (2004). "Signaling in myxobacteria". Annu Rev Microbiol. 58: 75–98. doi:10.1146/annurev.micro.58.030603.123620. PMID 15487930.
104. Kerfeld CA, Sawaya MR, Tanaka S, Nguyen CV, Phillips M, Beeby M, Yeates TO (2005). "Protein structures forming the shell of primitive bacterial organelles". Science. 309 (5736): 936–8. Bibcode:2005Sci...309..936K. doi:10.1126/science.1113397. PMID 16081736.
105. Khachatourians GG (1998). "Agricultural use of antibiotics and the evolution and transfer of antibiotic-resistant bacteria". CMAJ. 159 (9): 1129–36. PMC 1229782Freely accessible. PMID 9835883.
106. Koch AL (2002). "Control of the bacterial cell cycle by cytoplasmic growth". Crit Rev Microbiol. 28 (1): 61–77. doi:10.1080/1040-840291046696. PMID 12003041.
107. Koch AL (2003). "Bacterial wall as target for attack: past, present, and future research". Clin Microbiol Rev. 16 (4): 673–87. doi:10.1128/CMR.16.4.673-687.2003. PMC 207114Freely accessible. PMID 14557293.
108. Kojima S, Blair DF (2004). "The bacterial flagellar motor: structure and function of a complex molecular machine". Int Rev Cytol. International Review of Cytology. 233: 93–134. doi:10.1016/S0074-7696(04)33003-2. ISBN 978-0-12-364637-8. PMID 15037363.
109. Kooijman SA, Auger P, Poggiale JC, Kooi BW (2003). "Quantitative steps in symbiogenesis and the evolution of homeostasis". Biol Rev Camb Philos Soc. 78 (3): 435–63. doi:10.1017/S1464793102006127. PMID 14558592.
110. Lang BF, Gray MW, Burger G (1999). "Mitochondrial genome evolution and the origin of eukaryotes". Annu Rev Genet. 33: 351–97. doi:10.1146/annurev.genet.33.1.351. PMID 10690412.
111. LEF.org > Bacterial Infections Updated: 19 January 2006. Retrieved on 11 April 2009
112. Liese A, Filho MV (1999). "Production of fine chemicals using biocatalysis". Current Opinion in Biotechnology. 10 (6): 595–603. doi:10.1016/S0958-1669(99)00040-3. PMID 10600695.
113. Lonhienne TG, Sagulenko E, Webb RI, Lee KC, Franke J, Devos DP, Nouwens A, Carroll BJ, Fuerst JA (2010). "Endocytosis-like protein uptake in the bacterium Gemmata obscuriglobus". Proceedings of the National Academy of Sciences of the United States of America. 107 (29): 12883–12888. Bibcode:2010PNAS..10712883L. doi:10.1073/pnas.1001085107. PMC 2919973Freely accessible. PMID 20566852.
114. Louie M, Louie L, Simor AE (8 August 2000). "The role of DNA amplification technology in the diagnosis of infectious diseases". CMAJ. 163 (3): 301–9. PMC 80298Freely accessible. PMID 10951731.
115. Lux R, Shi W (2004). "Chemotaxis-guided movements in bacteria". Crit Rev Oral Biol Med. 15 (4): 207–20. doi:10.1177/154411130401500404. PMID 15284186.

116. Macnab RM (1 December 1999). "The bacterial flagellum: reversible rotary propellor and type III export apparatus". J. Bacteriol. 181 (23): 7149–53. PMC 103673Freely accessible. PMID 10572114.

117. Martin MO (2002). "Predatory prokaryotes: an emerging research opportunity". Journal of Microbiology and Biotechnology. 4 (5): 467–77. PMID 12432957.

118. McFadden GI (1999). "Endosymbiosis and evolution of the plant cell". Current Opinion in Plant Biology. 2 (6): 513–9. doi:10.1016/S1369-5266(99)00025-4. PMID 10607659.

119. Merz A, So M, Sheetz M (2000). "Pilus retraction powers bacterial twitching motility". Nature. 407 (6800): 98–102. Bibcode:2000Natur.407...98M. doi:10.1038/35024105. PMID 10993081.

120. Michod RE, Bernstein H, Nedelcu AM (2008). "Adaptive value of sex in microbial pathogens" (PDF). Infect. Genet. Evol. 8 (3): 267–85. doi:10.1016/j.meegid.2008.01.002. PMID 18295550.

121. Miller MB, Bassler BL (2001). "Quorum sensing in bacteria". Annu. Rev. Microbiol. 55: 165–99. doi:10.1146/annurev.micro.55.1.165. PMID 11544353.

122. Morel FM, Kraepiel AM, Amyot M (1998). "The chemical cycle and bioaccumulation of mercury". Annual Review of Ecology and Systematics. 29: 543–566. doi:10.1146/annurev.ecolsys.29.1.543.

123. Nakabachi A, Yamashita A, Toh H, Ishikawa H, Dunbar HE, Moran NA, Hattori M (2006). "The 160-kilobase genome of the bacterial endosymbiont Carsonella". Science. 314 (5797): 267. doi:10.1126/science.1134196. PMID 17038615.

124. Nealson KH (1999). "Post-Viking microbiology: new approaches, new data, new insights". Origins of Life and Evolution of Biospheres. 29 (1): 73–93. doi:10.1023/A:1006515817767. PMID 11536899.

125. Neves LC, Miyamura TT, Moraes DA, Penna TC, Converti A (2006). "Biofiltration methods for the removal of phenolic residues". Appl. Biochem. Biotechnol. 129–132: 130–52. doi:10.1385/ABAB:129:1:130. PMID 16915636.

126. Nicholson WL, Fajardo-Cavazos P, Rebeil R, Slieman TA, Riesenman PJ, Law JF, Xue Y (2002). "Bacterial endospores and their significance in stress resistance". Antonie Van Leeuwenhoek. 81 (1–4): 27–32. doi:10.1023/A:1020561122764. PMID 12448702.

127. Nicholson WL, Munakata N, Horneck G, Melosh HJ, Setlow P (2000). "Resistance of Bacillus endospores to extreme terrestrial and extraterrestrial environments". Microbiology and Molecular Biology Reviews. 64 (3): 548–72. doi:10.1128/MMBR.64.3.548-572.2000. PMC 99004Freely accessible. PMID 10974126.

128. Nicholson WL, Schuerger AC, Setlow P (2005). "The solar UV environment and bacterial spore UV resistance: considerations for Earth-to-Mars transport by natural processes and human spaceflight". Mutat Res. 571 (1–2): 249–64. doi:10.1016/j.mrfmmm.2004.10.012. PMID 15748651.

129. Norris V, den Blaauwen T, Cabin-Flaman A, Doi RH, Harshey R, Janniere L, Jimenez-Sanchez A, Jin DJ, Levin PA, Mileykovskaya E, Minsky A, Saier

M, Skarstad K (2007). "Functional taxonomy of bacterial hyperstructures". Microbiology and Molecular Biology Reviews. 71 (1): 230–53. doi:10.1128/MMBR.00035-06. PMC 1847379Freely accessible. PMID 17347523.

130. O'Brien SJ, Goedert JJ (1996). "HIV causes AIDS: Koch's postulates fulfilled". Current Opinion in Immunology. 8 (5): 613–8. doi:10.1016/S0952-7915(96)80075-6. PMID 8902385.
131. O'Hara AM, Shanahan F (2006). "The gut flora as a forgotten organ". EMBO Reports. 7 (7): 688–93. doi:10.1038/sj.embor.7400731. PMC 1500832Freely accessible. PMID 16819463.
132. Oliver J (2005). "The viable but nonculturable state in bacteria". J Microbiol. 43 Spec No: 93–100. PMID 15765062. Archived from the original on 28 September 2007.
133. Olsen GJ, Woese CR, Overbeek R (1994). "The winds of (evolutionary) change: breathing new life into microbiology". Journal of Bacteriology. 176 (1): 1–6. doi:10.2172/205047. PMC 205007Freely accessible. PMID 8282683.
134. Oskin B (14 March 2013). "Intraterrestrials: Life Thrives in Ocean Floor". LiveScience. Retrieved 17 March 2013.
135. Paerl HW, Fulton RS, Moisander PH, Dyble J (2001). "Harmful freshwater algal blooms, with an emphasis on cyanobacteria". ScientificWorldJournal. 1: 76–113. doi:10.1100/tsw.2001.16. PMID 12805693.
136. Poehlsgaard J, Douthwaite S (2005). "The bacterial ribosome as a target for antibiotics". Nature Reviews Microbiology. 3 (11): 870–81. doi:10.1038/nrmicro1265. PMID 16261170.
137. Poole AM, Penny D (2007). "Evaluating hypotheses for the origin of eukaryotes". BioEssays. 29 (1): 74–84. doi:10.1002/bies.20516. PMID 17187354.
138. Porter JR (1976). "Antony van Leeuwenhoek: tercentenary of his discovery of bacteria". Bacteriological Reviews. 40 (2): 260–9. PMC 413956Freely accessible. PMID 786250.
139. Pradella S, Hans A, Spröer C, Reichenbach H, Gerth K, Beyer S (2002). "Characterisation, genome size and genetic manipulation of the myxobacterium Sorangium cellulosum So ce56". Arch Microbiol. 178 (6): 484–92. doi:10.1007/s00203-002-0479-2. PMID 12420170.
140. Prats C, López D, Giró A, Ferrer J, Valls J (2006). "Individual-based modelling of bacterial cultures to study the microscopic causes of the lag phase". J Theor Biol. 241 (4): 939–53. doi:10.1016/j.jtbi.2006.01.029. PMID 16524598.
141. Psencík J, Ikonen TP, Laurinmäki P, Merckel MC, Butcher SJ, Serimaa RE, Tuma R (2004). "Lamellar organization of pigments in chlorosomes, the light harvesting complexes of green photosynthetic bacteria". Biophys. J. 87 (2): 1165–72. Bibcode:2004BpJ....87.1165P. doi:10.1529/biophysj.104.040956. PMC 1304455Freely accessible. PMID 15298919.
142. Rappé MS, Giovannoni SJ (2003). "The uncultured microbial majority". Annual Review of Microbiology. 57: 369–94. doi:10.1146/annurev.micro.57.030502.090759. PMID 14527284.

143. Reed JL, Vo TD, Schilling CH, Palsson BO (2003). "An expanded genome-scale model of Escherichia coli K-12 (iJR904 GSM/GPR)". Genome Biol. 4 (9): R54. doi:10.1186/gb-2003-4-9-r54. PMC 193654Freely accessible. PMID 12952533.

144. Robertson J, Gomersall M, Gill P (1975). "Mycoplasma hominis: growth, reproduction, and isolation of small viable cells". J Bacteriol. 124 (2): 1007–18. PMC 235991Freely accessible. PMID 1102522.

145. Saiman L (2004). "Microbiology of early CF lung disease". Paediatric Respiratory Reviews. 5 Suppl A: S367–9. doi:10.1016/S1526-0542(04)90065-6. PMID 14980298.

146. Saito Y, Taguchi H, Akamatsu T (2006). "Fate of transforming bacterial genome following incorporation into competent cells of Bacillus subtilis: a continuous length of incorporated DNA". J. Biosci. Bioeng. 101 (3): 257–62. doi:10.1263/jbb.101.257. PMID 16716928.

147. Salminen SJ, Gueimonde M, Isolauri E (1 May 2005). "Probiotics that modify disease risk". J Nutr. 135 (5): 1294–8. PMID 15867327.

148. Schloss PD, Handelsman J (2004). "Status of the microbial census". Microbiology and Molecular Biology Reviews. 68 (4): 686–91. doi:10.1128/MMBR.68.4.686-691.2004. PMC 539005Freely accessible. PMID 15590780.

149. Schopf JW (1994). "Disparate rates, differing fates: tempo and mode of evolution changed from the Precambrian to the Phanerozoic". Proceedings of the National Academy of Sciences of the United States of America. 91 (15): 6735–42. Bibcode:1994PNAS...91.6735S. doi:10.1073/pnas.91.15.6735. PMC 44277Freely accessible. PMID 8041691.

150. Schulz HN, Jorgensen BB (2001). "Big bacteria". Annu Rev Microbiol. 55: 105–37. doi:10.1146/annurev.micro.55.1.105. PMID 11544351.

151. Schwartz RS (2004). "Paul Ehrlich's magic bullets". N Engl J Med. 350 (11): 1079–80. doi:10.1056/NEJMp048021. PMID 15014180.

152. Schweinitzer T, Josenhans C (2010). "Bacterial energy taxis: a global strategy?". Arch Microbiol. 192 (7): 507–20. doi:10.1007/s00203-010-0575-7. PMC 2886117Freely accessible. PMID 20411245.

153. Sears CL (2005). "A dynamic partnership: celebrating our gut flora". Anaerobe. 11 (5): 247–51. doi:10.1016/j.anaerobe.2005.05.001. PMID 16701579.

154. Serres MH, Gopal S, Nahum LA, Liang P, Gaasterland T, Riley M (2001). "A functional update of the Escherichia coli K-12 genome". Genome Biology. 2 (9): research0035.1–research0035.7. doi:10.1186/gb-2001-2-9-research0035. PMC 56896Freely accessible. PMID 11574054.

155. Shapiro JA (1998). "Thinking about bacterial populations as multicellular organisms" (PDF). Annu. Rev. Microbiol. 52: 81–104. doi:10.1146/annurev.micro.52.1.81. PMID 9891794. Archived from the original (PDF) on 17 July 2011.

156. Shiba T, Tsutsumi K, Ishige K, Noguchi T (2000). "Inorganic polyphosphate and polyphosphate kinase: their novel biological functions and applications". Biochemistry (Mosc). 65 (3): 315–23. PMID 10739474.

157. Shih YL, Rothfield L (2006). "The bacterial cytoskeleton". Microbiology and Molecular Biology Reviews. 70 (3): 729–54. doi:10.1128/MMBR.00017-06. PMC 1594594Freely accessible. PMID 16959967.

158. Shimkets LJ (1999). "Intercellular signaling during fruiting-body development of Myxococcus xanthus". Annu Rev Microbiol. 53: 525–49. doi:10.1146/annurev.micro.53.1.525. PMID 10547700.

159. Silverman PM (1997). "Towards a structural biology of bacterial conjugation". Mol Microbiol. 23 (3): 423–9. doi:10.1046/j.1365-2958.1997.2411604.x. PMID 9044277.

160. Siunov AV, Nikitin DV, Suzina NE, Dmitriev VV, Kuzmin NP, Duda VI (1999). "Phylogenetic status of Anaerobacter polyendosporus, an anaerobic, polysporogenic bacterium" (PDF). Int J Syst Bacteriol. 49 (3): 1119–24. doi:10.1099/00207713-49-3-1119. PMID 10425769.

161. Solomon JM, Grossman AD (1996). "Who's competent and when: regulation of natural genetic competence in bacteria". Trends Genet. 12 (4): 150–5. doi:10.1016/0168-9525(96)10014-7. PMID 8901420.

162. Stams AJ, de Bok FA, Plugge CM, van Eekert MH, Dolfing J, Schraa G (2006). "Exocellular electron transfer in anaerobic microbial communities". Environ Microbiol. 8 (3): 371–82. doi:10.1111/j.1462-2920.2006.00989.x. PMID 16478444.

163. Stewart EJ, Madden R, Paul G, Taddei F (2005). "Aging and death in an organism that reproduces by morphologically symmetric division". PLoS Biol. 3 (2): e45. doi:10.1371/journal.pbio.0030045. PMC 546039Freely accessible. PMID 15685293.

164. Stokes RW, Norris-Jones R, Brooks DE, Beveridge TJ, Doxsee D, Thorson LM (2004). "The glycan-rich outer layer of the cell wall of Mycobacterium tuberculosis acts as an antiphagocytic capsule limiting the association of the bacterium with macrophages". Infect Immun. 72 (10): 5676–86. doi:10.1128/IAI.72.10.5676-5686.2004. PMC 517526Freely accessible. PMID 15385466.

165. Tanaka S, Kerfeld CA, Sawaya MR, Cai F, Heinhorst S, Cannon GC, Yeates TO (2008). "Atomic-level models of the bacterial carboxysome shell". Science. 319 (5866): 1083–6. Bibcode:2008Sci...319.1083T. doi:10.1126/science.1151458. PMID 18292340.

166. Thanbichler M, Wang SC, Shapiro L (2005). "The bacterial nucleoid: a highly organized and dynamic structure". J Cell Biochem. 96 (3): 506–21. doi:10.1002/jcb.20519. PMID 15988757.

167. The University of Waikato (March 25, 2014). "Bacterial DNA – the role of plasmids". Themes — Bacteria in biotech. Biotechnology Learning Hub. Retrieved 2014-09-03.

168. Thomson RB, Bertram H (2001). "Laboratory diagnosis of central nervous system infections". Infectious Disease Clinics of North America. 15 (4): 1047–71. doi:10.1016/S0891-5520(05)70186-0. PMID 11780267.

169. Thurston AJ (2000). "Of blood, inflammation and gunshot wounds: the history

of the control of sepsis". Aust N Z J Surg. 70 (12): 855–61. doi:10.1046/j.1440-1622.2000.01983.x. PMID 11167573.

170. van Heijenoort J (2001). "Formation of the glycan chains in the synthesis of bacterial peptidoglycan". Glycobiology. 11 (3): 25R–36R. doi:10.1093/glycob/11.3.25R. PMID 11320055.
171. van Leeuwenhoek A (1684). "An abstract of a letter from Mr. Anthony Leevvenhoek at Delft, dated Sep. 17, 1683, Containing Some Microscopical Observations, about Animals in the Scurf of the Teeth, the Substance Call'd Worms in the Nose, the Cuticula Consisting of Scales". Philosophical Transactions (1683–1775). 14 (155–166): 568–574. doi:10.1098/rstl.1684.0030.
172. van Leeuwenhoek A (1700). "Part of a Letter from Mr Antony van Leeuwenhoek, concerning the Worms in Sheeps Livers, Gnats, and Animalcula in the Excrements of Frogs". Philosophical Transactions (1683–1775). 22 (260–276): 509–518. doi:10.1098/rstl.1700.0013.
173. van Leeuwenhoek A (1702). "Part of a Letter from Mr Antony van Leeuwenhoek, F. R. S. concerning Green Weeds Growing in Water, and Some Animalcula Found about Them". Philosophical Transactions (1683–1775). 23 (277–288): 1304–11. doi:10.1098/rstl.1702.0042.
174. Velicer GJ, Mendes-Soares H (2009). "Bacterial predators". Current Biology. 19 (2): R55–6. doi:10.1016/j.cub.2008.10.043. PMID 19174136.
175. Velicer GJ, Stredwick KL (2002). "Experimental social evolution with Myxococcus xanthus". Antonie Van Leeuwenhoek. 81 (1–4): 155–64. doi:10.1023/A:1020546130033. PMID 12448714.
176. Velimirov B (2001). "Nanobacteria, Ultramicrobacteria and Starvation Forms: A Search for the Smallest Metabolizing Bacterium". Microbes and Environments. 16 (2): 67–77. doi:10.1264/jsme2.2001.67.
177. Vreeland RH, Rosenzweig WD, Powers DW (2000). "Isolation of a 250 million-year-old halotolerant bacterium from a primary salt crystal". Nature. 407 (6806): 897–900. Bibcode:2000Natur.407..897V. doi:10.1038/35038060. PMID 11057666.
178. Walsby AE (1994). "Gas vesicles". Microbiological Reviews. 58 (1): 94–144. PMC 372955Freely accessible. PMID 8177173.
179. Walsh FM, Amyes SG (2004). "Microbiology and drug resistance mechanisms of fully resistant pathogens". Current Opinion in Microbiology. 7 (5): 439–44. doi:10.1016/j.mib.2004.08.007. PMID 15451497.
180. Walsh G (2005). "Therapeutic insulins and their large-scale manufacture". Appl Microbiol Biotechnol. 67 (2): 151–9. doi:10.1007/s00253-004-1809-x. PMID 15580495.
181. Wanger G, Onstott TC, Southam G (2008). "Stars of the terrestrial deep subsurface: A novel 'star-shaped' bacterial morphotype from a South African platinum mine". Geobiology. 6 (3): 325–30. doi:10.1111/j.1472-4669.2008.00163.x. PMID 18498531.
182. Weinstein M (1994). "Clinical importance of blood cultures". Clin Lab Med.

14 (1): 9–16. PMID 8181237.

183. Whitman WB, Coleman DC, Wiebe WJ (1998). "Prokaryotes: the unseen majority". Proceedings of the National Academy of Sciences of the United States of America. 95 (12): 6578–83. Bibcode:1998PNAS...95.6578W. doi:10.1073/pnas.95.12.6578. PMC 33863Freely accessible. PMID 9618454.
184. Woese CR, Fox GE (1977). "Phylogenetic structure of the prokaryotic domain: the primary kingdoms". Proceedings of the National Academy of Sciences of the United States of America. 74 (11): 5088–90. Bibcode:1977PNAS...74.5088W. doi:10.1073/pnas.74.11.5088. PMC 432104Freely accessible. PMID 270744.
185. Woese CR, Kandler O, Wheelis ML (1990). "Towards a natural system of organisms: proposal for the domains Archaea, Bacteria, and Eucarya". Proceedings of the National Academy of Sciences of the United States of America. 87 (12): 4576–9. Bibcode:1990PNAS...87.4576W. doi:10.1073/pnas.87.12.4576. PMC 54159Freely accessible. PMID 2112744.
186. Woods GL, Walker DH (1996). "Detection of infection or infectious agents by use of cytologic and histologic stains". Clinical Microbiology Reviews. 9 (3): 382–404. PMC 172900Freely accessible. PMID 8809467.
187. Wright BE (2004). "Stress-directed adaptive mutations and evolution". Mol Microbiol. 52 (3): 643–50. doi:10.1111/j.1365-2958.2004.04012.x. PMID 15101972.
188. Wu M, Roberts J, Kim S, Koch D, DeLisa M (2006). "Collective bacterial dynamics revealed using a three-dimensional population-scale defocused particle tracking technique". Appl Environ Microbiol. 72 (7): 4987–94. doi:10.1128/AEM.00158-06. PMC 1489374Freely accessible. PMID 16820497.
189. Xu J (2006). "Microbial ecology in the age of genomics and metagenomics: concepts, tools, and recent advances". Mol Ecol. 15 (7): 1713–31. doi:10.1111/j.1365-294X.2006.02882.x. PMID 16689892.
190. Yeates TO, Kerfeld CA, Heinhorst S, Cannon GC, Shively JM (2008). "Protein-based organelles in bacteria: carboxysomes and related microcompartments". Nature Reviews Microbiology. 6 (9): 681–91. doi:10.1038/nrmicro1913. PMID 18679172.
191. Yeo M, Chater K (2005). "The interplay of glycogen metabolism and differentiation provides an insight into the developmental biology of Streptomyces coelicolor". Microbiology. 151 (Pt 3): 855–61. doi:10.1099/mic.0.27428-0. PMID 15758231.
192. Yonath A, Bashan A (2004). "Ribosomal crystallography: initiation, peptide bond formation, and amino acid polymerization are hampered by antibiotics". Annu Rev Microbiol. 58: 233–51. doi:10.1146/annurev.micro.58.030603.123822. PMID 15487937.
193. Young KD (2006). "The selective value of bacterial shape". Microbiol Mol Biol Rev. 70 (3): 660–703. doi:10.1128/MMBR.00001-06. PMC 1594593Freely accessible. PMID 16959965.
194. Zehr JP, Jenkins BD, Short SM, Steward GF (2003). "Nitrogenase gene

diversity and microbial community structure: a cross-system comparison". Environ Microbiol. 5 (7): 539–54. doi:10.1046/j.1462-2920.2003.00451.x. PMID 12823187.

195. Zillig W (1991). "Comparative biochemistry of Archaea and Bacteria". Current Opinion in Genetics & Development. 1 (4): 544–51. doi:10.1016/S0959-437X(05)80206-0. PMID 1822288.

196. Zoetendal EG, Vaughan EE, de Vos WM (2006). "A microbial world within us". Mol Microbiol. 59 (6): 1639–50. doi:10.1111/j.1365-2958.2006.05056.x. PMID 16553872.

197. Zumft WG (1 December 1997). "Cell biology and molecular basis of denitrification". Microbiol Mol Biol Rev. 61 (4): 533–616. PMC 232623Freely accessible. PMID 9409151.

198. βακτηρία in Liddell and Scott.

199. βακτήριον. Liddell, Henry George; Scott, Robert; A Greek–English Lexicon at the Perseus Project.

CHAPTER 2

Bacterial Cell Morphology

Chapter Contents

The first shape is called **coccus**, plural **cocci**. Cells that have a cocci shape are spherical, resembling tiny balls. The 'strep' in strep throat actually refers to the bacterium *Streptococcus*, which exists in tiny, spherical cells.

The second shape is **bacillus**, plural **bacilli**. These bacteria are shaped like small rods, longer than they are wide. A bacillus cell looks a lot like a pill. Have you ever heard of anthrax poisoning? Anthrax is caused by a rod-shaped bacteria called *Bacillus anthracis*. Some bacilli bacteria have round ends, while others are square. It is important to note that the term 'bacillus' can describe the cell shape as well as bacteria in the genus *Bacillus*.

INTRODUCTION

Bacteria are classified by direct examination with the light microscope through its morphology and aggregation.

The basic forms are spheres (coccus) and round-ended cylinders (bacillus). But there may be others such as helically twisted cylinders (spirochetes), cylinders curved in one plane

(Selenomonads) and unusual morphologies (such as the square Archaea Haloquadratum). They also conform diplos, tetrads, staphylos, streptos, palizadas, etc.

Coccus

A coccus (plural cocci, from the Latin coccinus (scarlet) and derived from the Greek kokkos (berry)) is any microorganism (usually bacteria) whose overall shape is spherical or nearly spherical. Describing a bacterium as a coccus, or sphere, distinguishes it from bacillus, or rod. This is the first of many taxonomic traits for identifying and classifying a bacterium according to binomial nomenclature.

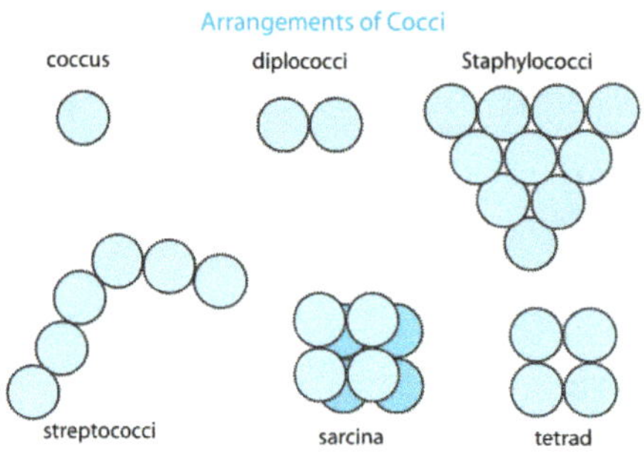

Arrangement of cocci bacteria

Aggregations

Aggregations of coccoid bacteria often occur and these forms have specific names as well;listed here are the basic forms as well as representative bacterial genera:

- pairs, or *diplococci* (*Neisseria*)
- groups of four or eight known as tetrads or *sarcina* (*Micrococci*)
- bead-like chains, or *streptococci* (*Streptococcus*)
- grapelike clusters, or *staphylococci* (*Staphylococcus*)

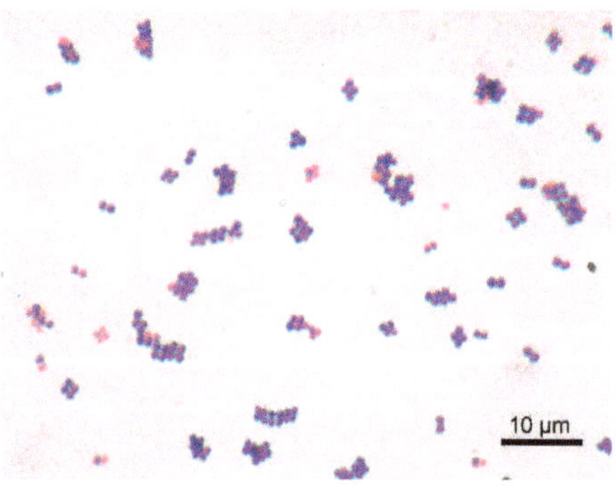

Staphylococcus bacteria

Diplococcus

A diplococcus (plural diplococci) is a round bacterium (a coccus) that typically occurs in pairs of two joined cells. Examples are Streptococcus pneumoniae, Moraxella catarrhalis, Neisseria gonorrhoeae and Neisseria meningitidis.

Its name comes from diplo, meaning double, and coccus, meaning berry. This is because berries are round, like a diplococcus, and diplococci come in pairs of two.

In former times, a bacterial genus Diplococcus was recognized, but it is not used anymore.

Coccobacillus

A coccobacillus (plural coccobacilli) is a type of rod-shaped bacteria. The word coccobacillus reflects an intermediate shape between coccus (spherical) and bacillus (elongated). Coccobacilli rods are so short and wide that they resemble cocci. Haemophilus influenzae and Chlamydia trachomatis are coccobacilli. Aggregatibacter actinomycetemcomitans is a gram negative coccobacillus which is prevalent in subgingival plaques. Acinetobacter strains may grow on solid media as coccobacilli.

Coxiella burnetti is also a coccobacillus.

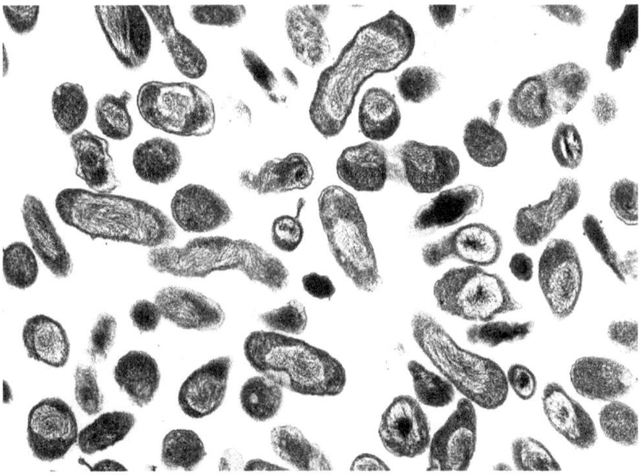

Coxiella burnetii (TEM)

Clinical Significance

Important human pathogens caused by coccoid bacteria those include staphylococci infections, some types of food poisoning, some urinary tract infections, toxic shock syndrome, gonorrhea, as well as some forms of meningitis, throat infections, pneumonias, and sinusitis.

Bacillus

A bacillus (plural bacilli) is a rod-shaped bacterium. Although Bacillus, capitalized and italicized, specifically refers to the genus, the word bacillus (plural bacilli) may also be used to describe any rod-shaped bacterium, and in this sense, bacilli are found in many different taxonomic groups of bacteria. There is no connection between the shape of a bacterium and its colors in the Gram staining.

Bacilli usually divide in the same plane and are solitary, but can combine to form diplobacilli, streptobacilli, and palisades.

- Diplobacilli: Two bacilli arranged side by side with each other.
- Streptobacilli: Bacilli arranged in chains.
- Coccobacillus: Oval and similar to coccus (circular shaped bacterium).

Spiral

Spiral bacteria form the third major bacterial cell morphology. Spiral bacteria can be sub-classified as spirilla, spirochetes, or vibrios based on the number of twists per cell, cell thickness, cell flexibility, and motility.

BACTERIAL MORPHOLOGICAL PLASTICITY

Bacterial morphological plasticity refers to changes in the shape and size that bacterial cells undergo when they encounter stressful environments. Although bacteria have evolved complex molecular strategies to maintain their shape, many are able to alter their shape as a survival strategy in response to protist predators, antibiotics, the immune response, and other threats.

Bacterial Shape and Size Under Selective Forces

Normally, bacteria have different shapes and sizes which include coccus, rod and helical/ spiral (among others less common) and that allow for their classification. For instance, rod shapes may allow bacteria to attach more readily in environments with shear stress (e.g., in flowing water). Cocci may have access to small pores, creating more attachment sites per cell and hiding themselves from external shear forces. Spiral bacteria combine some of the characteristics cocci (small footprints) and of filaments (more surface area on which shear forces can act) and the ability to form an unbroken set of cells to build biofilms. Several bacteria alter their morphology in response to the types and concentrations of external compounds. Bacterial morphology changes help to optimize interactions with cells and the surfaces to which they attach. This mechanism has been described in bacteria such as Escherichia coli and Helicobacter pylori.

Bacterial shape	Example	Changes under selective forces
Filamentation This allow bacteria to have more surface area for long-term attachments and can interlink themselves with porous surfaces.	Caulobacter crescentus: in their niche (freshwater), filament is the regular shape that contributes to their resistance to heat and survival.	Regular rod morphology of Escherichia coli versus SOS stress-induced filaments observed in the urinary tract infection model. Extended filamentous structures in Helicobacter pylori, which under normal conditions is a spiral-shaped bacteria.
Prosthecate Cells are more easily attached by placing adhesins on the tips of thin appendages or may insinuate these into pores or crevices in solid substrates.	Prosthecomicrobium pneumaticum	*Ancalomicrobium adetum*: Under high nutrients concentrations: road or spherical shape. Low nutrients: it prosthecaes to increase surface area for nutrients transport Ancalomicrobium adetumwith seven prosthecae
Bifid Y-shaped cell occurs most often in Gram positive, but also in Gram-negative bacteria. It is part of the normal cycle of several microorganisms, but could be induced by specific cues.	Bifidobacterium longum	Most of Bradyrhizobium japonicum cells swell and branch (changing to a Y shape) in culture by the addition of succinate or fumarate because these strains lack succinate dehydrogenase and do not progress through the cycle. Lactobacillus bifidus produces bifids and branched cells in the presence of cations or sodium salts.
Pleomorfic when bacteria grow adopting different forms under explicit genetic control and are associated with important physiological phenotypes (for example due to nutrient limitation).	Legionella pneumophila This bacteria have 3 shapes in vitro and 5 in vivo, including rods, cocci, filaments, and a form created by "fragmented" cell septation.	Campylobacter jejuni adopt different forms (commas, spirals, S shapes, dimpled cells and doughnut shapes), however there is a debate weather these forms are transitional or due to environmental stress.
Helical/spiral	*Leptospira spp*	Helical curvature in Escherichia coli artificially imposed by growing the cells in preformed cavities.

Bacterial Filamentation

Physiological Mechanisms

Oxidative stress, nutrient limitation, DNA damage and antibiotics exposure are some of stress conditions to which bacteria respond, altering their DNA replication and cell division. Filamentous bacteria have been considered to be over-stressed, sick and dying members of the population. However, the filamentous members of some communities have vital roles in the population′s continued existence, since the filamentous phenotype can confer protection against lethal environments. Filamentous E. coli can be up to 70 μm in length and has been identified playing an important role in pathogenesis in human cystitis. There are different mechanisms identified in some bacteria that are attributable to the development to filamentous forms.

- Base Excision Repair (BER) mechanism, as a strategy to repair DNA damage observed in *E. coli.* This involves two types of enzymes:
- *Bifunctional glycosylases*: the endonuclease III (encoded by *nth* gene)
- *Apurinic/Apirimidinic (AP)-endonucleases*: endonuclease IV (encoded by *nfo* gene) and exonuclease III (encoded by *xth* gene).

Under this mechanism, daughter cells are protected from receiving damaged copies of the bacterial chromosome, and at the same time promoting bacterial survival. A mutant for these genes lack BER activity and a strong formation of filamentous structures is observed.

- SulA/FtsZ mediated filamentation: This is a mechanism to halt cell division and repair DNA. In the presence of single-stranded DNA regions, due to the action of different external cues (that induce mutations), the major bacterial recombinase (RecA) binds to this DNA regions and is activated by the presence of free nucleotide triphosphates. This activated RecA stimulates the autoproteolysis of the SOS transcriptional repressor LexA. The LexA regulon includes a cell division inhibitor, SulA, that prevent the transmission of mutant DNA to the daughter cells. SulA is a dimer that binds FtsZ (a tubulin-like GTPase) in a 1:1 ratio and acts specifically on its polymerization which results in the formation of non-septated bacteria filaments. A similar mechanism may occur in *Mycobacterium tuberculosis*,which also elongates after being phagocytized.
- Ssd encoded by *rv3660c* promotes filamentation in *M. tuberculosis* in response to the stressful intracellular environment. Recently, septum site determining protein (Ssd) was discovered in this bacteria as a septum inhibitor, leading to elongated cells (not only in this specie but also in and in *Mycobacterium smegmatis*). The bacterial filament ultrastructure is consistent with inhibition of FtsZ polymerization (previously described). Ssd is believed to be part of a global regulatory mechanism in this bacteria that promotes a shift into an altered metabolic state.
- In *Helycobacter pylori*, a spriral-shaped Gram-negative bacterium, the filamentation mechanism are regulated by two mechanisms: the peptidases that

cause peptidoglycan relaxation and the coiled-coil-rich proteins (Ccrp) that are responsible for the helical cell shape *in vitro* as well as *in vivo.* A rod shape could have probably an advantage for motility than the regular helical shape. In this model, there is another protein Mre, which is not exactly involved in the maintenance of cell shape but in the cell cycle. It has been demotrated that mutant cells were highly elongated due to a delay in cell division and contained non-segregated chromosomes.

Environmental Cues

Immune Response

Some of the strategies for bacteria to bypass host defenses include the generation of filamentous structures. As it has been observed in other organisms (such as fungi), filamentous forms are resistant to phagocytosis. As an example of this, during urinary tract infection, filamentatious structures of uropathogenic E. coli (UPEC) start to develop in response to host innate immune response (more exactly in response to toll-like receptor 4-TLR4). TLR-4 is stimulated by the lipopolysaccharide (LPS) and recruits neutrophils (PMN) which are important leukocytes to eliminate these bacteria. Adopting filamentous structures, bacteria resist these phagocytic cells and their neutralizing activity (which include antimicrobial peptides, degradative enzyme and reactive oxygen species). It is believed that filamentation is induced as a response of DNA damage (by the mechanisms previously exposed), participating SulA mechanism and additional factors. Furthermore, the length of the filamentous bacteria could have a stronger attachment to the epithelial cells, with an increased number of adhesins participating in the interaction, making even harder the work for (PMN). The interaction between phagocyte cells and adopting filamentous-shape bacteria provide an advantage to their survival. In this relate, filamentation could be not only a virulence, but also a resistance factor in these bacteria.

Predator Protist

Bacteria exhibit a high degree of "morphological plasticity" that protects them from predation. Bacterial capture by protozoa is affected by size and irregularities in shape of bacteria. Oversized, filamentous, or prosthecate bacteria may be too large to be ingested. On the other hand, other factors such as extremely tiny cells, high-speed motility, tenacious attachment to surfaces, formation of biofilms and multicellular conglomerates may also reduce predation. Several phenotypic features of bacteria are adapted to escape protistan-grazing pressure.

Protistan grazing or bacterivory is a protozoan feeding on bacteria. It affects prokaryotic size and the distribution of microbial groups. There are several feeding mechanisms used to seek and capture prey, because the bacteria have to avoid being consumed from these factors. There are six feeding mechanisms listed by Kevin D. Young.

- ***Filter feeding***: transport water through a filter or sieve
- ***Sedimentation***: allows prey to settle into a capture device

- ***Interception***: capture by predator-induced current or motility and phagocytosis
- ***Raptorial***: predator craws and ingests prey through pharynx or by pseudopods
- ***Pallium***: prey engulfed e.g. by extrusion of feeding membrane
- ***Myzocytosis***: punctures prey and suck out cytoplasm and content

Bacterial responses are elicited depending on the predator and prey combinations because feeding mechanisms differ among the protists. Moreover, the grazing protists also produce the by-products, which directly lead to the morphological plasticity of prey bacteria. For example, the morphological phenotypes of Flectobacillus spp. were evaluated in the presence and absence of the flagellate grazer Orchromonas spp. in a laboratory that has environmental control within a chemostat. Without grazer and with adequate nutrient supply, the Flectobacillus spp. grew mainly in medium-sized rod (4-7 μm), remaining a typical 6.2 μm in length. With the predator, the Flectobacillus spp. size was altered to an average 18.6 μm and it is resistant to grazing. Interestingly, if the bacteria are exposed to the soluble by-products produced by grazing Orchromonas spp. and pass through a dialysis membrane, the bacterial length can increase to an average 11.4 μm. Filamentation occurs as a direct response to these effectors that are produced by the predator and there is a size preference for grazing that varies for each species of protist. The filamentous bacteria that are larger than 7 μm in length are generally inedible by marine protists. This morphological class is called grazing resistant. Thus, filamentation leads to the prevention of phagocytosis and killing by predator.

Bimodal Effect

Bimodal effect is a situation that bacterial cell in an intermediate size range are consumed more rapidly than the very large or the very small. The bacteria, which are smaller than 0.5 μm in diameter, are grazed by protists four to six times less than larger cells. Moreover, the filamentous cells or cells with diameters greater than 3 μm are often too large to ingest by protists or are grazed at substantially lower rates than smaller bacteria. The specific effects vary with the size ratio between predator and prey. Pernthaler et al. classified susceptible bacteria into four groups by rough size.

- Bacterial size $<$ 0.4 μm were not grazed well
- Bacterial size between 0.4 μm and 1.6 μm were “grazing vulnerable”
- Bacterial size between 1.6 μm and 2.4 μm were “grazing suppressed”
- Bacterial size $>$ 2.4 μm were “grazing resistant”

Filamentous preys are resistant to protist predation in a number of marine environments. In fact, there is no bacterium entirely safe. Some predators graze the larger filaments to some degree. Morphological plasticity of some bacterial strains is able to show at different growth conditions. For instance, at enhanced growth rates, some strains can form large thread-like morphotypes. While filament formation in subpopulations can occur during starvation or at suboptimal growth conditions. These morphological shifts could be triggered by external chemical cues that might be released by the predator itself.

Besides bacterial size, there are several factors affecting the predation of protists. Bacterial shape, the spiral morphology may play a defensive role towards predation feedings.

For example, Arthrospira may reduce its susceptibility to predation by altering its spiral pitch. This alteration inhibits some natural geometric feature of the protist's ingestion apparatus. Multicellular complexes of bacterial cells also change the ability of protist's ingestion. Cells in biofilms or microcolonies are often more resistant to predation. For instance, the swarm cells of Serratia liquefaciens resist predation by its predator, Tetrahymenu. Due to the normal-sized cells that first contact a surface are most susceptible, bacteria need elongating swarm cells to protect them from predation until the biofilm matures. For aquatic bacteria, they can produce a wide range of extracellular polymeric substances (EPS), which comprise protein, nucleic acids, lipids, polysaccharides and other biological macromolecules. EPS secretion protects bacteria from HNF grazing. The EPS-producing planktonic bacteria typically develop subpopulations of single cells and microcolonies that are embedded in an EPS matrix. The larger microcolonies are also protected from flagellate predation because of their size. The shift to the colonial type may be a passive consequence of selective feeding on single cells. However, the microcolony formation can be specifically induced in the presence of predators by cell-cell communication (quorum sensing).

As for bacterial motility, the bacteria with high-speed motility sometimes avoid grazing better than their nonmotile or slower strains especially the smallest, fastest bacteria. Moreover, a cell's movement strategy may be altered by predation. The bacteria move by run-and-reverse strategy, which help them to beat a hasty retreat before being trapped instead of moving by the run-and-tumble strategy. However, there is a study showed that the probability of random contacts between predators and prey increases with bacterial swimming, and motile bacteria can be consumed at higher rates by HNFs. In addition, bacterial surface properties affect predation as well as other factors. For example, there is an evidence shows that protists prefer gram-negative bacteria than gram-positive bacteria. Protists consume gram-positive cells at much lower rates than consuming gram-negative cells. The heterotrophic nanoflagellates actively avoid grazing on gram-positive actinobacteria as well. Grazing on gram-positive cells takes longer digestion time than on gram-negative cells. As a result of this, the predator cannot handle more prey until the previous ingested material is consumed or expelled. Moreover, bacterial cell surface charge and hydrophobicity have also been suggested that might reduce grazing ability. Another strategy that bacteria can use for avoiding the predation is to poison their predator. For example, certain bacteria such as Chromobacterium violaceum and Pseudomonas aeruginosa can secrete toxin agents related to quorum sensing to kill their predators.

Antibiotic

Antimicrobial agent has obvious implications for microbial infection therapeutics. The ability of bacteria to decrease their susceptibility to antimicrobial drugs importantly affects both bacterial ecology and the treatment of infectious diseases. From patients who are treated with antibiotics, filamentous organisms are commonly found in their clinical specimens. The filamentation contributes to a pathogen's resistance to this antimicrobial agent. The induction of bacterial filamentation by antibiotics can alter bacterial virulence, which would have important implications for the pathogenesis and treatment of the disease as well.

For Burkholderia pseudomallei, some clinical antibiotic agents that are used to treat its infection, mellioidosis, can induce morphological changes such as filamentation and physiological changes in this bacteria. These antibiotics are the β-lactam antibiotics, fluoroquinolones, and antibiotics that inhibit the synthesis of thymidine. The ability of some β-lactam antibiotics to induce filamentation in gram negative bacteria is to inhibit penicillin-binding proteins (PBPs). This inhibition stops the assembly of peptidoglycan network in bacterial cell wall. PBP-1 inhibition leads to rapid cell death. While PBP-2 and PBP-3 inhibition lead to morphological change, turn normal cells to spheroplasts and filamentous cells (elongated rods), respectively. PBP-3 forms the septum in dividing bacteria by involving transpeptidase so inhibition of this PBP-3 protein leads to the incomplete formation of septa in dividing bacteria resulting in the formation of long strands of bacteria (filaments). Kang Chen, et al. mentioned that the filament was induced by sublethal concentrations of ceftazidime, ofloxacin, or trimethoprim. At or below the minimal inhibitory concentration (MIC), filamentation occurred mainly at these concentration and bacteria remained as viable within the vacuoles of immortalized human macrophages, not rapidly killed. However, the B.pseudomallei filaments revert to normal forms when the antibiotics are removed. Moreover, bacillary daughter cells maintained cell-division capacity and viability despite re-exposure to antibiotics such as ceftazidime. Thus, this developmental alteration may provide additionally survival advantages to bacteria. Furthermore, for Pseudomonas aeruginosa, filamentation induced by antibiotics appears to trigger bacteria to change from a normal growth phase to a stationary growth phase. Filamentous bacteria are also associated with an increase in endotoxin (lipopolysaccharide, LPS) release and the immune system of patients needs to cope with this characteristic. Chloramphenicol antibiotic can induce the formation of filamentous cells, which contain multiple copies of unsegregated chromosomes. These chromosomes lead to the unsuccessful division of elongated cells, and the formation of bacterial filament. Moreover, the filamentation also depends on the expression levels of an efflux pump (MexAB-OprM) and the minimum inhibitory concentration of chloramphenicol.

The molecular correlate of the filament formation was described. The exposure to β-lactam antibiotics induced the SOS response in Escherichia coli. During repair of DNA damage, the SOS response aids bacterial propagation by inhibiting cell division. Moreover, both β-lactam antibiotics and genetic mutation induce SOS in E.coli through the DpiBA two-component signal transduction system leading to the inactivation of the ftsl gene product, penicillin binding protein 3 (PBP-3). The ftsl gene is a group of filamentous temperature-sensitive genes implicated in cell division. In addition, it is a membrane transpeptidase required for peptidoglycan synthesis at the septum generated by cell division. The event to inactivate ftsl gene product requires the SOS-promoting recA and lexA genes as well as dpiA and transiently inhibits bacterial cell division. Consequently, the bactericidal effects of β-lactam antibiotics are limited. The DpiA is the effector for the DpiB two-component system. Interaction of DpiA with replication origins competes with the binding of the replication proteins DnaA and DnaB. When overexpressed, DpiA can interrupt DNA replication and induce the SOS response resulting in inhibition of cell division.

Nutritional Stress

Nutritional stress can change bacterial morphology. A common shape alteration is filamentation which can be triggered by a limited availability of one or more substrates, nutrients or electron acceptors. Since the filament can increase a cell's uptake–surface area without significantly changing its volume appreciably. Moreover, the filamentation benefits bacterial cells attaching to a surface because it increases specific surface area in direct contact with the solid medium. In addition, the filamentation may allows bacterial cells to access nutrients by enhancing the possibility that part of the filament will contact a nutrient-rich zone and pass compounds to the rest of the cell's biomass. For example, Actinomyces israelii grows as filamentous rods or branched in the absence of phosphate, cysteine, or glutathione. However, it returns to a regular rod-like morphology when adding back these nutrients.

BACILLUS

Bacillus is a genus of gram-positive, rod-shaped bacteria and a member of the phylum Firmicutes. Bacillus species can be obligate aerobes (oxygen reliant), or facultative anaerobes (having the ability to be aerobic or anaerobic). They will test positive for the enzyme catalase when there has been oxygen used or present. Ubiquitous in nature, Bacillus includes both free-living (nonparasitic) and parasitic pathogenic species. Under stressful environmental conditions, the bacteria can produce oval endospores that are not true 'spores', but to which the bacteria can reduce themselves and remain in a dormant state for very long periods. These characteristics originally defined the genus, but not all such species are closely related, and many have been moved to other genera of the Firmicutes.

Many species of Bacillus can produce copious amounts of enzymes which are made use of in different industries. Some species can form intracellular inclusions of polyhydroxyalkanoates under certain adverse environmental conditions, as in a lack of elements such as phosphorus, nitrogen, or oxygen combined with an excessive supply of carbon sources.

B. subtilis has proved a valuable model for research. Other species of Bacillus are important pathogens, causing anthrax and food poisoning.

Industrial Significance

Many Bacillus species are able to secrete large quantities of enzymes. Bacillus amyloliquefaciens is the source of a natural antibiotic protein barnase (a ribonuclease), alpha amylase used in starch hydrolysis, the protease subtilisin used with detergents, and the BamH1 restriction enzyme used in DNA research.

A portion of the Bacillus thuringiensis genome was incorporated into corn (and cotton) crops. The resulting GMOs are therefore resistant to some insect pests.

Use as Model Organism

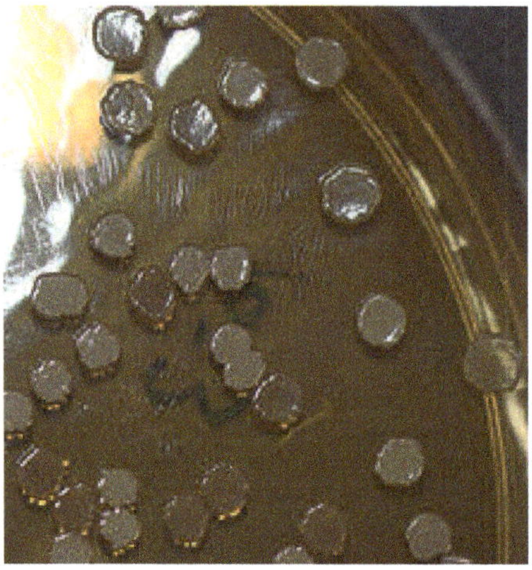

Colonies of the model species *Bacillus subtilis* on an agar plate.

Bacillus subtilis is one of the best understood prokaryotes, in terms of molecular and cellular biology. Its superb genetic amenability and relatively large size have provided the powerful tools required to investigate a bacterium from all possible aspects. Recent improvements in fluorescent microscopy techniques have provided novel insight into the dynamic structure of a single cell organism. Research on B. subtilis has been at the forefront of bacterial molecular biology and cytology, and the organism is a model for differentiation, gene/protein regulation, and cell cycle events in bacteria.

Ecological Significance

Bacillus species are almost ubiquitous in nature, e.g. in soil, but also occur in extreme environments such as high pH (B. alcalophilus), high temperature (B. thermophilus), or high salt (B. halodurans). B. thuringiensis produces a toxin that can kill insects and thus has been used as insecticide.

Clinical Significance

Two Bacillus species are considered medically significant: B. anthracis, which causes anthrax, and B. cereus, which causes food poisoning similar to that caused by Staphylococcus. A third species, B. thuringiensis, is an important insect pathogen, and is sometimes used to control insect pests. The type species is B. subtilis, an important model organism. It is also a notable food spoiler, causing ropiness in bread and related food. Some environmental and commercial strains of B. coagulans may play a role in food spoilage of highly acidic, tomato-based products.

An easy way to isolate Bacillus species is by placing nonsterile soil in a test tube with water, shaking, placing in melted mannitol salt agar, and incubating at room temperature for at least a day. Colonies are usually large, spreading, and irregularly shaped. Under the microscope, the Bacillus cells appear as rods, and a substantial portion of the cells usually contain oval endospores at one end, making it bulge.

Cell wall

The cell wall of Bacillus is a structure on the outside of the cell that forms the second barrier between the bacterium and the environment, and at the same time maintains the rod shape and withstands the pressure generated by the cell's turgor. The cell wall is composed of teichoic and teichuronic acids. B. subtilis is the first bacterium for which the role of an actin-like cytoskeleton in cell shape determination and peptidoglycan synthesis was identified, and for which the entire set of peptidoglycan-synthesizing enzymes was localised. The role of the cytoskeleton in shape generation and maintenance is important

Phylogeny

The genus Bacillus was named in 1835 by Christian Gottfried Ehrenberg, to contain rod-shaped (bacillus) bacteria. He had seven years earlier named the genus Bacterium. Bacillus was later amended by Ferdinand Cohn to further describe them as spore-forming, Gram-positive, aerobic or facultatively anaerobic bacteria. Like other genera associated with the early history of microbiology, such as Pseudomonas and Vibrio, the 266 species of Bacillus are ubiquitous. The genus has a very large ribosomal 16S diversity and is environmentally diverse.

Several studies have tried to reconstruct the phylogeny of the genus. The Bacillus-specific study with the most diversity covered is by Xu and Cote using 16S and the ITS regions, where they divide the genus into 10 groups, which includes the nested genera Paenibacillus, Brevibacillus, Geobacillus, Marinibacillus and Virgibacillus. However, the tree constructed by the living tree project, a collaboration between ARB-Silva and LPSN where a 16S (and 23S if available) tree of all validated species was constructed, the genus Bacillus contains a very large number of nested taxa and majorly in both 16S and 23S it is paraphyletic to the Lactobacillales (Lactobacillus, Streptococcus, Staphylococcus, Listeria, etc.), due to Bacillus coahuilensis and others. A gene concatenation study found similar results to Xu and Cote, but with a much more limited number of species in terms of groups, but used Listeria as an outgroup, so in light of the ARB tree, it may be "inside-out". One clade, formed by B. anthracis, B. cereus, B. mycoides, B. pseudomycoides, B. thuringiensis, and B. weihenstephanensis under current classification standards, should be a single species (within 97% 16S identity), but due to medical reasons, they are considered separate species,:34–35 an issue also present for four species of Shigella and Escherichia coli.

SPIRAL

Spiral bacteria form the third major bacterial cell morphology. Spiral bacteria can be sub-classified as spirilla, spirochetes, or vibrios based on the number of twists per cell, cell thickness, cell flexibility, and motility.

L-FORM BACTERIA

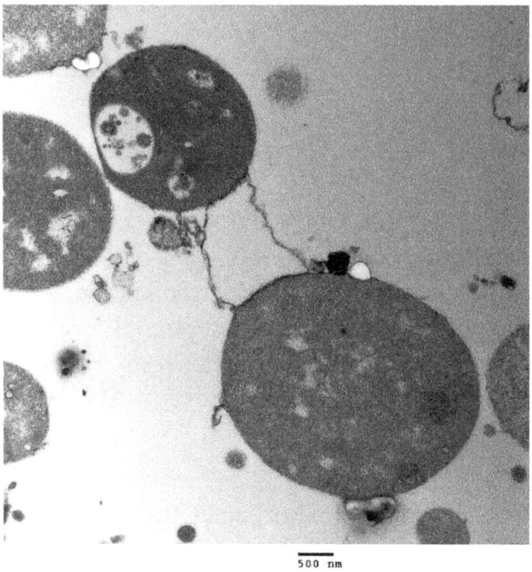

Transmission electron micrograph of L-form *Bacillus subtilis*. The cells lack the electron-dense cell wall of normal bacteria. Scale bar is 500 nanometers.

L-form bacteria, also known as L-phase bacteria, L-phase variants, and cell wall-deficient (CWD) bacteria, are strains of bacteria that lack cell walls. They were first isolated in 1935 by Emmy Klieneberger-Nobel, who named them "L-forms" after the Lister Institute in London where she was working.

Two types of L-forms are distinguished: *unstable L-forms*, spheroplasts that are capable of dividing, but can revert to the original morphology, and *stable L-forms*, L-forms that are unable to revert to the original bacteria.

Some parasitic species of bacteria, such as mycoplasma, also lack a cell wall, but these are not considered L-forms since they are not derived from bacteria that normally have cell walls.

Appearance and cell Division

Bacterial morphology is determined by the cell wall. Since the L-form has no cell wall, its morphology is different from that of the strain of bacteria from which it is derived. Typical L-form cells are spheres or spheroids. For example, L-forms of the rod-shaped bacterium Bacillus subtilis appear round when viewed by phase contrast microscopy or by transmission electron microscopy.

Although L-forms can develop from Gram-positive as well as from Gram-negative bacteria, in a Gram stain test, the L-forms always colour Gram-negative, due to the lack of a cell wall.

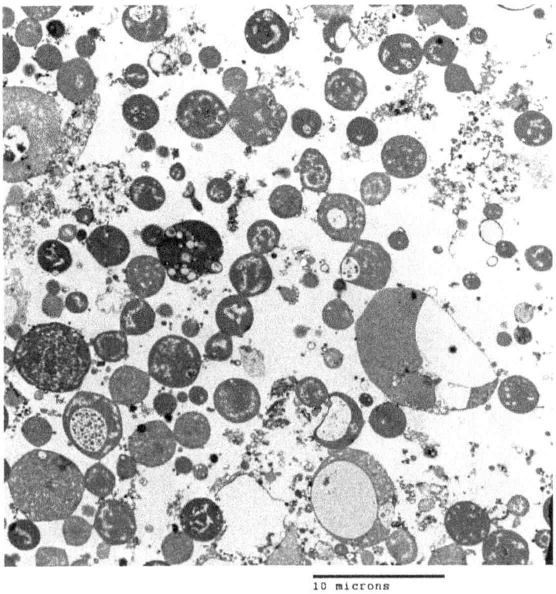

Transmission electron micrograph of a population of L-form *Bacillus subtilis*, showing a range of sizes. Scale bar is 10 micrometers.

The cell wall is important for cell division, which, in most bacteria, occurs by binary fission. This process usually requires a cell wall and components of the bacterial cytoskeleton such as FtsZ. The ability of L-form bacteria to grow and divide in the absence of both of these structures is highly unusual, and may represent a form of cell division that was important in early forms of life. This novel mode of division seems to involve the extension of thin protrusions from the cells surface and these protrusions then pinching off to form new cells. The lack of cell wall in L-forms means that division is disorganised, giving rise to a variety of cell sizes, from very tiny to very big.

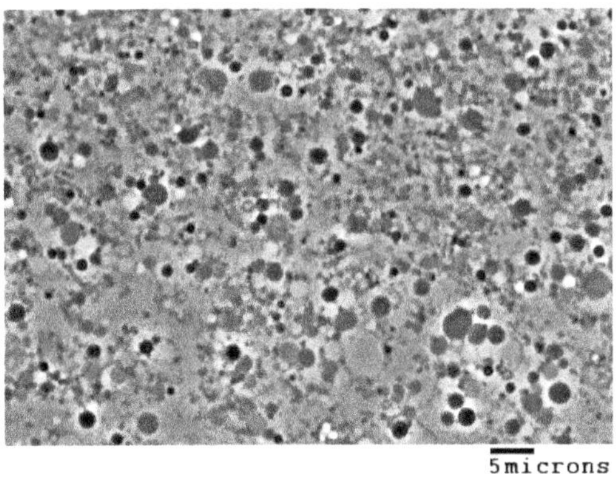

Phase contrast image of L-form cells from *Bacillus subtilis* showing a range of sizes. Scale bar is 5 micrometers.

Generation in Cultures

L-forms can be generated in the laboratory from many bacterial species that usually have cell walls, such as Bacillus subtilis or Escherichia coli. This is done by inhibiting peptidoglycan synthesis with antibiotics or treating the cells with lysozyme, an enzyme that digests cell walls. The L-forms are generated in a culture medium that is the same osmolarity as the bacterial cytosol (an isotonic solution), which prevents cell lysis by osmotic shock. L-form strains can be unstable, tending to revert to the normal form of the bacteria by regrowing a cell wall, but this can be prevented by long-term culture of the cells under the same conditions that were used to produce them.

Some studies have identified mutations that occur, as these strains are derived from normal bacteria. One such point mutation is in an enzyme involved in the mevalonate pathway of lipid metabolism that increased the frequency of L-form formation 1,000-fold. The reason for this effect is not known, but it is presumed that the increase is related to this enzyme's role in making a lipid important in peptidoglycan synthesis.

Another methodology of induction relies on nanotechnology and landscape ecology. Microfluidics devices can be built in order to challenge peptidoglycan synthesis by extreme spatial confinement. After biological dispersal through a constricted (sub-micrometre scale) biological corridor connecting adjacent micro habitat patches, L-form-like cells can be derived using a microfluifics-based (synthetic) ecosystem implementing an adaptive landscape selecting for shape-shifting phenotypes similar to L-forms. .

Significance and Applications

Some publications have suggested that L-form bacteria might cause diseases in humans, and other animals but, as the evidence that links these organisms to disease is fragmentary and frequently contradictory, this hypothesis remains controversial. The two extreme viewpoints on this question are that L-form bacteria are either laboratory curiosities of no clinical significance or important but unappreciated causes of disease. Research on L-form bacteria is continuing. For example, L-form organisms have been observed in mouse lungs after experimental inoculation with *Nocardia caviae*, and a recent study suggested that these organisms may infect immunosuppressed patients having undergone bone marrow transplants. The formation of strains of bacteria lacking cell walls has also been proposed to be important in the acquisition of bacterial antibiotic resistance.

L-form bacteria may be useful in research on early forms of life, and in biotechnology. These strains are being examined for possible uses in biotechnology as host strains for recombinant protein production. Here, the absence of a cell wall can allow production of large amounts of secreted proteins that would otherwise accumulate in the periplasmic space of bacteria.

PROTOPLAST

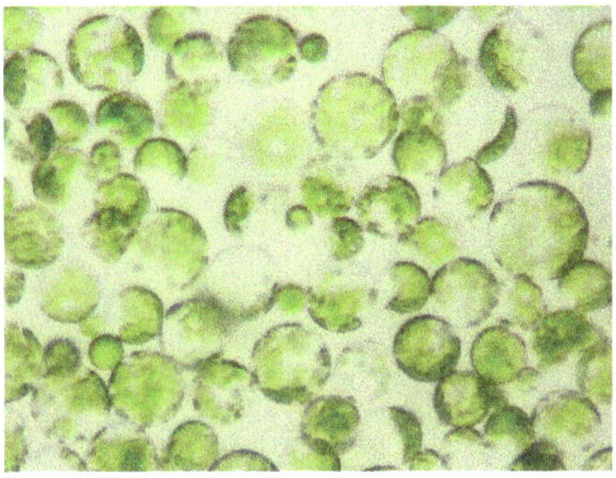

Protoplasts of cells from a petunia's leaf

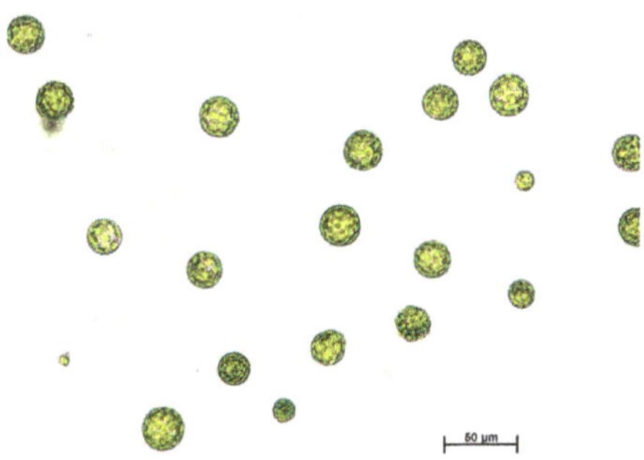

Protoplasts of the moss *Physcomitrella patens*

Protoplast, from ancient Greek πρωτόπλαστος (*prōtóplastos*, "first-formed"), in a religious context initially referred to the first human or, more generally, to the first organized body of a species.

In biology, it was proposed by Hanstein (1880) to refer to the entire cell, excluding the cell wall, but currently has several definitions:

- a plant, bacterial or fungal cell that had its cell wall completely or partially removed using either mechanical or enzymatic means. A further differentiation can be made for bacteria:
    - protoplasts: have their cell wall entirely removed and are derived from gram + (gram-positive)
    - spheroplasts: have their cell wall only partially removed and are gram - (gram-negative)
- more generally, a unit of biology which is composed of a cells nucleus and the surrounding protoplasmic materials.

Enzymes for the preparation of protoplasts

Cell walls are made of a variety of polysaccharides. Protoplasts can be made by degrading cell walls with a mixture of the appropriate polysaccharide-degrading enzymes:

Types of cell	**Enzyme**
Plant cells	Cellulase, pectinase, xylanase
Gram-positive bacteria	Lysozyme (+EDTA)
Fungal cells	Chitinase

During and subsequent to digestion of the cell wall, the protoplast becomes very sensitive to osmotic stress. This means cell wall digestion and protoplast storage must be done in an isotonic solution to prevent rupture of the plasma membrane.

Uses of Protoplasts

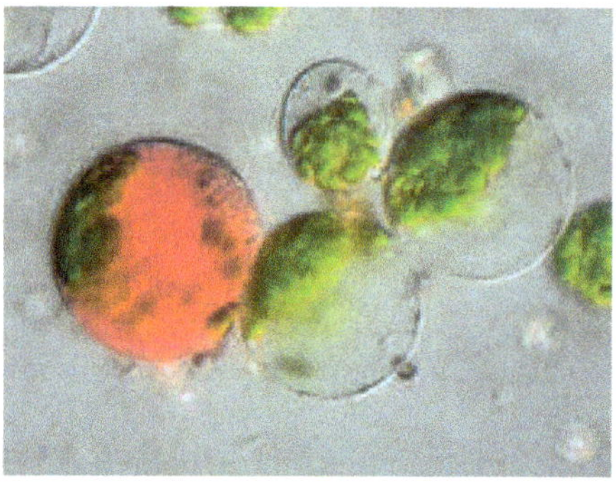

Fused protoplast (on left), containing both chloroplasts (from a leaf cell) as well as a coloured vacuole (from a petal).

Protoplasts can be used to study membrane biology, including the uptake of macromolecules and viruses . These are also used in somaclonal variation.

Protoplasts are widely used for DNA transformation (for making genetically modified organisms), since the cell wall would otherwise block the passage of DNA into the cell. In the case of plant cells, protoplasts may be regenerated into whole plants first by growing into a group of plant cells that develops into a callus and then by regeneration of shoots (caulogenesis) from the callus using plant tissue culture methods. Growth of protoplasts into callus and regeneration of shoots requires the proper balance of plant growth regulators in the tissue culture medium that must be customized for each species of plant. Unlike protoplasts from vascular plants, protoplasts from mosses, such as *Physcomitrella patens*, do not need phytohormones for regeneration, nor do they form a callus during regeneration. Instead, they regenerate directly into the filamentous protonema, mimicking a germinating moss spore.

Protoplasts may also be used for plant breeding, using a technique called protoplast fusion. Protoplasts from different species are induced to fuse by using an electric field or a solution of polyethylene glycol. This technique may be used to generate somatic hybrids in tissue culture.

Additionally, protoplasts of plants expressing fluorescent proteins in certain cells may be used for Fluorescence Activated Cell Sorting (FACS), where only cells fluorescing a selected wavelength are retained. Among other things, this technique is used to isolate specific cell types (e.g. guard cells from leaves, pericycle cells from roots) for further investigations, such as transcriptomics.

SPHEROPLAST

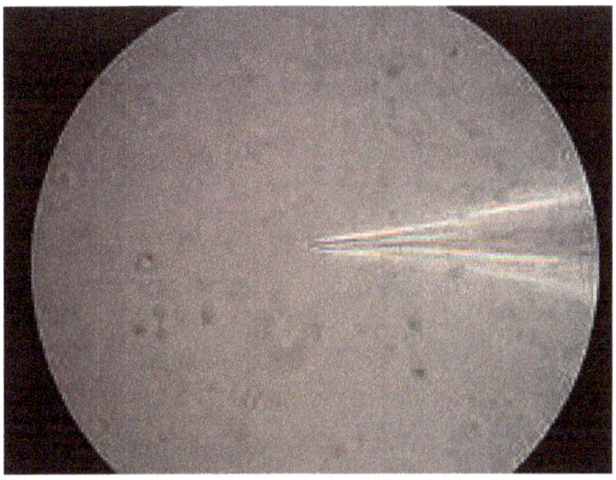

An *E. coli* spheroplast patched with a glass pipette.

A spheroplast is a cell from which the cell wall has been almost completely removed, as by the action of penicillin. The name stems from the fact that after a microbe's cell wall is digested, membrane tension causes the cell to acquire a characteristic spherical shape. Spheroplasts are osmotically fragile, and will lyse if transferred to a hypotonic solution.

Uses and Applications

Antibiotic discovery

From the 1960s into the 1990s Merck and Co. used a spheroplast screen as a primary method for discovery of antibiotics that inhibit cell wall biosynthesis. In this screen devised by Eugene Dulaney, growing bacteria were exposed to test substances under hypertonic conditions. Inhibitors of cell wall synthesis caused growing bacteria to form spheroplasts. This screen enabled the discovery of fosfomycin, cephamycin C, thienamycin and several carbapenems.

Patch Clamping

Specially prepared giant spheroplasts of Gram-negative bacteria can be used to study the function of bacterial ion channels through a technique called patch clamp, which was originally designed for characterizing the behavior of neurons and other excitable cells. To prepare giant spheroplasts, bacteria are grown in a medium containing chemicals that prevent the cells from dividing completely. This causes bacteria to form long "snakes" that share a single membrane and cytoplasm. After a period of time, the cell walls of the "snakes" are digested, and the bacteria collapse into very large spheres surrounded by a single lipid bilayer. The membrane can then be analyzed on a patch clamp apparatus to determine the phenotype of the ion channels embedded in it. It is also common to overexpress a particular channel to amplify its effect and make it easier to characterize.

The technique of patch clamping giant E. coli spheroplasts has been used extensively for studying the native mechanosensitive channels (MscL, MscS, and MscM) of E. coli since 1987. Recently, it has been extended to study other heterologously expressed ion channels and it has been shown that the giant E. coli spheroplast can be used as an ion-channel expression system comparable to the Xenopus oocyte.

Cell lysis

Yeast cells are normally protected by a thick cell wall which makes extraction of cellular proteins difficult. Enzymatic digestion of the cell wall with zymolyase, creating spheroplasts, renders the cells vulnerable to easy lysis with detergents or rapid osmolar pressure changes.

Transfection

Bacterial spheroplasts, with suitable recombinant DNA inserted into it, can be used to transfect animal cells. Spheroplasts with recombinant DNA are introduced into the media containing animal cells and are fused by polyethylene glycol (PEG). With this methodology, nearly 100% of the animal cells may take up the foreign DNA.

MYCOPLASMA PNEUMONIAE

Mycoplasma pneumoniae is a very small bacterium in the class Mollicutes. It is a human pathogen that causes the disease mycoplasma pneumonia, a form of atypical bacterial pneumonia related to cold agglutinin disease. M. pneumoniae is characterized by the absence of a peptidoglycan cell wall and resulting resistance to many antibacterial agents. The persistence of M. pneumoniae infections even after treatment is associated with its ability to mimic host cell surface composition.

In 1898, Nocard and Roux were the first to isolate a mycoplasma species in culture from bovine, however it wasnt until 1944 when *Mycoplasma pneumoniae*, known then as Eaton agent or Eaton's agent, was isolated and described from a patient with primary atypical pneumonia.

Initially M. pneumoniae was considered as a virus rather than a bacterium, when Eaton and colleagues cultured the causative agent of human primary atypical pneumonia (PAP) or walking pneumonia. The terms walking pneumonia and atypical pneumonia were coined to describe the unresponsiveness of pneumonia inducing M. pneumoniae infections to antibiotics like penicillin. Eaton's agent could be grown in chicken embryos and passed through a filter that excluded normal bacteria. Eaton suggested the possibility that the disease was caused by a mycoplasma, but the agent did not grow on the standard pleuropneumonia-like organism (PPLO) media of the time. These observations led to the conclusion that the causative agent of PAP was a virus. Researchers at that time showed that the cultured agent could induce disease in experimentally infected cotton rats and hamsters. In spite of controversy whether the researchers had truly isolated the causative agent of PAP (based largely on the unusual immunological response of patients with PAP), in retrospect their evidence along with that of colleagues and competitors appears to have been quite conclusive. There were reports linking Eaton agent to the PPLOs or mycoplasmas, well known then as parasites of cattle and rodents, due to sensitivity to antimicrobials. Studies that followed until 1963 determined that Eaton's agent was a bacterium that caused human lower respiratory tract infections.

Taxonomy and Classification

The term mycoplasma ("mykes", meaning fungus and "plasma", meaning formed) is derived from the fungal-like growth of some mycoplasma species. The mycoplasmas were classified as Mollicutes ("mollis", meaning soft and "cutis", meaning skin) in 1960 due to their small size and genome, lack of cell wall, low G+C content and unusual nutritional needs. M. pneumoniae has also been designated as an arginine nonfermenting species. Mycoplasmas are further classified by the sequence composition of 16s rRNA. All mycoplasmas of the pneumoniae group possess similar 16s rRNA variations unique to the group, of which M. pneumoniae has a 6.3% variation in the conserved regions, that suggest mycoplasmas formed by degenerative evolution from the gram-positive eubacterial group that includes bacilli, streptococci, and lactobacilli. M. pneumoniae is a member of the Mycoplasmataceae family and Mycoplasmatales order.

Cell Biology

Mycoplasmas, are among the smallest self-replicating organisms, are parasitic species that lack a cell wall and periplasmic space, have reduced genomes, and limited metabolic activity. Mycoplasma pneumoniae cells have an elongated shape that is approximately 0.1–0.2 μm (100-200 nm) in width and 1-2 μm (1000-2000 nm) in length.

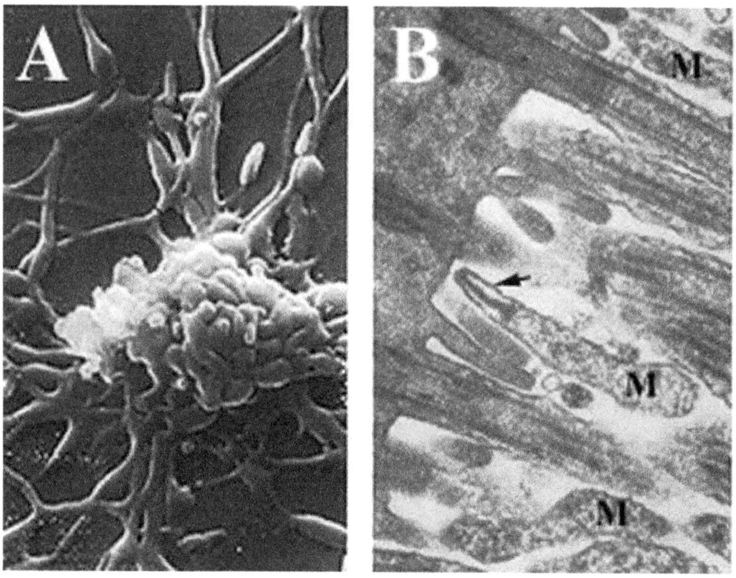

Filamentous *Mycoplasma pneumoniae* cells B) *M. pneumoniae* cells (M) attached to ciliated mucosal cells by the attachment organelle (indicated by arrow)

The extremely small cell size means they are incapable of being examined by light microscopy; a stereomicroscope is required for viewing the morphology of M. pneumoniae colonies, which are usually less than 100 μm in length. The inability to synthesize a peptidoglycan cell wall is due to the absence of genes encoding its formation and results in an increased importance in maintenance of osmotic stability to avoid desiccation.The lack of a cell wall also calls for increased support of the cell membrane(reinforced with sterols), which includes a rigid cytoskeleton composed of an intricate protein network and, potentially, an extracellularcapsule to facilitate adherence to the host cell. M. pneumoniae are the only bacterial cells that possess cholesterol in their cell membrane (obtained from the host) and possess more genes that encode for membrane lipoprotein variations than other mycoplasmas, which are thought to be associated with its parasitic lifestyle. M. pneumoniae cells also possess an attachment organelle, which is used in the gliding motility of the organism by an unknown mechanism.

Genomics and Metabolic Reconstruction

Sequencing of the M. pneumoniae genome in 1996 revealed it is 816,394 bp in size. The genome contains 687 genes that encode for proteins, of which about 56.6% code for essential metabolic enzymes; notably those involved in glycolysis and organic acid fermentation. M. pneumoniae is consequently very susceptible to loss of enzymatic function by gene mutations, as the only buffering systems against functional loss by point mutations are for maintenance of the pentose phosphate pathway and nucleotide metabolism. Loss of function in other pathways is suggested to be compensated by host cell metabolism. In addition to the potential for loss of pathway function, the reduced genome of M. pneumoniae outright lacks a number of pathways, including the TCA cycle, respiratory electron transport chain, and biosynthesis pathways for amino acids, fatty acids, cholesterol and purines and pyrimidines. These limitations make M. pneumoniae dependent upon import systems to acquire essential building blocks from their host or the environment that cannot be obtained through glycolytic pathways. Along with energy costly protein and RNA production, a large portion of energy metabolism is exerted to maintain proton gradients (up to 80%) due to the high surface area to volume ratio of M. pneumoniae cells. Only 12 – 29% of energy metabolism is directed at cell growth, which is unusually low for bacterial cells, and is thought to be an adaptation of its parasitic lifestyle. Unlike other bacteria, M. pneumoniae uses the codon UGA to code for tryptophan rather than using it as a stop codon.

Host and Reproduction

Mycoplasma pneumoniae exclusively parasitizes humans, and has never been isolated as a free-living organism due to its dependence upon the host for survival. Reproduction, therefore, is dependent upon attachment to a host cell. According to Waite and Talkington, specialized reproduction occurs by "binary fission, temporally linked with duplication of its attachment organelle, which migrates to the opposite pole of the cell during replication and before nucleoid separation".Mutations that affect the formation of the attachment organelle not only hinder motility and cell division, but also reduce the ability of M. pneumoniae cells to adhere to the host cell.

Pathogenicity

Mycoplasma pneumoniae parasitizes the respiratory tract epithelium of humans. Adherence to the respiratory epithelial cells is thought to occur via the attachment organelle, followed by evasion of host immune system by intracellular localization and adjustment of the cell membrane composition to mimic the host cell membrane.

Cytadherence

Adherence of M. pneumoniae to a host cell (usually a respiratory tract cell, but occasionally an erythrocyte or urogenital lining cell) is the initiating event for pneumonic disease and related symptoms. The specialized attachment organelle is a polar, electron dense and elongated cell extension that facilitates motility and cytadherence to host cells. It is composed of a central filament surrounded by an intracytoplasmic space, along with a number of adhesins and structural and accessory proteins localized at the tip of the organelle. A variety of proteins are known to contribute to the formation and functionality of the attachment organelle, including the accessory proteins HMW1–HMW5, P30, P56, and P90 that confer structure and adhesin support, and P1, P30 and P116 which are involved directly in attachment. This network of proteins participates not only in the initiation of attachment organelle formation and adhesion but also in motility. The P1 adhesin (trypsin-sensitive protein) is a 120 kDa protein highly clustered on the surface of the attachment organelle tip in virulent mycoplasmas. Both the presence of P1 and its concentration on the cell surface are required for the attachment of M. pneumoniae to the host cell. M. pneumoniae cells treated with monoclonal antibodies specific to the immunogenic C-terminus of the P1 adhesin have been shown to be inhibited in their ability to attach to the host cell surface by approximately 75%, suggesting P1 is a major component in cytadherence. These antibodies also decreased the ability of the cell to glide quickly, which may contribute to decreased adherence to the host by hindering their capacity to locate a host cell. Furthermore, mutations in P1 or degradation by trypsin treatment yield avirulent M. pneumoniae cells. Loss of proteins in the cytoskeleton involved in the localization of P1 in the tip structure, such as HMW1–HMW3, also cause avirulence due to the lack of adhesin clustering. Another protein considered to play an important role in cytadherence is P30, as M. pneumoniae cells with mutations in this protein or that have had antibodies raised against P30 are incapable of adhering to host cells. P30 is not involved in the localization of P1 in the tip structure since P1 is trafficked to the attachment organelle in P30 mutants, but rather it may function as a receptor-binding accessory adhesin. P30 mutants also display distinct morphological features such as multiple lobes and a rounded shape as opposed to elongated, which suggests P30 may interact with the cytoskeleton during formation of the attachment organelle. A number of eukaryotic cell surface components have been implicated in the adherence of M. pneumoniae cells to the respiratory tract epithelium. Among them are sialoglycoconjugates, sulfated glycolipids, glycoproteins, fibronectin, and neuraminic acid receptors. Lectins on the surface of the bacterial cells are capable of binding oligosaccharide chains on glycolipids and glycoproteins to facilitate attachment, in addition to the proteins TU and pyruvate dehydrogenase E1 β, which bind to fibronectin.

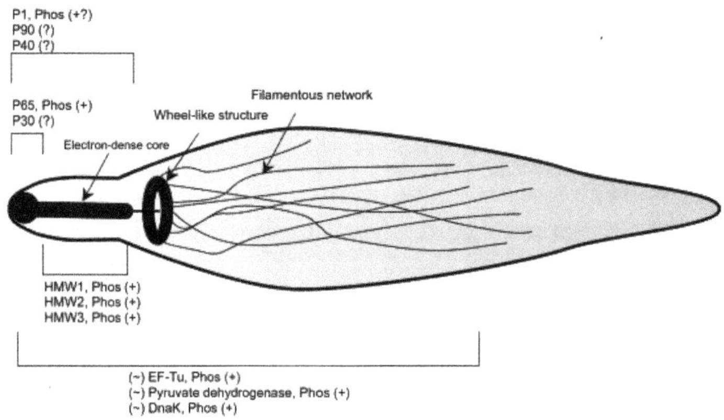

Schematic of the phosphorylated proteins in the attachment organelle of *Mycoplasma pneumoniae*

Intracellular Localization

Mycoplasma pneumoniae is known to evade host immune system detection, resist antibiotic treatment, and cross mucosal barriers, which may be due to its ability to fuse with host cells and survive intracellularly. In addition to the close physical proximity of M. pneumoniae and host cells, the lack of cell wall and peculiar cell membrane components, like cholesterol, may facilitate fusion (1). Internal localization may produce chronic or latent infections as M. pneumoniae is capable of persisting, synthesizing DNA, and replicating within the host cell even after treatment with antibiotics. The exact mechanism of intracellular localization is unknown, however the potential for cytoplasmic sequestration within the host explains the difficulty in completely eliminating M. pneumoniae infections in afflicted individuals.

Immune Response

In addition to evasion of host immune system by intracellular localization, M. pneumoniae can change the composition of its cell membrane to mimic the host cell membrane and avoid detection by immune system cells. M. pneumoniae cells possess a number of protein and glycolipid antigens that elicit immune responses, but variation of these surface antigens would allow the infection to persist long enough for M. pneumoniae cells to fuse with host cells and escape detection. The similarity between the compositions of M. pneumoniae and human cell membranes can also result in autoimmune responses in several organs and tissues.

Cytotoxicity and Organismal Effects

The main cytotoxic effect of M. pneumoniae is local disruption of tissue and cell structure along the respiratory tract epithelium due to its close proximity to host cells. Attachment of the bacteria to host cells can result in loss of cilia, a reduction in metabolism, biosynthesis, and import of macromolecules, and, eventually, infected cells may be shed from the epithelial lining. M. pneumoniae produces a unique virulence factor known as Community Acquired Respiratory Distress Syndrome (CARDS) toxin. The CARDS toxin most likely aids in the colonization and pathogenic pathways of M. pneumoniae, leading to inflammation and airway dysfunction. In addition, the formation of hydrogen peroxide is a key virulence factor in M. pneumoniae infections. Attachment of M. pneumoniae to erythrocytes permits diffusion of hydrogen peroxide from the bacteria to the host cell without detoxification by catalase or peroxidase, which can injure the host cell by reducing glutathione, damaging lipid membranes and causing protein denaturation. Local damage may also be a result of lactoferrin acquisition and subsequent hydroxyl radical, superoxide anion and peroxide formation. The cytotoxic effects of M. pneumoniae infections translate into common symptoms like coughing and lung irritation that may persist for months after infection has subsided. Local inflammation and hyperresponsiveness by infection induced cytokine production has been associated with chronic conditions such as bronchial asthma and has also been linked to progression of symptoms in individuals with cystic fibrosis and COPD.

Asthma-related Microbes

Epidemiology

The incidence of disease does not appear be related to season or geography, however infection tends to occur more frequently during the summer and fall months when other respiratory pathogens are less prevalent. Reinfection and epidemic cycling is thought to be a result of P1 adhesin subtype variation. Approximately 40% of community-acquired pneumonia is due to M. pneumoniae infections, with children and elderly individuals being most susceptible, however no personal risk factors for acquiring M. pneumoniae induced pneumonia have been determined. Transmission of M. pneumoniae can only occur through close contact and exchange of aerosols by coughing due to the increased susceptibility of the cell wall-lacking organism to desiccation. Outbreaks of M. pneumoniae infections tend to occur within groups of people in close and prolonged proximity, including schools, institutions, military bases, and households.

Symptoms of Infection

M. pneumoniae is known to cause a host of symptoms such as primary atypical pneumonia, tracheobronchitis, and upper respiratory tract disease. Primary atypical pneumonia is one of the most severe types of manifestation, with tracheobronchitis being the most common symptom and another 15% of cases, usually adults, remain asymptomatic. Symptomatic infections tend to develop over a period of several days and manifestation of pneumonia can be confused with a number of other bacterial pathogens and conditions that cause pneumonia. Tracheobronchitis is most common in children due to a reduced immune system capacity, and up to 18% of infected children require hospitalization. Common mild symptoms include sore throat, wheezing and coughing, fever, headache, coryza, myalgia and feelings of unease, in which symptom intensity and duration can be limited by early treatment with antibiotics. Rarely, M. pneumoniae pneumonia results in death due to lesions and ulceration of the epithelial lining, pulmonary edema, and bronchiolitis obliterans. Extrapulmonary symptoms such as autoimmune responses, central nervous system complications, and dermatological disorders have been associated with M. pneumoniae infections in up to 25% of cases.

Diagnosis

Diagnosis of Mycoplasma pneumoniae infections is complicated by the delayed onset of symptoms and the similarity of symptoms to other pulmonary conditions. Often, M. pneumoniae infections are diagnosed as other conditions and, occasionally, non-pathogenic mycoplasmas present in the respiratory tract are mistaken for M. pneumoniae. Historically, diagnosis of M. pneumoniae infections was made based on the presence of cold agglutinins and the ability of the infected material to reduce tetrazolium. Causative diagnosis is dependent upon laboratory testing, however these methods are more practical in epidemiological studies than in patient diagnosis. Culture tests are rarely used as diagnosic tools; rather immunoblotting, immunofluorescent staining, hemadsorption tests, tetrazolium reduction, metabolic inhibition tests, serological assays, and polymerase chain reaction (PCR) are used for diagnosis and characterization of bacterial pneumonic infections.PCR is the most rapid and effective way to determine the presence of M. pneumoniae, however the procedure does not indicate the activity or viability of the cells present. EIA serological assays are the most common method of M. pneumoniae detection used in patient diagnosis due to the low cost and relatively short testing time. One drawback of serology is that viable organisms are required, which may overstate the severity of infection. Neither of these methods, along with others, has been available to medical professionals in a rapid, efficient and inexpensive enough form to be used in routine diagnosis, leading to decreased ability of physicians to diagnose M. pneumoniae infections.

Treatment and Prevention

The difficulty in eradicating Mycoplasma pneumoniae infections is due to the ability of the bacterium to persist within an individual, as well as the lack of cell wall in M. pneumoniae, which renders multiple antibiotics directed at the bacterial cell wall ineffective in treating infections. M. pneumoniae therefore displays resistance to antimicrobials such as β-lactams, glycopeptides, sulfonamides, trimethoprim, polymixins, nalidixic acid, and rifampin. The majority of antibiotics used to treat M. pneumoniae infections are targeted at bacterial rRNA in ribosomal complexes, including macrolides, tetracycline, ketolides, and fluoroquinolone, many of which can be administered orally. Macrolides are capable of reducing hyperresponsiveness and protecting the epithelial lining from oxidative and structural damage, however they are capable only of inhibiting bacteria (bacteriostatic) and are not able to cause bacterial cell death. The most common macrolides used in the treatment of infected children in Japan are erythromycin and clarithromycin, which inhibit bacterial protein synthesis by binding 23S rRNA. Administration of antibiotics has been proven to reduce the longevity and intensity of M. pneumoniae infections in comparison to cases left untreated. Additionally, some high-dose steroid therapies have shown to reverse neurological effects in children with complicated infections. Antimicrobial drug resistance rates for Mycoplasma pneumoniae were determined in clinical specimens and isolates obtained during 2011–2012 in Ontario, Canada. Of 91 M. pneumoniae drug-resistant specimens, 11 (12.1%) carried nucleotide mutations associated with macrolide resistance in the 23S rRNA gene. None of the M. pneumoniae specimens were resistant to fluoroquinolones or tetracyclines. Vaccine design for M. pneumoniae has been focused primarily on prevention of host cell attachment, which would prevent initiation of cytotoxicity and subsequent symptoms. To date, vaccines targeted at the P1 adhesin have shown no reduction in the onset of infection, and some vaccine trials resulted in worsened symptoms due to immune system sensitization. Introduction of peptides that block adhesion receptors on the surface of the host cell may also be able to prevent attachment of M. pneumoniae.

Transmission of Mycoplasma pneumoniae infections is difficult to limit because of the several day period of infection before symptoms appear. The lack of proper diagnostic tools and effective treatment for the bacterium also contribute to the outbreak of infection. Using network theory, Meyers et al. analyzed the transmission of M. pneumoniae infections and developed control strategies based on the created model. They determined that cohorting is less effective due to the long incubation period, and so the best method of prevention is to limit caregiver-patient interactions and reduce the movement of caregivers to multiple wards.

REFERENCES

1. "Chapter 4: Functional Anatomy Of Prokaryotic And Eukaryotic Cells". Archived from the original on 23 September 2012.
2. "coccus" at Dorland's Medical Dictionary
3. "Dorlands Medical Dictionary:coccobacillus".
4. "persistent rickettsial disease".
5. Ammendola, Aldo; Otto Geisenberger; Jens Bo Andersen; Michael Givskov; Karl-Heinz Schleifer; Leo Eberl (July 1998). "Serratia liquefaciens swarm cells exhibit enhanced resistance to predation by Tetrahymena sp.". Microbiology Letters. 164 (1): 69–75. doi:10.1111/j.1574-6968.1998.tb13069.x.
6. Bacillus (shape)
7. Berg, H.C.; E. M. Purcell (November 1977). "Physics of chemoreception". Biophysical Journal. 20 (2): 193–219. doi:10.1016/S0006-3495(77)85544-6. PMC 1473391Freely accessible. PMID 911982.
8. Cordell, Suzanne C.; Elva J. H. Robinson; Jan Löwe (2003). "Crystal structure of the SOS cell division inhibitor SulA and in complex with FtsZ" (PDF). Proceedings of the National Academy of Sciences of the United States of America. 13. 110: 7889–7894. doi:10.1073/pnas.1330742100. PMC 164683Freely accessible. PMID 12808143. Retrieved 27 April 2012.
9. Corno, Gianluca; Klaus Jürgens (January 2006). "Direct and Indirect Effects of Protist Predation on Population Size Structure of a Bacterial Strain with High Phenotypic Plasticity". Applied and Environmental Microbiology. 72 (1): 78–86. doi:10.1128/AEM.72.1.78-86.2006.
10. Costa, Suelen B.; Ana Carolina C. Campos; Ana Claudia M. Pereira; Ana Luiza de Mattos-Guaraldi; Raphael Hirata Júnior; Ana Cláudia P. Rosa; Lídia M.B.O. Asad (2012). "The role of DNA base excision repair in filamentation in Escherichia coli K-12 adhered to epithelial HEp-2 cells" (PDF). Antonie van Leeuwenhoek. 101: 423–431. doi:10.1007/s10482-011-9649-z. Retrieved 18 April 2012.
11. Csuros, Maria (1999). Microbiological Examination of Water and Wastewater. Boca Raton, Florida: CRC Press. pp. 16–17. ISBN 9781566701792.
12. England, Kathleen; Rebecca Crew; Richard A Slayden (2011). "Mycobacterium tuberculosis septum site determining protein, Ssd encoded by rv3660c, promotes filamentation and elicits an alternative metabolic and dormancy stress response" (PDF). BMC Microbiology. 11 (79): 79. doi:10.1186/1471-2180-11-79. PMC 3095998Freely accessible. PMID 21504606. Retrieved 18 April 2012.
13. Harvey, Ronald W. (July 1997). "Microorganisms as tracers in groundwaterinjection and recovery experiments: areview". FEMS Microbiology Reviews. 20 (3-4): 461–472. doi:10.1111/j.1574-6976.1997.tb00330.x.
14. http://faculty.ccbcmd.edu/courses/bio141/lecguide/unit1/shape/shape.html
15. J. Iriberri; I. Azúa; Ainhoa Labirua-Iturburu; Itxaso Artolozaga; Isabel Barcina

(November 1994). "Differential elimination of enteric bacteria by protists in a freshwater system". Journal of Applied Microbiology. 77 (5): 476–483. doi:10.1111/j.1365-2672.1994.tb04390.x.

16. Janion, C; Sikora A; Nowosielka A; Grzesiuk E (2003). "E. coli BW535, a triple mutant for the DNA repair genes xthA, nth, nfo, chronically induces the SOS response". Environ Mol Mutagen. 41: 237–242. doi:10.1002/em.10154.
17. Jürgens, Klaus; Carsten Matz (2002). "Predation as a shaping force for the phenotypic and genotypic composition of planktonic bacteria". Antonie van Leeuwenhoek. 81 (1-4): 413–434. doi:10.1023/A:1020505204959.
18. Justice, Sheryl S.; Hunstad (2006). "Filamentation by Escherichia coli subverts innate defenses during urinary tract infection" (PDF). Proceedings of the National Academy of Sciences of the United States of America. 52. 103 (52): 19884–19889. doi:10.1073/pnas.0606329104. PMC 1750882Freely accessible. PMID 17172451. Retrieved 18 April 2012.
19. Justice, SS; Hunstad, DA; Cegelski, L; Hultgren, SJ (February 2008). "Morphological plasticity as a bacterial survival strategy.". Nature Reviews. Microbiology. 6 (2): 162–8. doi:10.1038/nrmicro1820. PMID 18157153.
20. Kang Chen; Guang Wen Sun; Kim Lee Chua; Yunn-Hwen Gan (March 2005). "Modified Virulence of Antibiotic-Induced Burkholderia pseudomallei Filaments". Antimicrobial Agents and Chemotherapy. 49 (3): 1002–1009. doi:10.1128/AAC.49.3.1002-1009.2005.
21. Madigan M; Martinko J, eds. (2005). Brock Biology of Microorganisms (11th ed.). Prentice Hall. ISBN 0-13-144329-1.
22. Matz, Carsten; Jens Boenigk; Hartmut Arndt; Klaus Jürgens (2002). "Role of bacterial phenotypic traits in selective feeding of the heterotrophic nanoflagellate Spumella sp.". Aquatic Microbial Ecology. 27 (2): 137–148. doi:10.3354/ame027137.
23. Matz, Carsten; Klaus Jürgens (February 2001). "Effects of hydrophobic and electrostatic cell surface properties of bacteria on feeding rates of heterotrophic nanoflagellates.". Applied and Environmental Microbiology. 67 (2): 814–820. doi:10.1128/AEM.67.2.814-820.
24. Matz, Carsten; Tanja Bergfeld; Scott A. Rice; Staffan Kjelleberg (March 2004). "Microcolonies, quorum sensing and cytotoxicity determine the survival of Pseudomonas aeruginosa biofilms exposed to protozoan grazing". Environmental Microbiology. 6 (3): 218–226. doi:10.1111/j.1462-2920.2004.00556.x.
25. Miller, Christine; Line Elnif Thomsen; Carina Gaggero; Ronen Mosseri; Hanne Ingmer; Stanley N. Cohen (September 2004). "SOS response induction by β-lactams and bacterial defense against antibiotic lethality". Science. 305 (5690): 1629–1631. doi:10.1126/science.1101630.
26. Pernthaler, Jakob (July 2005). "Predation on prokaryotes in the water column and its ecological implications". Nature Reviews Microbiology. 3 (7): 537–546. doi:10.1038/nrmicro1180.

27. Pernthaler, Jakob; Birgit Sattler; Karel Simek; Angela Schwarzenbacher; Roland Psenner (June 1996). "Top-down effects on the size-biomass distribution of a freshwater bacterioplankton community" (PDF). Aquatic Microbial Ecology. 10 (3): 255–263. doi:10.3354/ame010255. ISSN 1616-1564.
28. Pine, Leo; Clarence J. Boone (October 1967). "Comparative Cell Wall Analyses of Morphological Forms Within the Genus Actinomyces". 94 (4): 875–883.
29. Ryan KJ; Ray CG, eds. (2004). Sherris Medical Microbiology (4th ed.). McGraw Hill. ISBN 0-8385-8529-9.
30. Salton MRJ, Kim KS (1996). Baron S, et al., eds. Structure. In: Baron's Medical Microbiology (4th ed.). Univ of Texas Medical Branch. ISBN 0-9631172-1-1. (via NCBI Bookshelf).
31. Steel, Christina; Qian Wan; Xiao-Hong Nancy Xu (2004). "Single live cell imaging of chromosomes in chloramphenicol-induced filamentous Pseudomonas aeruginosa". Biochemistry. 43 (1): 175–182. doi:10.1021/bi035341e.
32. Waidner, Barbara; Mara Specht; Felix Dempwolff; Katharina Haeberer; Sarah Schaetzle; Volker Speth; Manfred Kist; Peter L. Graumann (2009). "A Novel System of Cytoskeletal Elements in the Human Pathogen Helicobacter pylori" (PDF). PLOS Pathog. 5 (11): 1–14. doi:10.1371/journal.ppat.1000669. PMC 2776988Freely accessible. PMID 19936218. Retrieved 20 April 2012.
33. Young, Kevin D. (September 2006). "The Selective Value of Bacterial Shape". Microbiology and Molecular Biology Reviews. 70 (3): 660–703. doi:10.1128/MMBR.00001-06. PMC 1594593Freely accessible. PMID 16959965.
34. Young, Kevin D. (September 2006). "The Selective Value of Bacterial Shape". Microbiology and Molecular Biology Reviews. 70 (3): 660–703. doi:10.1128/MMBR.00001-06. PMC 1594593Freely accessible. PMID 16959965.

CHAPTER 3

Bacterial Taxonomy

Chapter Contents

- **Introduction**
- **Bacterial Phyla**
- **Synechococcus**
- **Photosynthetic Picoplankton**
- **Cyanobacteria**
- **Archaea**

A bacterial species is a conceptual entity that is hard to define, despite its role as the basic taxonomic grouping. Bacteriologists accept the imprecision and recognize that a species represents a cluster of clones exhibiting some variations in minor properties. They have developed a formal approach to the description of the taxon while trying to solve the problems encountered in the process of recognizing and naming species.

INTRODUCTION

Bacterial taxonomy is the taxonomy, i.e. the rank-based classification, of bacteria.

In the scientific classification established by Carl von Linné, each species has to be assigned to a genus (binary nomenclature), which in turn is a lower level of a hierarchy of ranks (family, suborder, order, subclass, class, division/phyla, kingdom and domain). In the currently accepted classification of life, there are three domains (Eukaryotes, Bacteria and Archaea), which, in terms of taxonomy, despite following the same principles have several different conventions between them and between their subdivisions as are studied by different disciplines (botany, zoology, mycology and microbiology), for example in zoology there are type specimens, whereas in microbiology there are type strains.

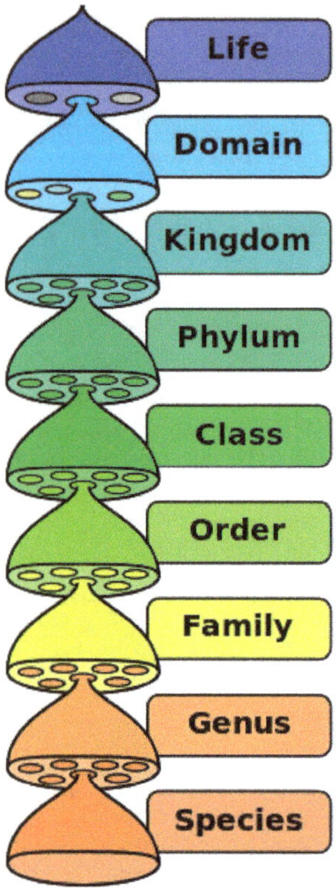

The hierarchy of biological classification's eight major taxonomic ranks. Intermediate minor rankings are not shown.

Diversity

Prokaryotes share many common features, such as lack of nuclear membrane, unicellularity, division by binary-fission and generally small size. The various species differ amongst each other based on several characteristics, allowing their identification and classification. Examples include:

- **Phylogeny**: All bacteria stem from a common ancestor and diversified since, consequently possess different levels of evolutionary relatedness (see Bacterial phyla and Timeline of evolution)
- **Metabolism**: Different bacteria may have different metabolic abilities (see Microbial metabolism)
- **Environment**: Different bacteria thrive in different environments, such as high/low temperature and salt (see Extremophiles)
- **Morphology**: There are many structural differences between bacteria, such as cell shape, Gram stain (number of lipid bilayers) or bilayer composition (see Bacterial cellular morphologies, Bacterial cell structure)

- **Pathogenicity**: Some bacteria are pathogenic to plants or animals (see Pathogenic bacteria)

Classification History

Bacteria were first observed by Antonie van Leeuwenhoek in 1676, using a single-lens microscope of his own design. He called them "animalcules and published his observations in a series of letters to the Royal Society. O. F. Müller (1773, 1786) described eight species of the genus Vibrio (in Infusoria), three of which were spirilliforms. The term Bacterium (a genus) was introduced much later, by Christian Gottfried Ehrenberg in 1838.

Classical Classification

Placement

Bacteria were first classified as plants constituting the class Schizomycetes, which along with the Schizophyceae (blue green algae/Cyanobacteria) formed the phylum Schizophyta.

Haeckel in 1866 placed the group in the phylum Moneres (from μονήρης: simple) in the kingdom Protista and defines them as completely structureless and homogeneous organisms, consisting only of a piece of plasma. He subdivided the phylum into two groups:

- die Gymnomoneren (no envelope)
  - *Protogenes*—such as *Protogenes primordialis*, now classed as a eukaryote and not a bacterium
  - *Protamaeba*—now classed as a eukaryote and not a bacterium
  - *Vibrio*—a genus of comma shaped bacteria first described in 1854)
  - *Bacterium*—a genus of rod shaped bacteria first described in 1828, that later gave its name to the members of the Monera, formerly referred to as "a moneron" (plural "monera") in English and "eine Moneren"(fem. plural "Moneres") in German
  - *Bacillus*—a genus of spore-forming rod shaped bacteria first described in 1835
  - *Spirochaeta*—thin spiral shaped bacteria first described in 1835
  - *Spirillum*—spiral shaped bacteria first described in 1832
- die Lepomoneren (with envelope)
  - *Protomonas*—now classed as a eukaryote and not a bacterium. The name was reused in 1984 for an unrelated genus of Bacteria
  - *Vampyrella*—now classed as a eukaryote and not a bacterium

The group was later reclassified as the Prokaryotes by Chatton.

The classification of Cyanobacteria (colloquially "blue green algae") has been fought between being algae or bacteria (for example, Haeckel classified Nostoc in the phylum Archephyta of Algae). in 1905 Erwin F. Smith accepted 33 valid different names of bacterial genera and over 150 invalid names, and in 1913 Vuillemin in a study concluded that all species of the Bacteria should fall into the genera Planococcus, Streptococcus, Klebsiella, Merista, Planomerista, Neisseria, Sarcina, Planosarcina, Metabacterium, Clostridium, Serratia, Bacterium and Spirillum.

Ferdinand Cohn recognized 4 tribes: Spherobacteria, Microbacteria, Desmobacteria, and Spirobacteria. Stanier and van Neil recognized the Kingdom Monera with 2 phyla, Myxophyta and Schizomycetae, the latter comprising classes Eubacteriae (3 orders), Myxobacteriae (1 order), and Spirochetae (1 order). Bisset distinguished 1 class and 4 orders: Eubacteriales, Actinomycetales, Streptomycetales, and Flexibacteriales. Migula, which was the most widely accepted system of its time and included all then-known species but was based only on morphology, contained the 3 basic groups, Coccaceae, Bacillaceae, and Spirillaceae but also Trichobacterinae for filamentous bacteria; Orla-Jensen established 2 orders: Cephalotrichinae (7 families) and Peritrichinae (presumably with only 1 family). Bergey et al presented a classification which generally followed the 1920 Final Report of the SAB(Society of American Bacteriologists) Committee (Winslow et al), which divided Class Schizomycetes into 4 orders: Myxobacteriales, Thiobacteriales, Chlamydobacteriales, and Eubacteriales, with a 5th group being 4 genera considered intermediate between bacteria and protozoans: *Spirocheta, Cristospira, Saprospira,* and *Treponema.*

However, different authors often reclassified the genera due to the lack of visible traits to go by, resulting in a poor state which was summarised in 1915 by Robert Earle Buchanan By then, the whole group received different ranks and names by different authors namely

- *Schizomycetes* (Naegeli 1857)
- *Bacteriaceae* (Cohn 1872,)
- *Bacteria* (Cohn 1872b,)
- *Schizomycetaceae* (DeToni and Trevisan 1889,)

Furthermore the families into which the class was subdivided, changed from author to author and for some such as Zipf the names where in German and not in Latin The first edition of the Bacteriological Code in 1947 sorted several problems out.

A.R. Prévot's system) had 4 subphyla and 8 classes as follows:

Eubacteriales (classes Asporulales and Sporulales) Mycobacteriales (classes Actinomycetales, Myxobacteriales, and Azotobacteriales) Algobacteriales (classes Siderobacteriales and Thiobacteriales) Protozoobacteriales (class Spirochetales)

Linnaeus 1735	Haeckel 1866	Chatton 1925	Copeland 1938	**Whittaker 1969**	Woese et al. 1990	Cavalier-Smith 1998
2 kingdoms	3 kingdoms	2 empires	4 kingdoms	5 kingdoms	3 domains	6 kingdoms

(not treated)	Protista	Prokaryota	Monera	Monera	Bacteria	Bacteria
					Archaea	
		Eukaryota	Protoctista	Protista	Eucarya	Protozoa
						Chromista
Vegetabilia	Plantae		Plantae	Plantae		Plantae
				Fungi		Fungi
Animalia	Animalia		Animalia	Animalia		Animalia

Subdivisions based on Gram staining

Despite there being little agreement on the major subgroups of the Bacteria, Gram staining results were most commonly used as a classification tool. Consequently, until the advent of molecular phylogeny, the Kingdom Prokaryotae was divided into four divisions, A classification scheme still formally followed by Bergey's manual of systematic bacteriology for tome order

- ***Gracilicutes*** (gram-negative)
    - *Photobacteria* (photosynthetic): class *Oxyphotobacteriae* (water as electron donor, includes the order *Cyanobacteriales*=blue-green algae, now phylum *Cyanobacteria*) and class *Anoxyphotobacteriae* (anaerobic phototrophs, orders: *Rhodospirillales* and *Chlorobiales*
    - *Scotobacteria* (non-photosynthetic, now the *Proteobacteria* and other gram-negative nonphotosynthetic phyla)
- ***Firmacutes*** [sic] (gram-positive, subsequently corrected to *Firmicutes*)
    - several orders such as *Bacillales* and *Actinomycetales* (now in the phylum *Actinobacteria*)
- ***Mollicutes*** (gram variable, e.g. *Mycoplasma*)
- ***Mendocutes*** (uneven gram stain, "methanogenic bacteria", now known as the *Archaea*)

Molecular Era

Woese argued that the bacteria, archaea, and eukaryotes represent separate lines of descent that diverged early on from an ancestral colony of organisms. However, a few biologists argue that the Archaea and Eukaryota arose from a group of bacteria. In any case, it is thought that viruses and archaea began relationships approximately two billion years ago, and that co-evolution may have been occurring between members of these groups. It is possible that the last common ancestor of the bacteria and archaea was a thermophile, which raises the possibility that lower temperatures are "extreme environments" in archaeal terms, and organisms that live in cooler environments appeared only later. Since the Archaea and Bacteria are no more related to each other than they are to eukaryotes, the term prokaryote's only surviving meaning is "not a eukaryote", limiting its value.

With improved methodologies it became clear that the methanogenic bacteria were profoundly different and were (erroneously) believed to be relics of ancient bacteria thus Carl Woese, regarded as the forerunner of the molecular phylogeny revolution, identified three primary lines of descent: the Archaebacteria, the Eubacteria, and the Urkaryotes, the latter now represented by the nucleocytoplasmic component of the Eukaryotes. These lineages were formalised into the rank Domain (regio in Latin) which divided Life into 3 domains: the Eukaryota, the Archaea and the Bacteria.This scheme is still followed today.

Subdivisions

In 1987 Carl Woese divided the Eubacteria into 11 divisions based on 16S ribosomal RNA (SSU) sequences, which with several additions are still used today.

Opposition

While the three domain system is widely accepted, some authors have opposed it for various reasons.

One prominent scientist who opposes the three domain system is Thomas Cavalier-Smith, who proposed that the Archaea and the Eukaryotes (the Neomura) stem from Gram positive bacteria (Posibacteria), which in turn derive from gram negative bacteria (Negibacteria) based on several logical arguments, which are highly controversial and generally disregarded by the molecular biology community (c.f. reviewers' comments on, e.g. Eric Bapteste is "agnostic" regarding the conclusions) and are often not mentioned in reviews (e.g.) due to the subjective nature of the assumptions made.

However, despite there being a wealth of statistically supported studies towards the rooting of the tree of life between the Bacteria and the Neomura by means of a variety of methods, including some that are impervious to accelerated evolution—which is claimed by Cavalier-Smith to be the source of the supposed fallacy in molecular methods—there are a few studies which have drawn different conclusions, some of which place the root in the phylum Firmicutes with nested archaea. Radhey Gupta's molecular taxonomy, based on conserved signature sequences of proteins, includes a monophyletic Gram negative clade, a monophyletic Gram positive clade, and a polyphyletic Archeota derived from Gram positives. Hori and Osawa's molecular analysis indicated a link between Metabacteria (=Archeota) and eukaryotes. The only cladistic analyses for bacteria based on classical evidence largely corroborate Gupta's results (see comprehensive mega-taxonomy).

James Lake presented a 2 primary kingdom arrangement (Parkaryotae + eukaryotes and eocytes + Karyotae) and suggested a 5 primary kingdom scheme (Eukaryota, Eocyta, Methanobacteria, Halobacteria, and Eubacteria) based on ribosomal structure and a 4 primary kingdom scheme (Eukaryota, Eocyta, Methanobacteria, and Photocyta), bacteria being classified according to 3 major biochemical innovations: photosynthesis (Photocyta), methanogenesis (Methanobacteria), and sulfur respiration (Eocyta). He has also discovered evidence that Gram-negative bacteria arose from a symbiosis between 2 Gram-positive bacteria.

Authorities

Classification is the grouping of organisms into progressively more inclusive groups based on phylogeny and phenotype, while nomenclature is the application of formal rules for naming organisms.

Nomenclature Authority

Despite there being no official and complete classification of prokaryotes, the names (nomenclature) given to prokaryotes are regulated by the International Code of Nomenclature of Bacteria (Bacteriological Code), a book which contains general considerations, principles, rules, and various notes, and advises in a similar fashion to the nomenclature codes of other groups.

Classification Authorities

The taxa which have been correctly described are reviewed in *Bergey's manual of Systematic Bacteriology*, which aims to aid in the identification of species and is considered the highest authority. An online version of the taxonomic outline of bacteria and archaea is available. LPSN is an online database which currently contains over two thousand accepted names with their references, etymologies and various notes.

Description of new species

The International Journal of Systematic Bacteriology/International Journal of Systematic and Evolutionary Microbiology (IJSB/IJSEM) is a peer reviewed journal which acts as the official international forum for the publication of new prokaryotic taxa. If a species is published in a different peer review journal, the author can submit a request to IJSEM with the appropriate description, which if correct, the new species will be featured in the Validation List of IJSEM.

Distribution

Microbial culture collections are depositories of strains which aim to safeguard them and to distribute them. The main ones being:

Collection Acronym	Name	Location
ATCC	American Type Culture Collection	Manassas, Virginia
NCTC	National Collection of Type Cultures	Public Health England, United Kingdom
BCCM	Belgium Coordinated Collection of Microorganisms	Ghent, Belgium
CIP	Collection d'Institut Pasteur	Paris, France

DSMZ	Deutsche Sammlung von Mikroorganismen und Zellkulturen	Braunschweig, Germany
JCM	Japan Collection of Microorganisms	Saitama, Japan
NCCB	Netherlands Culture Collection of Bacteria	Utrecht, Netherlands
NCIMB	National Collection of industrial, Marine and food bacteria	Aberdeen, Scotland
ICMP	International Collection of Microorganisms from Plants	Auckland, New Zealand

Analyses

Bacteria were at first classified based solely on their shape (vibrio, bacillus, coccus etc.), presence of endospores, gram stain, aerobic conditions and motility. This system changed with the study of metabolic phenotypes, where metabolic characteristics were used. Recently, with the advent of molecular phylogeny, several genes are used to identify species, the most important of which is the 16S rRNA gene, followed by 23S, ITS region, gyrB and others to confirm a better resolution. The quickest way to identify to match an isolated strain to a species or genus today is done by amplifying it's 16S gene with universal primers and sequence the 1.4kb amplicon and submit it to a specialised web-based identification database, namely either Ribosomal Database Project, which align the sequence to other 16S sequences using infernal, a secondary structure bases global alignment, or ARB SILVA, which aligns sequences via SINA (SILVA incremental aligner), which does a local alignment of a seed and extends it .

Several identification methods exists:

- Phenotypic analyses
  - fatty acid analyses
  - Growth conditions (Agar plate, Biolog multiwell plates)
- Genetic analyses
  - DNA-DNA hybridization
  - DNA profiling
  - Sequence
  - GC ratios
- Phylogenetic analyses
  - 16S-based phylogeny
  - phylogeny based on other genes
  - Multi-gene sequence analysis
  - Whole-genome sequence based analysis

New species

The minimal standards for describing a new species depend on which group the species belongs to. *c.f.*

Candidatus

Candidatus is a component of the taxonomic name for a bacterium that cannot be maintained in a Bacteriology Culture Collection. It is an interim taxonomic status for noncultivable organisms. e.g. "Candidatus Pelagibacter ubique

Species Concept

Bacteria divide asexually and for the most part do not show regionalisms ("Everything is everywhere"), therefore the concept of species, which works best for animals, becomes entirely a matter of judgement.

The number of named species of bacteria and archaea (approximately 13,000) is surprisingly small considering their early evolution, genetic diversity and residence in all ecosystems. The reason for this is the differences in species concepts between the bacteria and macro-organisms, the difficulties in growing/characterising in pure culture (a prerequisite to naming new species, vide supra) and extensive horizontal gene transfer blurring the distinction of species.

The most commonly accepted definition is the polyphasic species definition, which takes into account both phenotypic and genetic differences.However, a quicker diagnostic ad hoc threshold to separate species is less than 70% DNA–DNA hybridisation, which corresponds to less than 97% 16S DNA sequence identity. It has been noted that if this were applied to animal classification, the order primates would be a single species.

Pathology vs. phylogeny

Ideally, taxonomic classification should reflect the evolutionary history of the taxa, i.e. the phylogeny. Although some exceptions are present when the phenotype differs amongst the group, especially from a medical standpoint. Some examples of problematic classifications follow.

Escherichia Coli: Overly Large and Polyphyletic

In the Enterobacteriaceae family of the class Gammaproteobacteria, the species in the genus Shigella (S. dysenteriae, S. flexneri, S. boydii, S. sonnei) by an evolutionary point of view are strains of the species Escherichia coli (polyphyletic), but due to genetic differences cause different medical conditions in the case of the pathogenic strains., Escherichia coli is a badly classified species as some strains share only 20% of their genome. Being so diverse it should be given a higher taxonomic ranking. However, due to the medical conditions associated with the species, it will not be changed to avoid confusion in medical context.

Bacillus Cereus group: Close and Polyphyletic

In a similar way, the Bacillus species (=phylum Firmicutes) belonging to the "B. cereus group" (B. anthracis, B. cereus, B . thuringiensis, B. mycoides, B. pseudomycoides, B. weihenstephanensis and B. medusa) have 99-100% similar 16S rRNA sequence (97% is a commonly cited adequate species cut-off) and are polyphyletic, but for medical reasons (anthrax etc.) remain separate.

Yersinia Pestis: *Extremely Recent Species*

Yersinia pestis is in effect a strain of Yersinia pseudotuberculosis, but with a pathogenicity island that confer a drastically different pathology (Black plague and tuberculosis-like symptoms, respectively) which arose 15,000 to 20,000 years ago.

Nested Genera in Pseudomonas

In the gammaproteobacterial order Pseudomonadales, the genus Azotobacter and the species Azomonas macrocytogenes are actually members of the genus Pseudomonas, but were misclassified due to nitrogen fixing capabilities and the large size of the genus Pseudomonas which renders classification problematic. This will probably rectified in the close future.

Nested Genera in Bacillus

Another example of a large genus with nested genera is the Bacillus genus, in which the genera Paenibacillus and Brevibacillus are nested clades. There is insufficient genomic data at present to fully and effectively correct taxonomic errors in Bacillus.

Agrobacterium: *Resistance to Name Change*

the Agrobacterium species transferred to the Rhizobium genus (resulting in the following comp. nov.: Rhizobium radiobacter (formerly known as A. tumefaciens), R. rhizogenes, R. rubi, R. undicola and R. vitis) Given the plant pathogenic nature of Agrobacterium species, it was proposed to maintain the genus Agrobacterium and the latter was counter-argued

Nomenclature

Taxonomic names are written in italics (or underlined when handwritten) with a majuscule first letter with the exception of epithets for species and subspecies. Despite it being common in zoology, tautonyms (e.g. Bison bison) are not acceptable and names of taxa used in zoology, botany or mycology cannot be reused for Bacteria (Botany and Zoology do share names).

Nomenclature is the set of rules and conventions which govern the names of taxa. The difference in nomenclature between the various kingdoms/domains is reviewed in.

For Bacteria, valid names must have a Latin or Neolatin name and can only use basic latin letters (w and j inclusive, see History of the Latin alphabet for these), consequently hyphens, accents and other letters are not accepted and should be transliterated correctly (e.g. ß=ss).Ancient Greek being written in the Greek alphabet, needs to be transliterated into the Latin alphabet.

When compound words are created, a connecting vowel is needed depending on the origin of the preceding word, regardless of the word that follows, unless the latter starts with a vowel in which case no connecting vowel is added. If the first compound is Latin then the connecting vowel is an -i-, whereas if the first compound is Greek, the connecting vowel is an -o-.

For etymologies of names consult LPSN.

Rules for Higher Taxa

For the Prokaryotes (Bacteria and Archaea) the rank kingdom is not used (although some authors refer to phyla as kingdoms)

If a new or amended species is placed in new ranks, according to Rule 9 of the Bacteriologocal Code the name is formed by the addition of an appropriate suffix to the stem of the name of the type genus. For subclass and class the recommendation from is generally followed, resulting in a neutral plural, however a few names do not follow this and instead keep into account graeco-latin grammar (e.g. the female plurals Thermotogae, Aquificae and Chlamydiae, the male plurals Chloroflexi, Bacilli and Deinococci and the greek plurals Spirochaetes, Gemmatimonadetes and Chrysiogenetes).

Rank	Suffix	Example
Genus		*Elusimicrobium*
Subtribe (disused)	-inae	(*Elusimicrobiinae*)
Tribe (disused)	-inae	(*Elusimicrobiieae*)
Subfamily	-oideae	(*Elusimicrobioideae*)
Family	-aceae	*Elusimicrobiaceae*
Suborder	-ineae	(*Elusimicrobineae*)
Order	-ales	*Elusimicrobiales*
Subclass	-idae	(*Elusimicrobidae*)
Class	-ia	*Elusimicrobia*
Phylum	see text	*Elusimicrobia*

Phyla Endings

Phyla are not covered by the Bacteriological code, however, the scientific community generally follows the Ncbi and Lpsn taxonomy, where the name of the phylum is generally the plural of the type genus, with the exception of the Firmicutes, Cyanobacteria and Proteobacteria, whose names do not stem from a genus name. The higher taxa proposed by Cavalier-Smith are generally disregarded by the molecular phylogeny community (e.g.) (vide supra).

For the Archaea the suffix -archaeota is used. For bacterial phyla it was proposed that the suffix -bacteria be used for phyla.

Consequently for main phyla the name of the phyla is the same as the first described class:

- *Acidobacteria* (from *Acidobacterium*)
- *Actinobacteria* (from *Actinomyces*)
- *Caldisericia* (from *Caldisericum*)
- *Elusimicrobia* (from *Elusimicrobium*)
- *Fusobacteria* (from *Fusobacterium*)
- *Thermodesulfobacteria* (from *Thermodesulfobacterium*)
- *Thermotogae* (from *Thermotoga*)
- *Aquificae* (from *Aquifex*)
- *Chlamydiae* (from *Chlamydia*)
- *Chloroflexi* (from *Chloroflexus*)
- *Chrysiogenetes* (from *Chrysiogenes*)
- *Gemmatimonadetes* (from *Gemmatimonas*)
- *Deferribacteres* (from *Deferribacter*)

Whereas for others where the -ia suffix for class is used regardless of grammar they differ:

- phylum *Bacteroidetes* vs. class *Bacteroidia* from *Bacteroides*
- phylum *Chlorobi* vs. class *Chlorobia* from *Chlorobium*
- phylum *Verrucomicrobia* vs. class *Verrucomicrobiae* from *Verrucomicrobium* (anomalous class name)
- phylum *Dictyoglomi* versus class *Dictyoglomia* from *Dictyoglomus*
- phylum *Fibrobacteres* versus class *Fibrobacteria* from *Fibrobacter* (c.f. the suffix -bacter, note the difference with *Deferribacteres*)
- phylum *Lentisphaerae* versus class *Lentisphaeria* from *Lentisphaera*
- phylum *Nitrospira* or *Nitrospirae* versus class *Nitrospira* from *Nitrospira*
- phylum *Spirochaetes* versus class *Spirochaetae* from *Spirochaeta*
- phylum *Synergistetes* versus class *Synergistetia* from *Synergistes*
- phylum *Planctomycetes* versus *Planctomycea* from *Planctomyces*

An exception is the phylum *Deinococcus-Thermus*, which bears a hyphenated pair of genera —only non accented latin letters are accepted for valid names, but phyla are not officially recognised.

Names after People

Several species are named after people, either the discoverer or a famous person in the field of microbiology, for example Salmonella is after D.E. Salmon, who discovered it (albeit as "Bacillus typhi").

For the generic epithet, all names derived from people must be in the female nominative case, either by changing the ending to -a or to the diminutive -ella, depending on the name.

For the specific epithet, the names can be converted into either adjectival form (adding -nus (m.), -na (f.), -num (n.) according to the gender of the genus name) or the genitive of the latinised name.

Names after Places

Many species (the specific epithet) are named after the place they are present or found (e.g. Thiospirillum jenense). Their names are created by forming an adjective by joining the locality's name with the ending -ensis (m. or f.) or ense (n.) in agreement with the gender of the genus name, unless a classical Latin adjective exists for the place. However, names of places should not be used as nouns in the genitive case.

Vernacular Names

Despite the fact that some hetero/homogeneus colonies or biofilms of bacteria have names in English (e.g. dental plaque or Star jelly), no bacterial species has a vernacular/trivial/ common name in English.

For names in the singular form, plurals cannot be made (singulare tantum) as would imply multiple groups with the same label and not multiple members of that group (by analogy, in English, chairs and tables are types of furniture, which cannot be used in the plural form furnitures to describe both members), conversely names plural form are pluralia tantum. However, a partial exception to this is made by the use of vernacular names. However, to avoid repetition of taxonomic names which break the flow of prose, vernacular names of members of a genus or higher taxa are often used and recommended, these are formed by writing the name of the taxa in sentence case roman (standard in MS Office) type, therefore treating the proper noun as an English common noun (e.g. the salmonellas), although there is some debate about the grammar of plurals, which can either be regular plural by adding -(e)s (the salmonellas) or using the ancient Greek or Latin plural form (irregular plurals) of the noun (the salmonellae); the latter is problematic as the plural of - bacter would be -bacteres, while the plural of myces (N.L. masc. n. from Gr. masc. n. mukes) is mycetes.

Customs are present for centain names, such as those ending in -monas are converted into -monad (one pseudomonad, two aeromonads and not -monades).

Bacteria which are the etiological cause for a disease are often referred to by the disease name followed by a describing noun (bacterium, bacillus, coccus, agent or the name of their phylum) e.g. cholera bacterium (Vibrio cholerae) or Lyme disease spirochete (Borrelia burgdorferi) , note also rickettsialpox (Rickettsia akari) (for more see).

Treponema is converted into treponeme and the plural is treponemes and not treponemata.

Some unusual bacteria have special names such as Quin's oval (*Quinella ovalis*) and Walsby's square (*Haloquadratum walsbyi*).

Before the advent of molecular phylogeny, many higher taxonomic groupings had only trivial names, which are still used today, some of which are polyphyletic, such as Rhizobacteria. Some higher taxonomic trivial names are:

- Blue-green algae are members of the phylum *Cyanobacteria*
- Green non-sulfur bacteria are members of the phylum *Chloroflexi*
- Green sulfur bacteria are members of the *Chlorobi*
- Purple bacteria are some, but not all, members of the phylum Proteobacteria
- Purple sulfur bacteria are members of the order *Chromatiales*
- low G+C Gram-positive bacteria are members of the phylum *Firmicutes*, regardless of GC content
- high G+C Gram-positive bacteria are members of the phylum *Actinobacteria*, regardless of GC content
- Rhizobacteria are members of various genera of proteobacteria
- Rhizobia are members of the order *Rhizobiales*
- Lactic streptococci are members of the genus *Lactococcus*
- Coryneform bacteria are members of the family *Corynebacteriaceae*
- Fruiting gliding bacteria or myxobacteria are members of the order *Myxococcales*
- Enterics are members of the order Enterobacteriales, although the term is avoided if they do not live in the intestines, such as *Pectobacterium*
- Acetic acid bacteria are members of the family *Acetobacteraceae*

Terminology

- The abbreviation for species is **sp.** (plural **spp.**) and is used after a generic epithet to indicate a species of that genus. Often used to denote a strain of a genus for which the species is not known either because has the organism has not been described yet as a species or insufficient tests were conducted to identify it. For example *Halomonas* sp. GFAJ-1
- If a bacterium is known and well-studied but not culturable, it is given the term Candidatus in its name
- A basonym is original name of a new combination, namely the first name given to a taxa before it was reclassified
- A synonym is an alternative name for a taxa, i.e. a taxa was erroneusly described twice
- When a taxon is transferred it becomes a new combination (comb. nov.) or nomina nova (nom. nov.)
- paraphyly, monophyly and polyphyly

BACTERIAL PHYLA

Phylogenetic tree showing the diversity of bacteria, compared to other organisms. Eukaryotes are colored red, archaea green and bacteria blue.

The bacterial phyla are the major lineages, known as phyla or divisions, of the domain Bacteria.

In the scientific classification established by Carl von Linné, each bacterial strain has to be assigned to a species (binary nomenclature), which is a lower level of a hierarchy of ranks. Currently, the most accepted mega-classification system is under the three-domain system, which is based on molecular phylogeny. In that system, bacteria are members of the domain Bacteria and "phylum" is the rank below domain, since the rank "kingdom" is disused at present in bacterial taxonomy. When bacterial nomenclature was controlled under the Botanical Code, the term division was used, but now that bacterial nomenclature (with the exception of cyanobacteria) is controlled under the Bacteriological Code, the term phylum is preferred.

In this classification scheme, Bacteria is (unofficially) subdivided into 30 phyla with representatives cultured in a lab. Many major clades of bacteria that cannot currently be cultured are known solely and somewhat indirectly through metagenomics, the analysis of bulk samples from the environment. If these possible clades, candidate phyla, are included, the number of phyla is 52 or higher. Therefore, the number of major phyla has increased from 12 identifiable lineages in 1987, to 30 in 2014, or over 50 including candidate phyla. The total number has been estimated to exceed 1,000 bacterial phyla.

At the base of the clade Bacteria, close to the last universal common ancestor of all living things, some scientists believe there may be a definite branching order, whereas other scientists, such as Norman Pace, believe there was a large hard polytomy, a simultaneous multiple speciation event.

Molecular Phylogenetics

Traditionally, phylogeny was inferred and taxonomy established based on studies of morphology. Recently molecular phylogenetics has been used to allow better elucidation of the evolutionary relationship of species by analysing their DNA and protein sequences, for example their ribosomal DNA. The lack of easily accessible morphological features, such as those present in animals and plants, hampered early efforts of classification and resulted in erroneous, distorted and confused classification, an example of which, noted Carl Woese, is Pseudomonas whose etymology ironically matched its taxonomy, namely "false unit".

Initial Sub-Division

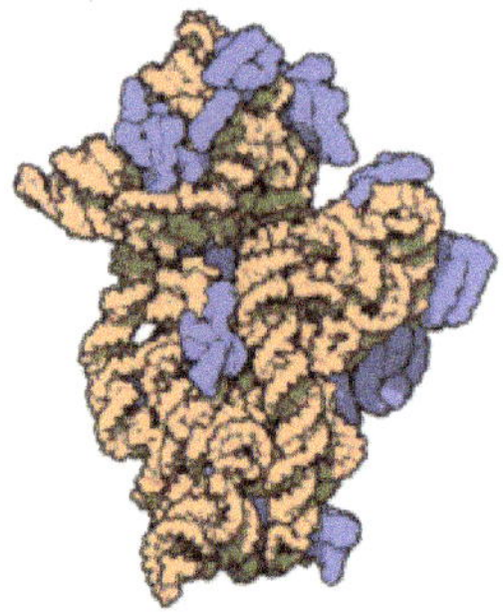

Atomic structure of the 30S ribosomal Subunit from *Thermus thermophilus* of which 16S makes up a part. Proteins are shown in blue and the single RNA strand in orangeish.

In 1987, Carl Woese, regarded as the forerunner of the molecular phylogeny revolution, divided Eubacteria into 11 divisions based on 16S ribosomal RNA (SSU) sequences:

- **Purple Bacteria and their relatives** (later renamed Proteobacteria)
  - alpha subdivision (purple non-sulfur bacteria, rhizobacteria, *Agrobacterium*, *Rickettsiae*, *Nitrobacter*)
  - beta subdivision (*Rhodocyclus*, (some) *Thiobacillus*, *Alcaligenes*, *Spirillum*, *Nitrosovibrio*)
  - gamma subdivision (enterics, fluorescent pseudomonads, purple sulfur bacteria, *Legionella*, (some) *Beggiatoa*)
  - delta subdivision (Sulfur and sulfate reducers (*Desulfovibrio*), Myxobacteria, *Bdellovibrio*)
- Gram-positive Eubacteria
  - High-G+C species (later renamed Actinobacteria) (*Actinomyces*, *Streptomyces*, *Arthrobacter*, *Micrococcus*, *Bifidobacterium*)
  - Low-G+C species (later renamed Firmicutes) (*Clostridium*, *Peptococcus*, *Bacillus*, *Mycoplasma*)
  - Photosynthetic species (*Heliobacterium*)
  - Species with Gram-negative walls (*Megasphaera*, *Sporomusa*)
- **Cyanobacteria and chloroplasts** (*Aphanocapsa*, *Oscillatoria*, *Nostoc*, *Synechococcus*, *Gloeobacter*, *Prochloron*)
- Spirochetes and relatives
  - Spirochetes (*Spirochaeta*, *Treponema*, *Borrelia*)
  - Leptospiras (*Leptospira*, *Leptonema*)

- **Green sulfur bacteria** (*Chlorobium*, *Chloroherpeton*)
- **Bacteroides, Flavobacteria and relatives** (later renamed Bacteroidetes
  - Bacteroides (*Bacteroides*, *Fusobacterium*)
  - Flavobacterium group (*Flavobacterium*, *Cytophaga*, *Saprospira*, *Flexibacter*)
- **Planctomyces and relatives** (later renamed Planctomycetes)
  - Planctomyces group (*Planctomyces*, *Pasteuria* [*sic*])
  - Thermophiles (*Isocystis pallida*)
- **Chlamydiae** (*Chlamydia psittaci*, *Chlamydia trachomatis*)
- **Radioresistant micrococci and relatives** (now commonly referred to as Deinococcus–Thermus or Thermi)
  - Deinococcus group (*Deinococcus radiodurans*)
  - Thermophiles (*Thermus aquaticus*)
- **Green non-sulfur bacteria and relatives** (later renamed Chloroflexi)
  - Chloroflexus group (*Chloroflexus*, *Herpetosiphon*)
  - Thermomicrobium group (*Thermomicrobium roseum*)
- **Thermotogae** (*Thermotoga maritima*)

New cultured phyla

New species have been cultured since 1987, when Woese's review paper was published, that are sufficiently different that they warrant a new phylum. Most of these are thermophiles and often also chemolithoautotrophs, such as Aquificae, which oxidises hydrogen gas. Other non-thermophiles, such as Acidobacteria, a ubiquitous phylum with divergent physiologies, have been found, some of which are chemolithotrophs, such as Nitrospira (nitrile-oxidising) or Leptospirillum (Fe-oxidising)., some proposed phyla however do not appear in LPSN as they were insufficiently described or are awaiting approval or it is debated if they may belong to a pre-existing phylum. An example of this is the genus Caldithrix, consisting of C. palaeochoryensis and C. abyssi, which is considered Deferribacteres,however, it shares only 81% similarity with the other Deferribacteres (Deferribacter species and relatives) and is considered a separate phylum by Rappé and Giovannoni. Additionally the placement of the genus Geovibrio in the phylum Deferribacteres is debated.

Uncultivated Phyla and metagenomics

With the advent of methods to analyse environmental DNA (metagenomics), the 16S rRNA of an extremely large number of undiscovered species have been found, showing that there are several whole phyla which have no known cultivable representative and that some phyla lack in culture major subdivisions as is the case for Verrucomicrobia and Chloroflexi. The term Candidatus is used for proposed species for which the lack of information prevents it to be validated, such as where the only evidence is DNA sequence data, even if the whole genome has been sequenced. When the species are members of a whole phylum it is called a candidate division (or candidate phylum) and in 2003 there were 26 candidate phyla out of 52. A candidate phylum was defined by Hugenholtz and Pace in 1998, as a set of 16S ribosomal RNA sequences with less than 85% similarity to already-described phyla. More recently an even lower threshold of 75% was proposed. Three candidate phyla were known before 1998, prior to the 85% threshold definition by Hugenholtz and Pace:

- OS-K group (from Octopus spring, Yellowstone National Park)
- Marine Group A (from Pacific ocean)
- Termite Group 1 (from a *Reticulitermes speratus* termite gut, now Elusimicrobia)

Since then several other candidate phyla have been identified:)

- OP1, OP3, OP5 (now Caldiserica), OP8, OP9 (now Atribacteria), OP10 (now Armatimonadetes), OP11 (obsidian pool, Yellowstone National Park)
- WS2, WS3, WS5, WS6 (Wurtsmith contaminated aquifer)
- SC3 and SC4 (from arid soil)
- vadinBE97 (now Lentisphaerae)
- NC10 (from flooded caves)
- BRC1 (from bulk soil and rice roots)
- ABY1 (from sediment)
- Guyamas1 (from hydrothermal vents)
- GN01, GN02, GN04 (from a Guerrero Negro hypersaline microbial mat)
- NKB19 (from activated sludge)
- SBR1093 (from activated sludge)
- TM6 and TM7 (Torf, Mittlere Schicht ["peat, middle layer"])

Since then a candidate phylum called Poribacteria was discovered, living in symbiosis with sponges and extensively studied. (Note: the divergence of the major bacterial lineages predates sponges) Another candidate phylum, called Tectomicrobia, was also found living in symbiosis with sponges. And Nitrospina gracilis, which had long eluded phylogenetic placement, was proposed to belong to a new phylum, Nitrospinae.

Other candidate phyla that have been the center of some studies are TM7, the genomes of organisms of which have even been sequenced (draft), WS6and Marine Group A.

Two species of the candidate phylum OP10, which is now called Armatimonadetes, where recently cultured: Armatimonas rosea isolated from the rhizoplane of a reed in a lake in Japan and Chthonomonas calidirosea from an isolate from geothermally heated soil at Hell's Gate, Tikitere, New Zealand.

One species, *Caldisericum exile*, of the candidate phylum OP5 was cultured, leading to it being named Caldiserica.

The candidate phylum VadinBE97 is now known as Lentisphaerae after Lentisphaera araneosa and Victivallis vadensis were cultured.

More recently several candidate phyla have been given provisional names despite the fact that they have no cultured representatives:

- Candidate phylum ACD58 was renamed Berkelbacteria
- Candidate phylum CD12 (also known as candidate phylum BHI80-139) was renamed Aerophobetes
- Candidate phylum EM19 was renamed Calescamantes
- Candidate phylum GN02 (also known as candidate phylum BD1-5) was renamed Gracilibacteria
- Candidate phylum KSB3 was renamed Modulibacteria
- Candidate phylum NKB19 was renamed Hydrogenedentes
- Candidate phylum OctSpa1-106 was renamed Fervidibacteria
- Candidate phylum OD1 was renamed Parcubacteria
- Candidate phylum OP1 was renamed Acetothermia
- Candidate phylum OP3 was renamed Omnitrophica
- Candidate phylum OP8 was renamed Aminicenantes
- Candidate phylum OP9 (also known as candidate phylum JS1) was renamed Atribacteria
- Candidate phylum OP11 was renamed Microgenomates
- Candidate phylum PER was renamed Perigrinibacteria
- Candidate phylum SAR406 (also known as candidate phylum Marine Group A) was renamed Marinimicrobia
- Candidate phylum SR1 was renamed Absconditabacteria
- Candidate phylum TM6 was renamed Dependentiae
- Candidate phylum TM7 was renamed Saccharibacteria
- Candidate phylum WS3 was renamed Latescibacteria
- Candidate phylum WWE1 was renamed Cloacimonetes
- Candidate phylum WWE3 was renamed Katanobacteria
- Candidate phylum ZB1 was renamed Ignavibacteriae

Despite these lineages not being officially recognised (due to the ever-increasing number of sequences belonging to undescribed phyla) the ARB-Silva database lists 67 phyla, including 37 candidate phyla (Acetothermia, Aerophobetes, Aminicenantes, aquifer1, aquifer2, Atribacteria, Calescamantes, CKC4, Cloacimonetes, GAL08, GOUTA4, Gracilibacteria, Fermentibacteria (Hyd24-12), Hydrogenedentes, JL-ETNP-Z39, Kazan-3B-09, Latescibacteria, LCP-89, LD1-PA38, Marinimicrobia, Microgenomates, OC31, Omnitrophica, Parcubacteria, PAUC34f, RsaHF231, S2R-29, Saccharibacteria, SBYG-2791, SHA-109, SM2F11, SR1, TA06, TM6, WCHB1-60, WD272, and WS6), the Ribosomal Database Project 10, lists 49 phyla, including 20 candidate phyla (Acetothermia, Aminicenantes, Atribacteria, BRC1, Calescamantes, Cloacimonetes, Hydrogenedentes, Ignavibacteriae, Latescibacteria, Marinimicrobia, Microgenomates, Nitrospinae, Omnitrophica, Parcubacteria, Poribacteria, SR1, Saccharibacteria, WPS-1, WPS-2, and ZB3), and NCBI lists 120 phyla, including 90 candidate phyla (AC1, Acetothermia,

Aerophobetes, Aminicenantes, Atribacteria, Berkelbacteria, BRC1, CAB-I, Calescamantes, CPR1, CPR2, CPR3, EM 3, Fervidibacteria, GAL15, GN01, GN03, GN04, GN05, GN06, GN07, GN08, GN09, GN10, GN11, GN12, GN13, GN14, GN15, Gracilibacteria, Fermentibacteria (Hyd24-12), Hydrogenedentes, JL-ETNP-Z39, KD3-62, kpj58rc, KSA1, KSA2, KSB1, KSB2, KSB3, KSB4, Latescibacteria, marine group A, Marinimicrobia, Microgenomates, MSBL2, MSBL3, MSBL4, MSBL5, MSBL6, NC10, Nitrospinae, NPL-UPA2, NT-B4, Omnitrophica, OP2, OP4, OP6, OP7, OS-K, Parcubacteria, Peregrinibacteria, Poribacteria, RF3, Saccharibacteria, SAM, SBR1093, Sediment-1, Sediment-2, Sediment-3, Sediment-4, SPAM, SR1, TA06, TG2, TM6, VC2, WOR-1, WOR-3, WPS-1, WPS-2, WS1, WS2, WS4, WS5, WS6, WWE3, WYO, ZB3, and Zixibacteria).

Superphyla

Despite the unclear branching order for most bacterial phyla, several groups of phyla have clear clustering and are referred to as superphyla.

The FCB Group

Main article: FCB group

The FCB group includes Bacteroidetes, the unplaced genus Caldithrix, Chlorobi, candidate phylum Cloacimonetes, Fibrobacteres, Gemmatimonadates, candidate phylum Ignavibacteriae, candidate phylum Latescibacteria, candidate phylum Marinimicrobia, and candidate phylum Zixibacteria.

The PVC Group

Main article: PVC group

The PVC group includes Chlamydiae, Lentisphaerae, candidate phylum Omnitrophica, Planctomycetes, candidate phylum Poribacteria, and Verrucomicrobia.

Patescibacteria

The proposed superphylum, Patescibacteria, includes candidate phyla Gracilibacteria, Microgenomates, Parcubacteria, and Saccharibacteria and possibly Dependentiae. These same candidate phyla, along with candidate phyla Berkelbacteria, CPR2, CPR3, Kazan, Perigrinibacteria, SM2F11, WS6, and WWE3 were more recently proposed to belong to the larger CPR Group. To complicate matters, it has been suggested that several of these phyla are themselves actually superphyla (see the section on cryptic superphyla below).

Terrabacteria

The proposed superphylum, Terrabacteria, includes Actinobacteria, Cyanobacteria, Deinococcus–Thermus, Chloroflexi, Firmicutes, and candidate phylum OP10.

Proteobacteria as superphylum

It has been proposed that several of the classes of the phylum Proteobacteria are phyla in their own right, which would make Proteobacteria a superphylum.

Cryptic Superphyla

Several candidate phyla (Microgenomates, Omnitrophica, Parcubacteria, and Saccharibacteria) and several accepted phyla (Elusimicrobia, Caldiserica, and Armatimonadetes) have been suggested to actually be superphyla that were incorrectly described as phyla because rules for defining a bacterial phylum are lacking. For example, it is suggested that candidate phylum Microgenomates is actually a superphylum that encompasses 28 subordinate phyla and that phylum Elusimocrobia is actually a superphylum that encompasses 7 subordinate phyla.

Overview of phyla

For the origin of each phylum name, see Bacterial taxonomy § Phylum endings.

As of January 2016, there are 30 phyla in the domain "Bacteria" accepted by LPSN. There are no fixed rules to the nomenclature of bacterial phyla. It was proposed that the suffix "-bacteria" be used for phyla, but generally the name of the phylum is generally the plural of the type genus, with the exception of the *Firmicutes*, *Cyanobacteria*, and *Proteobacteria*, whose names do not stem from a genus name (*Actinobacteria* instead is from *Actinomyces*).

Acidobacteria

Main article: Acidobacteria

The Acidobacteria (diderm Gram negative) is most abundant bacterial phylum in many soils, but its members are mostly uncultured. Additionally, they phenotypically diverse and include not only acidophiles, but also many non-acidophiles. Generally its members divide slowly, exhibit slow metabolic rates under low-nutrient conditions and can tolerate well fluctuations in soil hydration.

Actinobacteria

Main article: Actinobacteria

The Actinobacteria is a phylum of monoderm Gram positive bacteria, many of which notable secondary metabolite producers. There are only two phyla of monoderm Gram positive bacteria, the other being the Firmicutes; the actinobacteria generally have higher GC content so are sometimes called "high-CG Gram positive bacteria". Notable genera/species include Streptomyces (antibiotic production), Propionibacterium acnes (odorous skin commensal) and Propionibacterium freudenreichii (holes in Emmental)

Aquificae

Main article: Aquificae

The Aquificae (diderm Gram negative) contains only 14 genera (including Aquifex and Hydrogenobacter). The species are hyperthermophiles and chemolithotrophs (sulphur). According to some studies may be one of the most deep branching phyla.

Armatimonadetes

Main article: Armatimonadetes

Bacteroidetes

Main article: Bacteroidetes

The *Bacteroidetes* (diderm Gram negative) is a member of the FBC superphylum. Some species are opportunistic pathogens, while other are the most common human gut commensal bacteria. Gained notoriety in the non-scientific community with the urban myth as a bacterial weight loss powder.

Caldiserica

Main article: Caldiserica

This phylum was formerly known as candidate phylum OP5, *Caldisericum exile* is the sole representative.

Chlamydiae

Main article: Chlamydiae

The *Chlamydiae* (diderms, weakly Gram negative) is a phylum of the PVC superphylum. It is composed of only 6 genera of obligate intracellular pathogens with a complex life cycle. Species include *Chlamydia trachomatis* (chlamydia infection).

Chlorobi

Main article: Chlorobi

Chlorobi is a member of the FBC superphylum. It contains only 7 genera of obligately anaerobic photoautotrophic bacteria, known colloquially as Green sulfur bacteria. The reaction centre for photosynthesis in Chlorobi and Chloroflexi (another photosynthetic group) is formed by a structures called the chlorosome as opposed to phycobilisomes of cyanobacteria (another photosynthetic group).

Chloroflexi

Main article: Chloroflexi (phylum)

Chloroflexi,diverse phylum including thermophiles and halorespirers, known colloquially as Green non-sulfur bacteria.

Chrysiogenetes

Main article: Chrysiogenetes

Chrysiogenetes, only 3 genera (*Chrysiogenes arsenatis*, *Desulfurispira natronophila*, *Desulfurispirillum alkaliphilum*)

Cyanobacteria

Main article: Cyanobacteria

Cyanobacteria, major photosynthetic clade believed to have caused Earth's oxygen atmosphere, also known as the blue-green algae

Deferribacteres

Main article: Deferribacteres

Deferribacteres

Deinococcus–Thermus

Main article: Deinococcus–Thermus

Deinococcus–Thermus, *Deinococcus radiodurans* and *Thermus aquaticus* are "commonly known" species of this phylum.

Dictyoglomi

Main article: Dictyoglomi

Dictyoglomi

Elusimicrobia

Main article: Elusimicrobia

Elusimicrobia, formerly candidate phylum Termite Group 1

Fibrobacteres

Main article: Fibrobacteres

Fibrobacteres, member of the FBC superphylum.

Firmicutes

Main article: Firmicutes

Firmicutes, Low-G+C Gram positive species most often spore-forming, in two/three classes: the class Bacilli such as the *Bacillus* spp. (e.g. *B. anthracis*, a pathogen, and *B. subtilis*, biotechnologically useful), lactic acid bacteria (e.g. *Lactobacillus casei* in yoghurt, *Oenococcus oeni* in malolactic fermentation, *Streptococcus pyogenes*, pathogen), the class Clostridia of mostly anaerobic sulphite-reducing saprophytic species, includes the genus *Clostridium* (e.g. the pathogens *C. dificile, C. tetani, C. botulinum* and the biotech *C. acetobutylicum*)

Fusobacteria

Main article: Fusobacteria

Fusobacteria

Gemmatimonadetes

Main article: Gemmatimonadetes

Gemmatimonadetes, member of the FBC superphylum.

Lentisphaerae

Main article: Lentisphaerae

Lentisphaerae, formerly clade VadinBE97, member of the PVC superphylum.

Nitrospirae

Main article: Nitrospirae

Nitrospirae

Planctomycetes

Main article: Planctomycetes

Planctomycetes, member of the PVC superphylum.

Proteobacteria

Main article: Proteobacteria

Proteobacteria, contains most of the "commonly known" species, such as *Escherichia coli* and *Pseudomonas aeruginosa.*

Spirochaetes

Main article: Spirochaetes

Spirochaetes, notable for compartmentalisation and species include *Borrelia burgdorferi*, which causes Lyme disease.

Synergistetes

Main article: Synergistetes

The *Synergistetes* is a phylum whose members are diderm Gram negative, rod-shaped obligate anaerobes, some of which are human commensals.

Tenericutes

Main article: Tenericutes

The *Tenericutes* includes the class *Mollicutes*, formerly/debatedly of the phylum *Firmicutes* (sister clades). Despite their monoderm Gram-positive relatives, they lack peptidoglycan. Notable genus: *Mycoplasma.*

Thermodesulfobacteria

Main article: Thermodesulfobacteria

The *Thermodesulfobacteria* is a phylum composed of only three genera in the same family (*Thermodesulfobacteriaceae*: *Caldimicrobium*, *Thermodesulfatator* and *Thermodesulfobacterium*). The members of the phylum are thermophilic sulphate-reducers.

Thermomicrobia

Main article: Thermomicrobia

Thermomicrobia

Thermotogae

Main article: Thermotogae

The *Thermotogae* is a phylum of whose members possess an unusual outer envelope called the toga and are mostly hyperthermophilic obligate anaerobic fermenters.

Verrucomicrobia

Main article: Verrucomicrobia

Verrucomicrobia is a phylum of the PVC superphylum. Like the Planctomycetes species, its members possess a compartmentalised cell plan with a condensed nucleoid and the ribosomes pirellulosome (enclosed by the intracytoplasmic membrane) and paryphoplasm compartment between the intracytoplasmic membrane and cytoplasmic membrane.

SYNECHOCOCCUS

Synechococcus (from the Greek synechos, in succession, and the Greek kokkos, granule) is a unicellular cyanobacterium that is very widespread in the marine environment. Its size varies from 0.8 to 1.5 μm. The photosynthetic coccoid cells are preferentially found in well–lit surface waters where it can be very abundant (generally 1,000 to 200,000 cells per ml). Many freshwater species of Synechococcus have also been described.

The genome of S. elongatus strain PCC7002 has a size of 3008047 bp, whereas the oceanic strain WH8102 has a genome of size 2.4 Mbp.

Synechococcus is one of the most important components of the prokaryotic autotrophic picoplankton in the temperate to tropical oceans. The genus was first described in 1979, and was originally defined to include "small unicellular cyanobacteria with ovoid to cylindrical cells that reproduce by binary traverse fission in a single plane and lack sheaths". This definition of the genus Synechococcus contained organisms of considerable genetic diversity and was later subdivided into subgroups based on the presence of the accessory pigment phycoerythrin. The marine forms of Synechococcus are coccoid cells between 0.6 and 1.6 μm in size. They are Gram-negative cells with highly structured cell walls that may contain projections on their surface. Electron microscopy frequently reveals the presence of phosphate inclusions, glycogen granules, and more importantly, highly structured carboxysomes. Cells are known to be motile by a gliding method and a novel uncharacterized, nonphototactic swimming method that does not involve flagellar motion. While some cyanobacteria are capable of photoheterotrophic or even chemoheterotrophic growth, all marine Synechococcus strains appear to be obligate photoautotrophs that are capable of supporting their nitrogen requirements using nitrate, ammonia, or in some cases urea as a sole nitrogen source. Marine Synechococcus species are traditionally not thought to fix nitrogen.

Pigments

The main photosynthetic pigment in *Synechococcus* is chlorophyll a, while its major accessory pigments are phycobilliproteins. The four commonly recognized phycobilins are phycocyanin, allophycocyanin, allophycocyanin B and phycoerythrin. In addition *Synechococcus* also contains zeaxanthin but no diagnostic pigment for this organism is known. Zeaxanthin is also found in *Prochlorococcus*, red algae and as a minor pigment in some chlorophytes and eustigmatophytes. Similarly, phycoerythrin is also found in rhodophytes and some cryptomonads.

Phylogeny

Phylogenetic description of Synechococcus is difficult. Isolates are morphologically very similar, yet exhibit a G+C content ranging from 39 to 71%, illustrating the large genetic diversity of this provisional taxon. Initially, attempts were made to divide the group into three subclusters, each with a specific range of genomic G+C content. The observation that open-ocean isolates alone nearly span the complete G+C spectrum, however, indicates that Synechococcus is composed of at least several species. Bergey's Manual (Herdman et al. 2001) now divides Synechococcus into five clusters (equivalent to genera) based on morphology, physiology, and genetic traits.

Cluster 1 includes relatively large (1–1.5 μm) nonmotile obligate photoautotrophs that exhibit low salt tolerance. Reference strains for this cluster are PCC6301 (formerly Anacycstis nidulans) and PCC6312, which were isolated from fresh water in Texas and California, respectively. Cluster 2 also is characterized by low salt tolerance. Cells are obligate photoautrotrophs, lack phycoerythrin, and are thermophilic. The reference strain PCC6715 was isolated from a hot spring in Yellowstone National Park. Cluster 3 includes phycoerythrin-lacking marine Synechococcus species that are euryhaline, i.e. capable of growth in both marine and freshwater environments. Several strains, including the reference strain PCC7003, are facultative heterotrophs and require vitamin B12 for growth. Cluster 4 contains a single isolate, PCC7335. This strain is obligate marine. This strain contains phycoerthrin and was first isolated from the intertidal zone in Puerto Peñasco, Mexico. The last cluster contains what had previously been referred to as 'marine A and B clusters' of Synechococcus. These cells are truly marine and have been isolated from both the coastal and the open ocean. All strains are obligate photoautrophs and are around 0.6–1.7 µm in diameter. This cluster is, however, further divided into a population that either contains (cluster 5.1) or does not contain (cluster 5.2) phycoerythrin. The reference strains are WH8103 for the phycoerythrin-containing strains and WH5701 for those strains that lack this pigment. More recently, Badger et al. (2002) proposed the division of the cyanobacteria into a α- and a β-subcluster based on the type of rbcL (large subunit of ribulose 1,5-bisphosphate carboxylase/oxygenase) found in these organisms. α-cyanobacteria were defined to contain a form IA, while β-cyanobacteria were defined to contain a form IB of this gene. In support for this division Badger et al. analyze the phylogeny of carboxysomal proteins, which appear to support this division. Also, two particular bicarbonate transport systems appear to only be found in α-cyanobacteria, which lack carboxysomal carbonic anhydrases.

The complete phylogenetic tree of 16S rRNA sequences of Synechococcus revealed at least 12 groups, which morphologically correspond to Synechococcus, but they have not derived from the common ancestor. Moreover, it has been estimated based on molecular dating that the first Synechococcus lineage has appeared 3 billion years ago in thermal springs with subsequent radiation to marine and freshwater environments.

Ecology and Distribution

Synechococcus has been observed to occur at concentrations ranging between a few cells to 106 cells per ml in virtually all regions of oceanic euphotic zone except in samples from the McMurdo Sound and Ross Ice Shelf in Antarctica. Cells are generally much more abundant in nutrient-rich environments than in the oligotrophic ocean and prefer the upper, well-lit portion of the euphotic zone. Synechococcus has also been observed to occur at high abundances in environments with low salinities and/or low temperatures. It is usually far outnumbered by Prochlorococcus in all environments where they co-occur. Exceptions to this rule are areas of permanently enriched nutrients such as upwelling areas and coastal watersheds. In the nutrient-depleted areas of the oceans, such as the central gyres, Synechococcus is apparently always present, although only at low concentrations, ranging from a few to 4×10^3 cells per ml. Vertically Synechococcus is usually relatively equitably distributed throughout the mixed layer and exhibits an affinity for the higher-light areas. Below the mixed layer, cell concentrations rapidly decline. Vertical profiles are strongly influenced by hydrologic conditions and can be very variable both seasonally and spatially. Overall, Synechococcus abundance often parallels that of Prochlorococcus in the water column. In the Pacific high-nutrient, low-chlorophyll zone and in temperate open seas where stratification was recently established both profiles parallel each other and exhibit abundance maxima just about the subsurface chlorophyll maximum.

The factors controlling the abundance of Synechococcus still remain poorly understood, especially considering that even in the most nutrient-depleted regions of the central gyres, where cell abundances are often very low, population growth rates are often high and not drastically limited. Factors such as grazing, viral mortality, genetic variability, light adaptation, and temperature, as well as nutrients are certainly involved, but remain to be investigated on a rigorous and global scale. Despite the uncertainties, a relationship probably exists between ambient nitrogen concentrations and Synechococcus abundance, with an inverse relationship to Prochlorococcus in the upper euphotic zone, where light is not limiting. One environment where Synechococcus thrives particularly well is coastal plumes of major rivers. Such plumes are coastally enriched with nutrients such as nitrate and phosphate, which drives large phytoplankton blooms. High productivity in coastal river plumes is often associated with large populations of Synechococcus and elevated form IA (cyanobacterial) rbcL mRNA.

Prochlorococcus is thought to be at least 100 times more abundant than Synechococcus in warm oligotrophic waters. Assuming average cellular carbon concentrations, it has thus been estimated that Prochlorococcus accounts for at least 22 times more carbon in these waters, thus may be of much greater significance to the global carbon cycle than Synechococcus.

PHOTOSYNTHETIC PICOPLANKTON

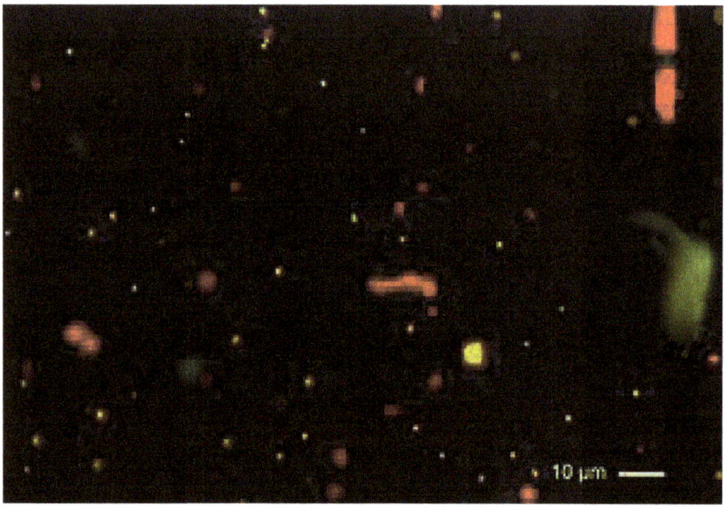

Picoplankton observed by epifluorescence

Photosynthetic picoplankton is the fraction of the phytoplankton performing photosynthesis composed by cells between 0.2 and 2 µm (picoplankton). It is especially important in the central oligotrophic regions of the world oceans that have very low concentration of nutrients.

Methods of Study

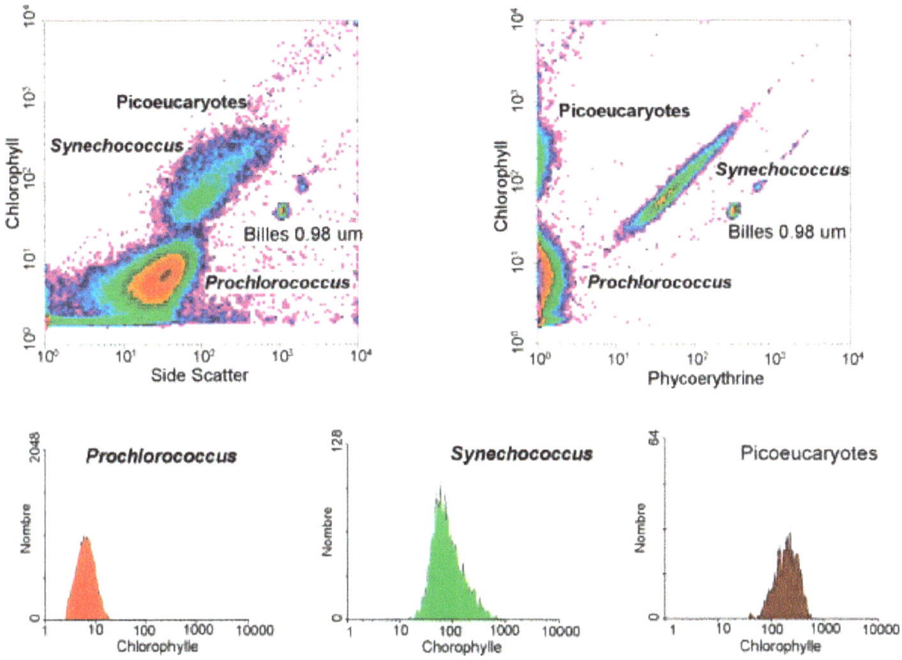

Analysis of Picoplankton by Flow Cytometry

Because of its very small size, picoplankton is difficult to study by classic methods such as optical microscopy. More sophisticated methods are needed.

- Epifluorescence microscopy allows to detect certain groups of cells possessing fluorescent pigments such as *Synechococcus* which possess phycoerythrin.
- Flow cytometry measures the size (" forward scatter ") and fluorescence of 1,000 in 10,000 cells per second. It allows one to determine very easily the concentration of the various picoplankton populations on marine samples. Three groups of cells (*Prochlorococcus,Synechococcus* and picoeukaryotes) can be distinguished. For example *Synechococcus* is characterized by the double fluorescence of its pigments: orange for phycoerythrin and red for chlorophyll. Flow cytometry also allows to sort out specific populations (for example *Synechococcus*) in order put them in culture, or to make more detailed analyses.
- Analysis of photosynthetic pigments such as chlorophyll or carotenoids by high precision chromatography (HPLC) allows to determine the various groups of algae present in a sample.
- Molecular biology techniques:
- Cloning and sequencing of genes such as that of ribosomal RNA, which allows to determine total diversity within a sample
- DGGE (Denaturing Gel Electrophoresis), that is faster than the previous approach allows to have an idea of the global diversity within a sample

- In situ hybridization (FISH) uses fluorescent probes recognizing specific taxon, for example a species, a genus or a class. This original description as a species is now thought to be composed of a number of different cryptic species, a finding that has been confirmed by a genome sequencing project of two strains led by researchers at the Monterey Bay Aquarium Research Institute
- Quantitative PCR can be used, as FISH, to determine, the abundance of specific groups. It has the main advantage to allow the rapid analysis of a large number of samples simultaneously, but requires more sophisticated controls and calibrations.

Composition

Three major groups of organisms constitute photosynthetic picoplankton.

- Cyanobacteria belonging to the genus *Synechococcus* of a size of 1 μm (micrometer) were first discovered in 1979 by J. Waterbury (Woods Hole Oceanographic Institution). They are quite ubiquitous, but most abundant in relatively mesotrophic waters.
- Cyanobacteria belonging to the genus *Prochlorococcus* are particularly remarkable. With a typical size of 0.6 μm, *Prochlorococcus* was discovered only in 1988 by two American researchers, Sallie W. (Penny) Chisholm (Massachusetts Institute of Technology) and R.J. Olson (Woods Hole Oceanographic Institution). In spite of its small size, this photosynthetic organism is undoubtedly the most abundant of the planet: indeed its density can reach up to 100 million cells per liter and it can be found down to a depth of 150 m in all the intertropical belt.
- Picoplanktonic eukaryotes are the least well known, as demonstrated by the recent discovery of major groups. Andersen created in 1993 a new class of brown algae, the Pelagophyceae. More surprising still, the discovery in 1994 of a eukaryote of very small size, *Ostreococcus tauri*, dominating the phytoplanktonic biomass of a French brackish lagoon (étang de Thau), shows that these organisms can also play a major ecological role in coastal environments. In 1999, yet a new class of alga was discovered, the Bolidophyceae, very close genetically of diatoms, but quite different morphologically. At the present time, about 50 species are known belonging to several classes.

Algal classes containing picoplankton species	
Classes	**Picoplanktonic genera**
Chlorophyceae	*Nannochloris*
Prasinophyceae	*Micromonas, Ostreococcus, Pycnococcus*
Prymnesiophyceae	*Imantonia*
Pelagophyceae	*Pelagomonas*
Bolidophyceae	*Bolidomonas*
Dictyochophyceae	*Florenciella*

The use of molecular approaches implemented since the 1990s for bacteria, were applied to the photosynthetic picoeukaryotes only 10 years later around 2000. They revealed a very wide diversity and brought to light the importance of the following groups in the picoplankton :

- Prasinophyceae

- Haptophyta
- Cryptophyta

In temperate coastal environment, the genus Micromonas (Prasinophyceae) seems dominant. However, in numerous oceanic environments, the dominant species of eukaryotic picoplankton remain still unknown.

Ecology

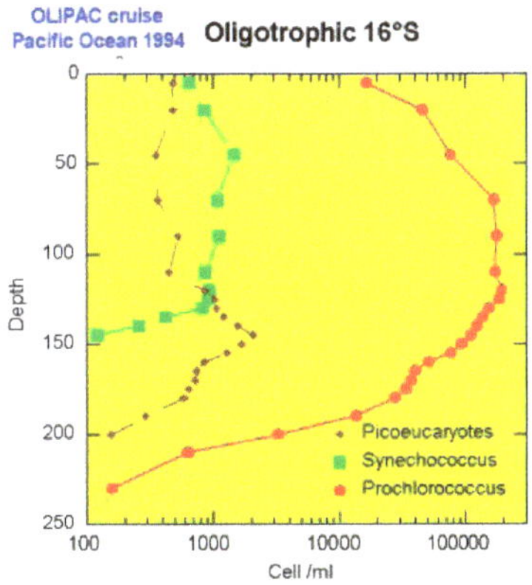

Vertical distribution of picoplankton in the Pacific Ocean

Each picoplanktonic population occupies a specific ecological niche in the oceanic environment.

- The *Synechococcus* cyanobacterium is generally abundant in mesotrophic environments, for example in the vicinity of the equatorial upwelling or in coastal regions.
- The *Prochlorococcus* cyanobacterium replaces it when the waters becomes impoverished in nutrients (i.e. oligotrophic). On the other hand in temperate region (for example in the North Atlantic Ocean),*Prochlorococcus* is absent because the cold waters prevent its development.
- The diversity of eukaryotes, corresponds undoubtedly to a big variety of environments. In oceanic regions, they are often observed at depth at the base of the well-lit layer (the euphotic layer). In coastal regions, certain sorts of picoeukaryotes such as Micromonas dominate. Their abundance follows a seasonal cycle, as the plankton of bigger size, with a maximum in summer.

Thirty years ago, it was hypothesized that the speed of division for micro-organisms in central oceanic ecosystems was very slow, of the order of one week or one month. This hypothesis was consolidated by the fact that the biomass (estimated for example by the contents of chlorophyll) was very stable over time. However with the discovery of the picoplankton, it was found that the system was much more dynamic than previously thought. In particular, small predators of a size of a few micrometres which ingest picoplanktonic algae as quickly as they were produced, were found to be ubiquitous.

This extremely sophisticated predator-prey system is practically always at equilibrium and results in a quasi-constant picoplankton biomass. This perfect equivalence between production and consumption makes it however extremely difficult to measure precisely the speed at which the system turns over.

In 1988, two American researchers, Carpenter and Chang, had suggested estimating the speed of cell division of phytoplankton by following the course of DNA replication by microscopy. By replacing the microscope by a flow cytometer, it is possible to follow the DNA content of picoplankton cells over time. This allowed to establish that picoplankton cells are extremely synchronous: they replicate their DNA and then divide all at the same time at the end of the day. This synchronization could be due to the presence of an internal biological clock.

Genomics

In the 2000s, genomics allowed to cross a supplementary stage. Genomics consists in determining the complete sequence of genome of an organism and to list every gene present. It is then possible to get an idea of the metabolic capacities of the targeted organisms and understand how it adapts to its environment. To date, the genomes of several types of Prochlorococcus and Synechococcus, and of a strain of Ostreococcus have been determined. The complete genomes of two different Micromonas strains revealed that they were quite different (different species) - and had similarities with land plants. Several other cyanobacteria and of small eukaryotes (Bathycoccus, Pelagomonas) are under sequencing. In parallel, genome analyses begin to be done directly from oceanic samples (ecogenomics or métagenomics), allowing us to access to large sets of gene for uncultivated organisms.

Genomes of photosynthetic picoplankton strains that have been sequenced to date			
Genus	**Strain**	**Sequencing center**	**Remark**
Prochlorococcus	MED4	JGI	
	SS120	Genoscope	
	MIT9312	JGI	
	MIT9313	JGI	
	NATL2A	JGI	
	CC9605	JGI	
	CC9901	JGI	
Synechococcus	WH8102	JGI	
	WH7803	Genoscope	
	RCC307	Génoscope	
	CC9311	TIGR	
Ostreococcus	OTTH95	Genoscope	
Micromonas	RCC299 and CCMP1545	JGI	

CYANOBACTERIA

Cyanobacteria, also known as Cyanophyta, is a phylum of bacteria that obtain their energy through photosynthesis. The name cyanobacteria comes from the color of the bacteria (Greek: κυανός (kyanós) = blue). Sometimes, they are called blue-green algae, and incorrectly so, because cyanobacteria are prokaryotes and the term "algae is reserved for eukaryotes.

Like other prokaryotes, cyanobacteria have no membrane-sheathed organelles. Photosynthesis is performed in distinctive folds in the outer membrane of the cell (unlike green plants which use organelles adapted for this specific role, called chloroplasts). Biologists commonly agree that chloroplasts found in eukaryotes, have their ancestry in cyanobacteria, via a process called endosymbiosis.

By producing oxygen as a byproduct of photosynthesis, cyanobacteria are thought to have converted the early oxygen-poor, reducing atmosphere, into an oxidizing one, causing the "rusting of the Earth" and the Great Oxygenation Event, that dramatically changed the composition of life forms and led to the near-extinction of anaerobic organisms.

Cyanobacteria are a group of photosynthetic, nitrogen fixing bacteria that live in a wide variety of habitats such as moist soils and in water. They may be free-living or form symbiotic relationships with plants or with lichen-forming fungi as in the lichen genus Peltigera. They range from unicellular to filamentous and include colonial species. Colonies may form filaments, sheets, or even hollow balls. Some filamentous species can differentiate into several different cell types: vegetative cells, the normal, photosynthetic cells that are formed under favorable growing conditions; akinetes, climate-resistant spores that may form when environmental conditions become harsh; and thick-walled heterocysts, which contain the enzyme nitrogenase, vital for nitrogen fixation.

Nitrogen fixation

Cyanobacteria can fix atmospheric nitrogen in anaerobic conditions by means of specialized cells called heterocysts. Heterocysts may also form under the appropriate environmental conditions (anoxic) when fixed nitrogen is scarce. Heterocyst-forming species are specialized for nitrogen fixation and are able to fix nitrogen gas into ammonia (NH3), nitrites (NO−2) or nitrates (NO−3), which can be absorbed by plants and converted to protein and nucleic acids (atmospheric nitrogen is not bioavailable to plants, except for those having endosymbiotic nitrogen-fixing bacteria, especially the Fabaceae family, among others). Most importantly they are unicellular.

Free-living cyanobacteria are present in the water column in rice paddies, and cyanobacteria can be found growing as epiphytes on the surfaces of the green alga, Chara, where they may fix nitrogen. Cyanobacteria such as (Anabaena, a symbiont of the aquatic fern Azolla), can provide rice plantations with biofertilizer.

Morphology

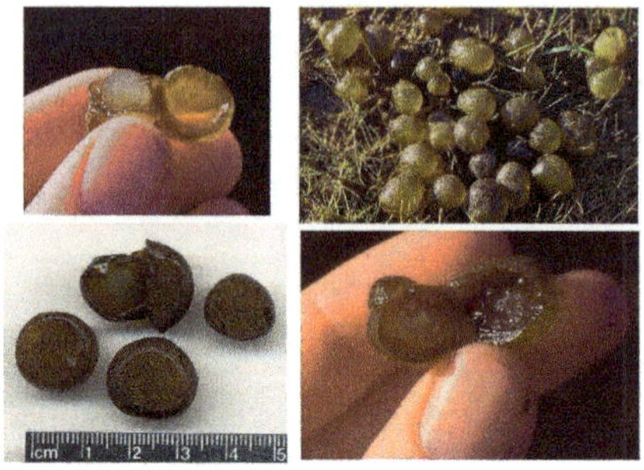

Colonies of *Nostoc pruniforme*

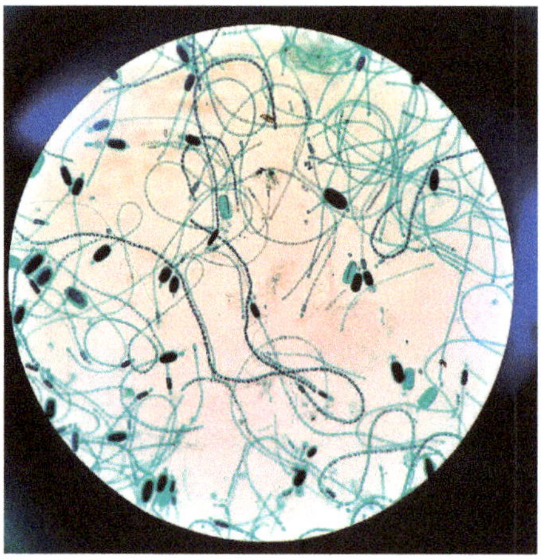

Cylindrospermum sp.

Many cyanobacteria form motile filaments of cells, called hormogonia, that travel away from the main biomass to bud and form new colonies elsewhere. The cells in a hormogonium are often thinner than in the vegetative state, and the cells on either end of the motile chain may be tapered. To break away from the parent colony, a hormogonium often must tear apart a weaker cell in a filament, called a necridium.

Each individual cell of a cyanobacterium typically has a thick, gelatinous cell wall. They lack flagella, but hormogonia of some species can move about by gliding along surfaces. Many of the multicellular filamentous forms of Oscillatoria are capable of a waving motion; the filament oscillates back and forth. In water columns, some cyanobacteria float by forming gas vesicles, as in archaea. These vesicles are not organelles as such. They are not bounded by lipid membranes, but by a protein sheath.

Ecology

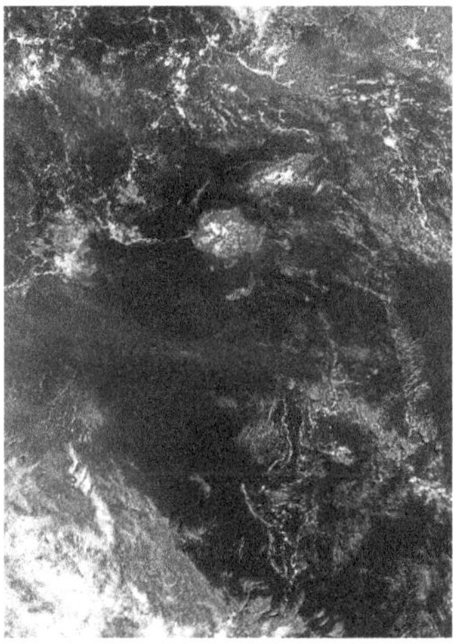

Cyanobacterial Bloom Near Fiji

Cyanobacteria can be found in almost every terrestrial and aquatic habitat—oceans, fresh water, damp soil, temporarily moistened rocks in deserts, bare rock and soil, and even Antarctic rocks. They can occur as planktonic cells or form phototrophic biofilms. They are found in almost every endolithic ecosystem. A few are endosymbionts in lichens, plants, various protists, or sponges and provide energy for the host. Some live in the fur of sloths, providing a form of camouflage.

Aquatic cyanobacteria are known for their extensive and highly visible blooms that can form in both freshwater and marine environments. The blooms can have the appearance of blue-green paint or scum. These blooms can be toxic, and frequently lead to the closure of recreational waters when spotted. Marine bacteriophages are significant parasites of unicellular marine cyanobacteria.

Cyanobacteria prefer calm waters, such as those provided by ponds and lakes. Their life cycles are disrupted when the water naturally or artificially mixes from churning currents caused by the flowing water of streams or the churning water of fountains. For this reason blooms of cyanobacteria seldom occur in rivers unless the water is flowing slowly. When the bacteria are found in rivers, they have usually come from the outfall of lakes upstream from the sampling point. Cyanobacteria are a growing concern for drinking water utilities who use lakes and rivers as their source water. The bacteria can interfere with treatment in various ways, primarily by plugging filters (often large beds of sand and similar media), and by producing cyanotoxins, which have the potential of causing serious illness if consumed.

Some of these organisms contribute significantly to global ecology and the oxygen cycle. The tiny marine cyanobacterium Prochlorococcus was discovered in 1986 and accounts for more than half of the photosynthesis of the open ocean. Many cyanobacteria even display the circadian rhythms that were once thought to exist only in eukaryotic cells (see bacterial circadian rhythms). Cyanobacteria are arguably the most successful group of microorganisms on earth. They are the most genetically diverse; they occupy a broad range of habitats across all latitudes, widespread in freshwater, marine, and terrestrial ecosystems, and they are found in the most extreme niches such as hot springs, salt works, and hypersaline bays. Photoautotrophic, oxygen-producing cyanobacteria created the conditions in the planet's early atmosphere that directed the evolution of aerobic metabolism and eukaryotic photosynthesis. Cyanobacteria fulfill vital ecological functions in the world's oceans, being important contributors to global carbon and nitrogen budgets. – Stewart and Falconer

Photosynthesis

While contemporary cyanobacteria are linked to the plant kingdom as descendants of the endosymbiotic progenitor of the chloroplast, there are several features which are unique to this group.

Carbon Fixation

Cyanobacteria use the energy of sunlight to drive photosynthesis, a process where the energy of light is used to split water molecules into oxygen, protons, and electrons. Because they are aquatic organisms, they typically employ several strategies which are collectively known as a "carbon concentrating mechanism" to aid in the acquisition of inorganic carbon (CO2 or bicarbonate). Among the more specific strategies is the widespread prevalence of the bacterial microcompartments known as carboxysomes. These icosahedral structures are composed of hexameric shell proteins that assemble into cage-like structures that can be several hundreds of nanometers in diameter. It is believed that these structures tether the CO2-fixing enzyme, RuBisCO, to the interior of the shell, as well as the enzyme carbonic anhydrase, using the paradigm of metabolic channeling to enhance the local CO2 concentrations and thus increase the efficiency of the RuBisCO enzyme.

Electron Transport

In contrast to chloroplast-containing eukaryotes, cyanobacteria lack compartmentalization of their thylakoid membranes, which are contiguous with the plasma membrane. Thus, the protein complexes involved in respiratory energy metabolism share several mobile energy carrier pools (e.g., the Quinone pool, cytochrome c, ferredoxins), so photosynthetic and respiratory metabolism interact with each other. Furthermore, there is a tremendous diversity among the respiratory components between species. Thus cyanobacteria can be said to have a "branched electron transport chain", analogous to the situation in purple bacteria.

While most of the high-energy electrons derived from water are used by the cyanobacterial cells for their own needs, a fraction of these electrons may be donated to the external environment via electrogenic activity.

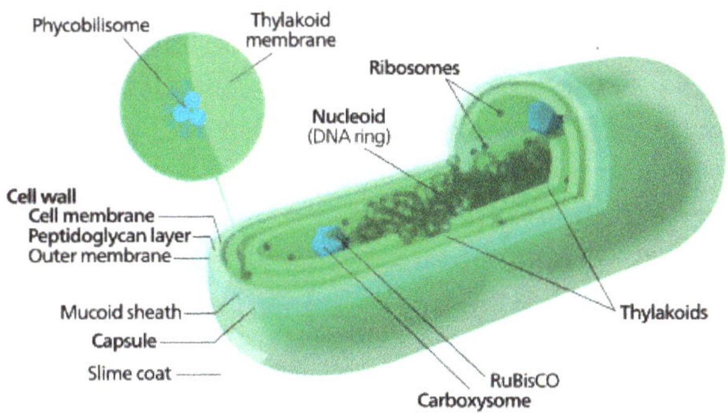

Diagram of a typical cyanobacterial cell

Metabolism and Organelles

As prokaryotes, cyanobacteria do not have nuclei or an internal membrane system. In most forms, the photosynthetic machinery is embedded into folds of the external cell membrane, called thylakoids. Cyanobacteria get their colour from the bluish pigment phycocyanin, which they use to capture light for photosynthesis. In general, photosynthesis in cyanobacteria uses water as an electron donor and produces oxygen as a byproduct, though some may also use hydrogen sulfide a process which occurs among other photosynthetic bacteria such as the purple sulfur bacteria. Carbon dioxide is reduced to form carbohydrates via the Calvin cycle.The large amounts of oxygen in the atmosphere are considered to have been first created by the activities of ancient cyanobacteria. They are often found as symbionts with a number of other groups of organisms such as fungi (lichens), corals, pteridophytes (Azolla), angiosperms (Gunnera), etc.

Many cyanobacteria are able to reduce nitrogen and carbon dioxide under aerobic conditions, a fact that may be responsible for their evolutionary and ecological success. The water-oxidizing photosynthesis is accomplished by coupling the activity of photosystem (PS) II and I (Z-scheme). In anaerobic conditions, they are able to use only PS I—cyclic photophosphorylation—with electron donors other than water (hydrogen sulfide, thiosulphate, or even molecular hydrogen) just like purple photosynthetic bacteria. Furthermore, they share an archaeal property, the ability to reduce elemental sulfur by anaerobic respiration in the dark. Their photosynthetic electron transport shares the same compartment as the components of respiratory electron transport. Their plasma membrane contains only components of the respiratory chain, while the thylakoid membrane hosts an interlinked respiratory and photosynthetic electron transport chain. The terminal oxidases in the thylakoid membrane respiratory/photosynthetic electron transport chain are essential for survival to rapid light changes, although not for dark maintenance under conditions where cells are not light stressed.

Attached to the thylakoid membrane, phycobilisomes act as light-harvesting antennae for the photosystems. The phycobilisome components (phycobiliproteins) are responsible for the blue-green pigmentation of most cyanobacteria. The variations on this theme are due mainly to carotenoids and phycoerythrins that give the cells their red-brownish coloration. In some cyanobacteria, the color of light influences the composition of phycobilisomes. In green light, the cells accumulate more phycoerythrin, whereas in red light they produce more phycocyanin. Thus, the bacteria appear green in red light and red in green light. This process of complementary chromatic adaptation is a way for the cells to maximize the use of available light for photosynthesis. A few genera lack phycobilisomes and have chlorophyll b instead (Prochloron, Prochlorococcus, Prochlorothrix). These were originally grouped together as the prochlorophytes or chloroxybacteria, but appear to have developed in several different lines of cyanobacteria. For this reason, they are now considered as part of the cyanobacterial group.

There are some groups capable of heterotrophic growth, while others are parasitic, causing diseases in invertebrates or eukaryotic algae (e.g., the black band disease).

Relationship to Chloroplasts

Cladogram showing plastids (chloroplasts and similar) and basal cyanobacteria

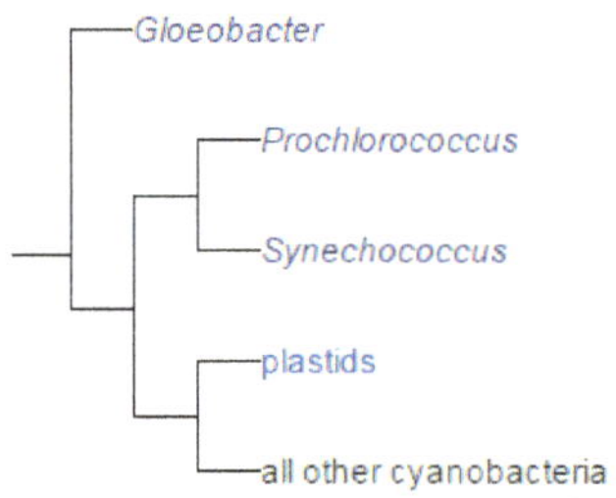

Chloroplasts found in eukaryotes (algae and plants) appear to have evolved from an endosymbiotic relation with cyanobacteria. This endosymbiotic theory is supported by various structural and genetic similarities. Primary chloroplasts are found among the "true plants or green plants – species ranging from sea lettuce to evergreens and flowers that contain chlorophyll b – as well as among the red algae and glaucophytes, marine species that contain phycobilins. It now appears that these chloroplasts probably had a single origin, in an ancestor of th

Classification

Historically, bacteria were first classified as plants constituting the class Schizomycetes, which along with the Schizophyceae (blue-green algae/Cyanobacteria) formed the phylum Schizophyta, then in the phylum Monera in the kingdom Protista by Haeckel in 1866, comprising Protogens, Protamaeba, Vampyrella, Protomonae, and Vibrio, but not Nostoc and other cyanobacteria, which were classified with algae, later reclassified as the Prokaryotes by Chatton.

The cyanobacteria were traditionally classified by morphology into five sections, referred to by the numerals I-V. The first three – Chroococcales, Pleurocapsales, and Oscillatoriales – are not supported by phylogenetic studies. The latter two – Nostocales and Stigonematales – are monophyletic, and make up the heterocystous cyanobacteria.

The members of Chroococales are unicellular and usually aggregate in colonies. The classic taxonomic criterion has been the cell morphology and the plane of cell division. In Pleurocapsales, the cells have the ability to form internal spores (baeocytes). The rest of the sections include filamentous species. In Oscillatoriales, the cells are uniseriately arranged and do not form specialized cells (akinetes and heterocysts). In Nostocales and Stigonematales, the cells have the ability to develop heterocysts in certain conditions. Stigonematales, unlike Nostocales, include species with truly branched trichomes.

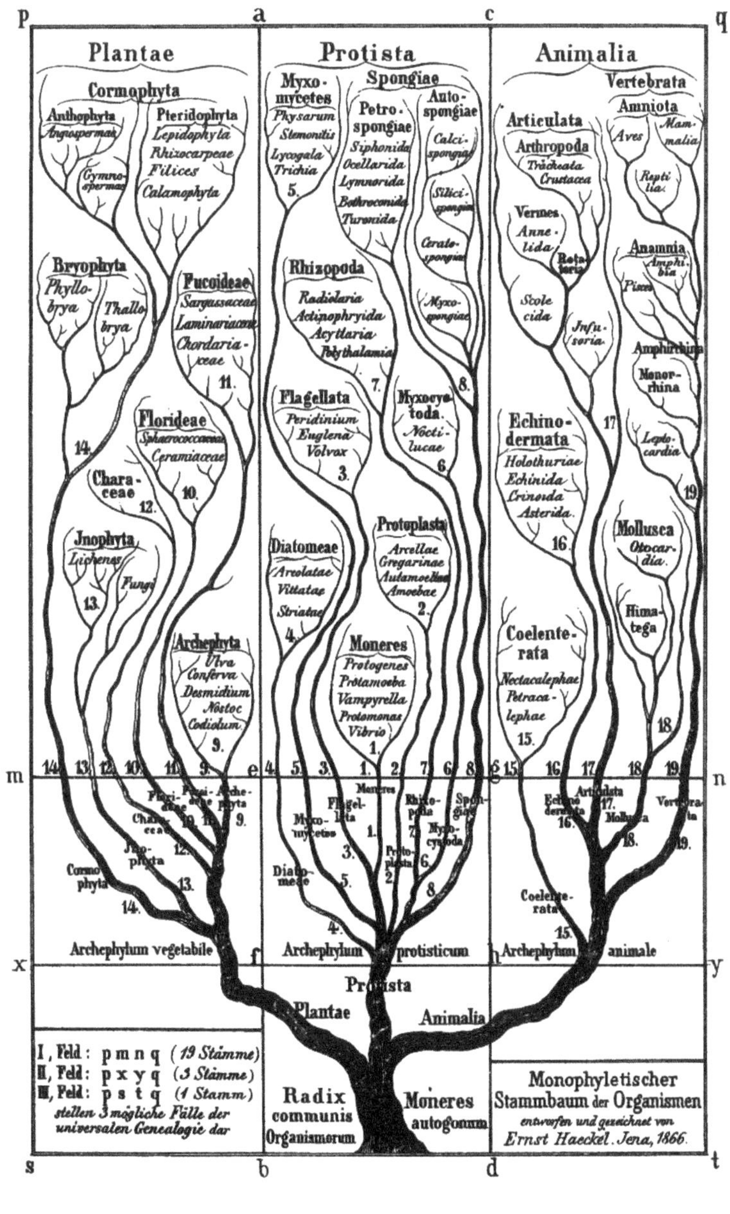

Tree of Life in Generelle Morphologie der Organismen (1866). Note the location of the genus Nostoc with algae and not with bacteria (kingdom "Monera")

Most taxa included in the phylum or division Cyanobacteria have not yet been validly published under the Bacteriological Code, except:

- The classes Chroobacteria, Hormogoneae, and Gloeobacteria
- The orders Chroococcales, Gloeobacterales, Nostocales, Oscillatoriales, Pleurocapsales, and Stigonematales
- The families Prochloraceae and Prochlorotrichaceae
- The genera *Halospirulina, Planktothricoides, Prochlorococcus, Prochloron*, and *Prochlorothrix*

The remainder are validly published under the International Code of Nomenclature for algae, fungi, and plants.

Formerly, some bacteria, like *Beggiatoa*, were thought to be colorless Cyanobacteria.

Earth History

Stromatolites are layered biochemical accretionary structures formed in shallow water by the trapping, binding, and cementation of sedimentary grains by biofilms (microbial mats) of microorganisms, especially cyanobacteria.

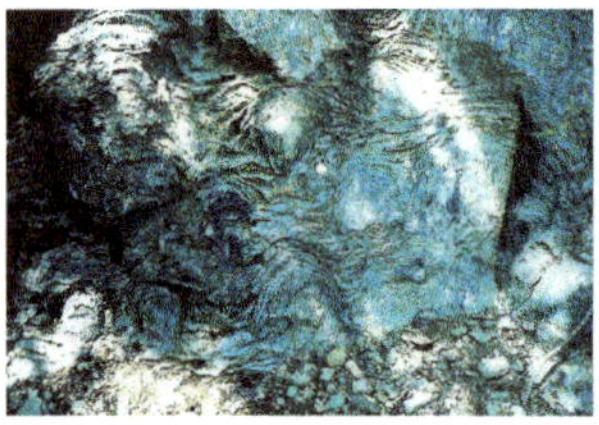

Stromatolites left behind by cyanobacteria are the oldest known fossils of life on Earth. This one-billion-year-old fossil is from Glacier National Park in Montana.

During the Precambrian, stromatolite communities of microorganisms grew in most marine and non-marine environments in the photic zone. After the Cambrian explosion of marine animals, grazing on the stromatolite mats by herbivores greatly reduced the occurrence of the stromatolites in marine environments. Since then, they are found mostly in hypersaline conditions where grazing invertebrates cannot live (e.g. Shark Bay, Western Australia). Stromatolites provide ancient records of life on Earth by fossil remains which might date from more than 3.5 Ga ago, but this is disputed. As of 2010 the oldest undisputed evidence of cyanobacteria is from 2.1 Ga ago, but there is some evidence for them as far back as 2.7 Ga ago. Oxygen levels in the atmosphere remained around or below 1% of today's level until 2.4 Ga ago (the Great Oxygenation Event). The rise in oxygen may have caused a fall in methane levels, and triggered the Huronian glaciation from around 2.4 to 2.1 Ga ago. In this way, cyanobacteria may have killed off much of the other bacteria of the time.

Oncolites are sedimentary structures composed of oncoids, which are layered structures formed by cyanobacterial growth. Oncolites are similar to stromatolites, but instead of forming columns, they form approximately spherical structures that were not attached to the underlying substrate as they formed. The oncoids often form around a central nucleus, such as a shell fragment, and a calcium carbonate structure is deposited by encrusting microbes. Oncolites are indicators of warm waters in the photic zone, but are also known in contemporary freshwater environments. These structures rarely exceed 10 cm in diameter.

Biotechnology and Applications

The unicellular cyanobacterium Synechocystis sp. PCC6803 was the third prokaryote and first photosynthetic organism whose genome was completely sequenced. It continues to be an important model organism. Cyanothece ATCC 51142 is an important diazotrophic model organism. The smallest genomes have been found in Prochlorococcus spp. (1.7 Mb) and the largest in Nostoc punctiforme (9 Mb). Those of Calothrix spp. are estimated at 12–15 Mb, as large as yeast.

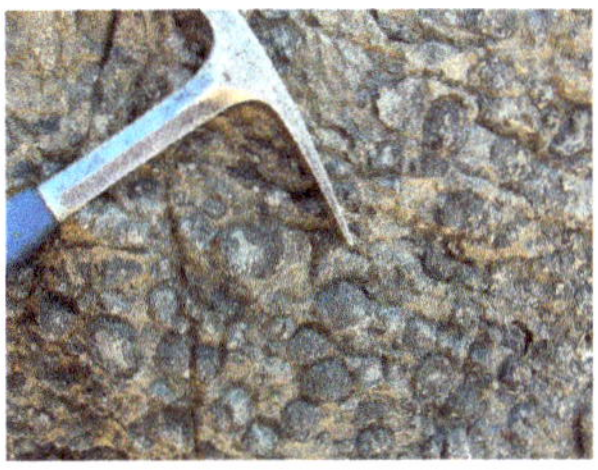

Oncolites from the Late Devonian Alamo bolide impact in Nevada

Recent research has suggested the potential application of cyanobacteria to the generation of renewable energy by converting sunlight into electricity. Internal photosynthetic pathways can be coupled to chemical mediators that transfer electrons to external electrodes. Currently, efforts are underway to commercialize algae-based fuels such as diesel, gasoline, and jet fuel.

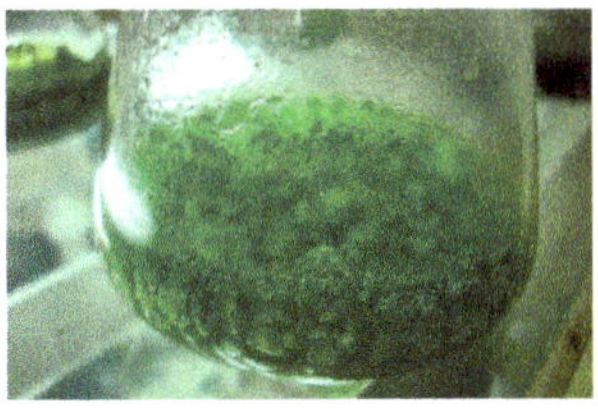

Cyanobacteria cultured in specific media: Cyanobacteria can be helpful in agriculture as they have the ability to fix atmospheric nitrogen in soil.

Researchers from a company called Algenol have cultured genetically modified cyanobacteria in sea water inside a clear plastic enclosure so they first make sugar (pyruvate) from CO2 and the water via photosynthesis. Then, the bacteria secrete ethanol from the cell into the salt water. As the day progresses, and the solar radiation intensifies, ethanol concentrations build up and the ethanol itself evaporates onto the roof of the enclosure. As the sun recedes, evaporated ethanol and water condense into droplets, which run along the plastic walls and into ethanol collectors, from where it is extracted from the enclosure with the water and ethanol separated outside the enclosure. As of March 2013, Algenol was claiming to have tested its technology in Florida and to have achieved yields of 9,000 US gallons per acre per year. This could potentially meet US demands for ethanol in gasoline in 2025, assuming a B30 blend, from an area of around half the size of California's San Bernardino County, requiring less than one-tenth of the area than ethanol from other biomass, such as corn, and only very limited amounts of fresh water.

Cyanobacteria may possess the ability to produce substances that could one day serve as anti-inflammatory agents and combat bacterial infections in humans.

Spirulina's extracted blue color is used as a natural food coloring in gum and candy.

Researchers from several space agencies argue that cyanobacteria could be used for producing goods for human consumption (food, oxygen...) in future manned outposts on Mars, by transforming materials available on this planet.

Health Risks

Cyanobacteria can produce neurotoxins, cytotoxins, endotoxins, and hepatotoxins (i.e. the microcystin-producing bacteria species microcystis), and are called cyanotoxins.

Specific toxins include, anatoxin-a, anatoxin-as, aplysiatoxin, cyanopeptolin, cylindrospermopsin, domoic acid, nodularin R (from Nodularia), neosaxitoxin, and saxitoxin. Cyanobacteria reproduce explosively under certain conditions. This results in algal blooms, which can become harmful to other species, and pose a danger to humans and animals, if the cyanobacteria involved produce toxins. Several cases of human poisoning have been documented, but a lack of knowledge prevents an accurate assessment of the risks.

Recent studies suggest that significant exposure to high levels of cyanobacteria producing toxins such as BMAA can cause amyotrophic lateral sclerosis (ALS). People living within a half-mile of cyanobacterially contaminated lakes have had a 2.3 times greater risk of developing ALS than the rest of the population; people around New Hampshire's Lake Mascoma had an up to 25 times greater risk of ALS than the expected incidence. BMAA from desert crusts found throughout Qatar might have contributed to higher rates of ALS in Gulf War veterans.

Chemical Control

Several chemicals can eliminate blue-green algal blooms from water-based systems. They include: calcium hypochlorite, copper sulphate, cupricide, and simazine. The calcium hypochlorite amount needed varies depending on the cyanobacteria bloom, and treatment is needed periodically. According to the Department of Agriculture Australia, a rate of 12 g of 70% material in 1000 l of water is often effective to treat a bloom. Copper sulfate is also used commonly, but no longer recommended by the Australian Department of Agriculture, as it kills livestock, crustaceans, and fish. Culpricide is a chelated copper product that eliminates blooms with lower toxicity risks than copper sulfate. Dosage recommendations vary from 190 ml to 4.8 l per 1000 m^2. Ferric alum treatments at the rate of 50 mg/l will reduce algae blooms. Simazine, which is also a herbicide, will continue to kill blooms for several days after an application. Simazine is marketed at different strengths (25, 50, and 90%), the recommended amount needed for one cubic meter of water per product is 25% product 8 ml; 50% product 4 ml; or 90% product 2.2 ml.

Dietary Supplementation

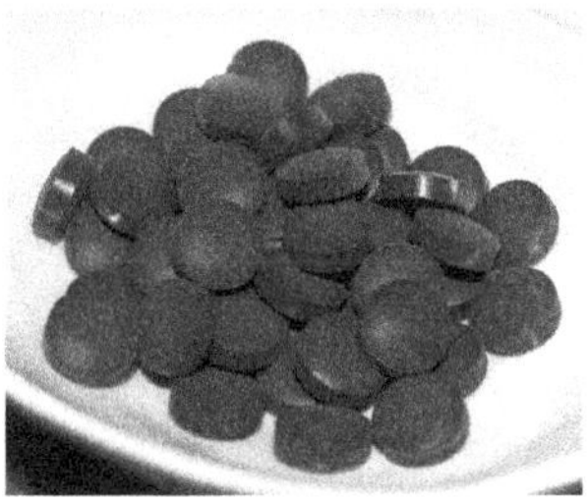

Spirulina tablets

Some cyanobacteria are sold as food, notably Aphanizomenon flos-aquae and Arthrospira platensis (Spirulina).

Despite the associated toxins which many of the members of this phylum produce, some microalgae also contain substances of high biological value, such as polyunsaturated fatty acids, amino acids (proteins), pigments, antioxidants, vitamins, and minerals. Edible blue-green algae reduce the production of pro-inflammatory cytokines by inhibiting NF-κB pathway in macrophages and splenocytes.Sulfate polysaccharides exhibit immunomodulatory, antitumor, antithrombotic, anticoagulant, anti-mutagenic, anti-inflammatory, antimicrobial, and even antiviral activity against HIV, herpes, and hepatitis.

ARCHAEA

The Archaea constitute a domain and kingdom of single-celled microorganisms. These microbes (archaea; singular archaeon) are prokaryotes, meaning that they have no cell nucleus or any other membrane-bound organelles in their cells.

Archaea were initially classified as bacteria, receiving the name archaebacteria (in the Archaebacteria kingdom), but this classification is outdated. Archaeal cells have unique properties separating them from the other two domains of life, Bacteria and Eukaryota. The Archaea are further divided into multiple recognized phyla. Classification is difficult because the majority have not been isolated in the laboratory and have only been detected by analysis of their nucleic acids in samples from their environment.

Archaea and bacteria are generally similar in size and shape, although a few archaea have very strange shapes, such as the flat and square-shaped cells of Haloquadratum walsbyi. Despite this morphological similarity to bacteria, archaea possess genes and several metabolic pathways that are more closely related to those of eukaryotes, notably the enzymes involved in transcription and translation. Other aspects of archaeal biochemistry are unique, such as their reliance on ether lipids in their cell membranes, including archaeols. Archaea use more energy sources than eukaryotes: these range from organic compounds, such as sugars, to ammonia, metal ions or even hydrogen gas. Salt-tolerant archaea (the Haloarchaea) use sunlight as an energy source, and other species of archaea fix carbon; however, unlike plants and cyanobacteria, no known species of archaea does both. Archaea reproduce asexually by binary fission, fragmentation, or budding; unlike bacteria and eukaryotes, no known species forms spores.

Archaea were initially viewed as extremophiles living in harsh environments, such as hot springs and salt lakes, but they have since been found in a broad range of habitats, including soils, oceans, marshlands and the human colon, oral cavity, and skin. Archaea are particularly numerous in the oceans, and the archaea in plankton may be one of the most abundant groups of organisms on the planet. Archaea are a major part of Earth's life and may play roles in both the carbon cycle and the nitrogen cycle. No clear examples of archaeal pathogens or parasites are known, but they are often mutualists or commensals. One example is the methanogens that inhabit human and ruminant guts, where their vast numbers aid digestion. Methanogens are also used in biogas production and sewage treatment, and enzymes from extremophile archaea that can endure high temperatures and organic solvents are exploited in biotechnology.

Classification

New Domain

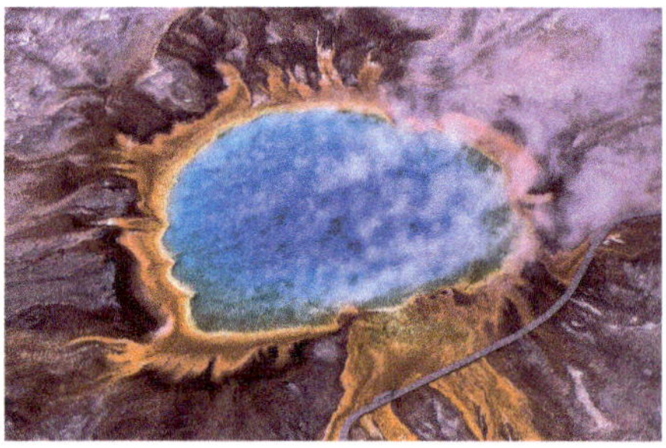

Archaea were first found in extreme environments, such as volcanic hot springs. Pictured here is Grand Prismatic Spring of Yellowstone National Park.

For much of the 20th century, prokaryotes were regarded as a single group of organisms and classified based on their biochemistry, morphology and metabolism. For example, microbiologists tried to classify microorganisms based on the structures of their cell walls, their shapes, and the substances they consume. In 1965, Emile Zuckerkandl and Linus Pauling proposed instead using the sequences of the genes in different prokaryotes to work out how they are related to each other. This approach, known as phylogenetics, is the main method used today.

Archaea were first classified as a separate group of prokaryotes in 1977 by Carl Woese and George E. Fox in phylogenetic trees based on the sequences of ribosomal RNA (rRNA) genes. These two groups were originally named the Archaebacteria and Eubacteria and treated as kingdoms or subkingdoms, which Woese and Fox termed Urkingdoms. Woese argued that this group of prokaryotes is a fundamentally different sort of life. To emphasize this difference, Woese later proposed a new natural system of organisms with three separate Domains: the Eukarya, the Bacteria and the Archaea, in what is now known as "The Woesian Revolution".

The word archaea comes from the Ancient Greek ἀρχαῖα,, meaning ancient things, as the first representatives of the domain Archaea were methanogens and it was assumed that their metabolism reflected Earth's primitive atmosphere and the organism's antiquity. For a long time, archaea were seen as extremophiles that only exist in extreme habitats such as hot springs and salt lakes. However, as new habitats were studied, more organisms were discovered. Extreme halophilic and hyperthermophilic microbes were also included in the Archaea. By the end of the 20th century, archaea had been identified in non-extreme environments as well. Today, they are known to be a large and diverse group of organisms that are widely distributed in nature and are common in all habitats. This new appreciation of the importance and ubiquity of archaea came from using polymerase chain reaction (PCR) to detect prokaryotes from environmental samples (such as water or soil) by multiplying their ribosomal genes. This allows the detection and identification of organisms that have not been cultured in the laboratory.

Current Classification

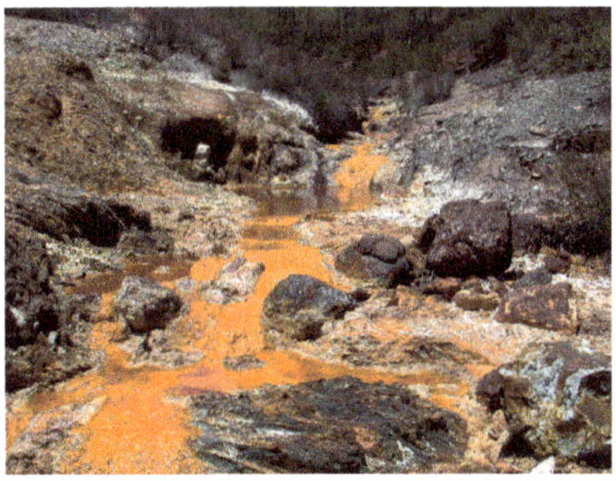

The ARMAN are a new group of archaea recently discovered in acid mine drainage.

The classification of archaea, and of prokaryotes in general, is a rapidly moving and contentious field. Current classification systems aim to organize archaea into groups of organisms that share structural features and common ancestors. These classifications rely heavily on the use of the sequence of ribosomal RNA genes to reveal relationships between organisms (molecular phylogenetics). Most of the culturable and well-investigated species of archaea are members of two main phyla, the Euryarchaeota and Crenarchaeota. Other groups have been tentatively created. For example, the peculiar species Nanoarchaeum equitans, which was discovered in 2003, has been given its own phylum, the Nanoarchaeota.

A new phylum Korarchaeota has also been proposed. It contains a small group of unusual thermophilic species that shares features of both of the main phyla, but is most closely related to the Crenarchaeota. Other recently detected species of archaea are only distantly related to any of these groups, such as the Archaeal Richmond Mine acidophilic nanoorganisms (ARMAN), which were discovered in 2006 and are some of the smallest organisms known.

A superphylum - TACK - has been proposed that includes the Thaumarchaeota, Aigarchaeota, Crenarchaeota, and Korarchaeota. This superphylum may be related to the origin of eukaryotes.

Concept of Species

The classification of archaea into species is also controversial. Biology defines a species as a group of related organisms. The familiar exclusive breeding criterion (organisms that can breed with each other but not with others) is of no help here because archaea reproduce asexually.

Archaea show high levels of horizontal gene transfer between lineages. Some researchers suggest that individuals can be grouped into species-like populations given highly similar genomes and infrequent gene transfer to/from cells with less-related genomes, as in the genus Ferroplasma. On the other hand, studies in Halorubrum found significant genetic transfer to/from less-related populations, limiting the criterion's applicability. A second concern is to what extent such species designations have practical meaning.

Current knowledge on genetic diversity is fragmentary and the total number of archaeal species cannot be estimated with any accuracy.Estimates of the number of phyla range from 18 to 23, of which only 8 have representatives that have been cultured and studied directly. Many of these hypothesized groups are known from a single rRNA sequence, indicating that the diversity among these organisms remains obscure. The Bacteria also contain many uncultured microbes with similar implications for characterization.

Origin and Evolution

The age of the Earth is about 4.54 billion years. Scientific evidence suggests that life began on Earth at least 3.5 billion years ago.The earliest evidence for life on Earth is graphite found to be biogenic in 3.7 billion-year-old metasedimentary rocks discovered in Western Greenland and microbial mat fossils found in 3.48 billion-year-old sandstone discovered in Western Australia. More recently, in 2015, remains of biotic life were found in 4.1 billion-year-old rocks in Western Australia. An unrelated researcher, S. Blair Hedges, wrote in an email about the study saying, If life arose relatively quickly on Earth ... then it could be common in the universe.

Although probable prokaryotic cell fossils date to almost 3.5 billion years ago, most prokaryotes do not have distinctive morphologies and fossil shapes cannot be used to identify them as archaea. Instead, chemical fossils of unique lipids are more informative because such compounds do not occur in other organisms. Some publications suggest that archaeal or eukaryotic lipid remains are present in shales dating from 2.7 billion years ago; such data have since been questioned. Such lipids have also been detected in even older rocks from west Greenland. The oldest such traces come from the Isua district, which include Earth's oldest known sediments, formed 3.8 billion years ago. The archaeal lineage may be the most ancient that exists on Earth.

Woese argued that the bacteria, archaea, and eukaryotes represent separate lines of descent that diverged early on from an ancestral colony of organisms. One possibility is that this occurred before the evolution of cells, when the lack of a typical cell membrane allowed unrestricted lateral gene transfer, and that the common ancestors of the three domains arose by fixation of specific subsets of genes. It is possible that the last common ancestor of the bacteria and archaea was a thermophile, which raises the possibility that lower temperatures are extreme environments in archaeal terms, and organisms that live in cooler environments appeared only later. Since the Archaea and Bacteria are no more related to each other than they are to eukaryotes, the term *prokaryote*'s only surviving meaning is "not a eukaryote", limiting its value.

Comparison to Other Domains

The following table compares some major characteristics of the three domains, to illustrate their similarities and differences. Many of these characteristics are also discussed below.

Property	Archaea	Bacteria	Eukarya
Cell Membrane	Ether-linked lipids, pseudopeptidoglycan	Ester-linked lipids, peptidoglycan	Ester-linked lipids, various structures
Gene Structure	Circular chromosomes, similar translation and transcription to Eukarya	Circular chromosomes, unique translation and transcription	Multiple, linear chromosomes, similar translation and transcription to Archaea
Internal Cell Structure	No membrane-bound organelles or nucleus	No membrane-bound organelles or nucleus	Membrane-bound organelles and nucleus
Metabolism	Various, with methanogenesis unique to Archaea	Various, including photosynthesis, aerobic and anaerobic respiration, fermentation, and autotrophy	Photosynthesis and cellular respiration
Reproduction	Asexual reproduction, horizontal gene transfer	Asexual reproduction, horizontal gene transfer	Sexual and asexual reproduction

Archaea were split off as a third domain because of the large differences in their ribosomal RNA structure. The particular RNA molecule sequenced, known as 16s rRNA, is present in all organisms and always has the same vital function, the production of proteins. Because this function is so central to life, organisms with mutations of its 16s rRNA are unlikely to survive, leading to great stability in the structure of this nucleotide over many generations. 16s rRNA is also large enough to retain organism-specific information, but small enough to be sequenced in a manageable amount of time. In 1977, Carl Woese, a microbiologist studying the genetic sequencing of organisms, developed a new sequencing method that involved splitting the RNA into fragments that could be sorted and compared to other fragments from other organisms. The more similar the patterns between species were, the more closely related the organisms.

Woese used his new rRNA comparison method to categorize and contrast different organisms. He sequenced a variety of different species and happened upon a group of methanogens that had vastly different patterns than any known prokaryotes or eukaryotes. These methanogens were much more similar to each other than they were to other organisms sequenced, leading Woese to propose the new domain of Archaea.One of the interesting results of his experiments was that the Archaea were more similar to eukaryotes than prokaryotes, even though they were more similar to prokaryotes in structure. This led to the conclusion that Archaea and Eukarya shared a more recent common ancestor than Eukarya and Bacteria in general. The development of the nucleus occurred after the split between Bacteria and this common ancestor.Although Archaea are prokaryotic, they are more closely related to Eukarya and thus cannot be placed within either the Bacteria or Eukarya domains.

One property unique to Archaea is the abundant use of ether-linked lipids in their cell membranes. Ether linkages are more chemically stable than the ester linkages found in Bacteria and Eukarya, which may be a contributing factor to the ability of many Archaea to survive in extreme environments that place heavy stress on cell membranes, such as extreme heat and salinity. Another unique feature of Archaea is that no other known organisms are capable of methanogenesis (the metabolic production of methane). Methanogenic Archaea play a pivotal role in ecosystems with organisms that derive energy from oxidation of methane, many of which are Bacteria, as they are often a major source of methane in such environments and can play a role as primary producers. Methanogens also play a critical role in the carbon cycle, breaking down organic carbon into methane, which is also a major greenhouse gas.

Relationship to other Prokaryotes

Phylogenetic tree showing the relationship between the Archaea and other domains of life. Eukaryotes are colored red, archaea green and bacteria blue. Adapted from Ciccarelli, et al. (2006).

The relationship between the three domains is of central importance for understanding the origin of life. Most of the metabolic pathways, which comprise the majority of an organism's genes, are common between Archaea and Bacteria, while most genes involved in genome expression are common between Archaea and Eukarya.Within prokaryotes, archaeal cell structure is most similar to that of gram-positive bacteria, largely because both have a single lipid bilayer and usually contain a thick sacculus (exoskeleton) of varying chemical composition. In some phylogenetic trees based upon different gene/protein sequences of prokaryotic homologs, the archaeal homologs are more closely related to those of gram-positive bacteria.Archaea and gram-positive bacteria also share conserved indels in a number of important proteins, such as Hsp70 and glutamine synthetase I; however, the phylogeny of these genes was interpreted to reveal interdomain gene transfer,and might not reflect the organismal relationship(s).

It has been proposed that the archaea evolved from gram-positive bacteria in response to antibiotic selection pressure. This is suggested by the observation that archaea are resistant to a wide variety of antibiotics that are primarily produced by gram-positive bacteria, and that these antibiotics primarily act on the genes that distinguish archaea from bacteria. The proposal is that the selective pressure towards resistance generated by the gram-positive antibiotics was eventually sufficient to cause extensive changes in many of the antibiotics' target genes, and that these strains represented the common ancestors of present-day Archaea. The evolution of Archaea in response to antibiotic selection, or any other competitive selective pressure, could also explain their adaptation to extreme environments (such as high temperature or acidity) as the result of a search for unoccupied niches to escape from antibiotic-producing organisms; Cavalier-Smith has made a similar suggestion.This proposal is also supported by other work investigating protein structural relationships and studies that suggest that gram-positive bacteria may constitute the earliest branching lineages within the prokaryotes.

Relation to Eukaryotes

The evolutionary relationship between archaea and eukaryotes remains unclear. Aside from the similarities in cell structure and function that are discussed below, many genetic trees group the two.

Complicating factors include claims that the relationship between eukaryotes and the archaeal phylum Crenarchaeota is closer than the relationship between the Euryarchaeota and the phylum Crenarchaeota and the presence of archaea-like genes in certain bacteria, such as Thermotoga maritima, from horizontal gene transfer. The standard hypothesis states that the ancestor of the eukaryotes diverged early from the Archaea, and that eukaryotes arose through fusion of an archaean and eubacterium, which became the nucleus and cytoplasm; this explains various genetic similarities but runs into difficulties explaining cell structure. An alternative hypothesis, the eocyte hypothesis, posits that Eukaryota emerged relatively late from the Archaea.

A recently discovered lineage of archaea, Lokiarchaeum, named for a hydrothermal vent called Loki's Castle in the Arctic Ocean, has been found to be most closely related to eukaryotes. It has been called a transitional organism between prokaryotes and eukaryotes.

Morphology

Individual archaea range from 0.1 micrometers (μm) to over 15 μm in diameter, and occur in various shapes, commonly as spheres, rods, spirals or plates. Other morphologies in the Crenarchaeota include irregularly shaped lobed cells in Sulfolobus, needle-like filaments that are less than half a micrometer in diameter in Thermofilum, and almost perfectly rectangular rods in Thermoproteus and Pyrobaculum. Haloquadratum walsbyi are flat, square archaea that live in hypersaline pools. These unusual shapes are probably maintained both by their cell walls and a prokaryotic cytoskeleton. Proteins related to the cytoskeleton components of other organisms exist in archaea, and filaments form within their cells, but in contrast to other organisms, these cellular structures are poorly understood. In Thermoplasma and Ferroplasma the lack of a cell wall means that the cells have irregular shapes, and can resemble amoebae.

Some species form aggregates or filaments of cells up to 200 μm long. These organisms can be prominent in biofilms. Notably, aggregates of Thermococcus coalescens cells fuse together in culture, forming single giant cells. Archaea in the genus Pyrodictium produce an elaborate multicell colony involving arrays of long, thin hollow tubes called cannulae that stick out from the cells' surfaces and connect them into a dense bush-like agglomeration. The function of these cannulae is not settled, but they may allow communication or nutrient exchange with neighbors. Multi-species colonies exist, such as the "string-of-pearls" community that was discovered in 2001 in a German swamp. Round whitish colonies of a novel Euryarchaeota species are spaced along thin filaments that can range up to 15 centimetres (5.9 in) long; these filaments are made of a particular bacteria species.

Structure, Composition Development, and Operation

Archaea and bacteria have generally similar cell structure, but cell composition and organization set the archaea apart. Like bacteria, archaea lack interior membranes and organelles. Like bacteria, archaea cell membranes are usually bounded by a cell wall and they swim using one or more flagella. Structurally, archaea are most similar to gram-positive bacteria. Most have a single plasma membrane and cell wall, and lack a periplasmic space; the exception to this general rule is Ignicoccus, which possess a particularly large periplasm that contains membrane-bound vesicles and is enclosed by an outer membrane.

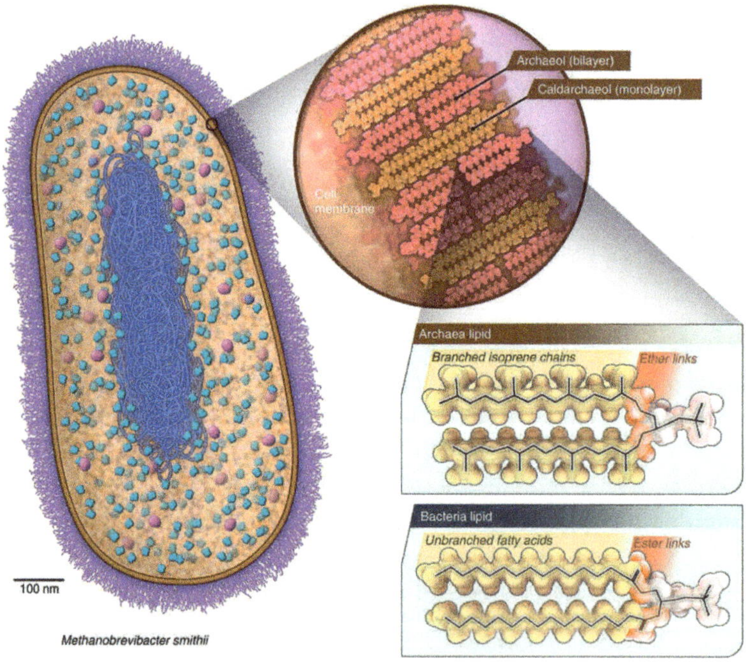

Diagrammatic view of *Methanobrevibacter smithii*, showing the cell membrane (ochre, with inset) and cell wall (purple).

Cell wall and flagella

Most archaea (but not Thermoplasma and Ferroplasma) possess a cell wall. In most archaea the wall is assembled from surface-layer proteins, which form an S-layer. An S-layer is a rigid array of protein molecules that cover the outside of the cell (like chain mail).This layer provides both chemical and physical protection, and can prevent macromolecules from contacting the cell membrane. Unlike bacteria, archaea lack peptidoglycan in their cell walls. Methanobacteriales do have cell walls containing pseudopeptidoglycan, which resembles eubacterial peptidoglycan in morphology, function, and physical structure, but pseudopeptidoglycan is distinct in chemical structure; it lacks D-amino acids and N-acetylmuramic acid.

Archaea flagella operate like bacterial flagella—their long stalks are driven by rotatory motors at the base. These motors are powered by the proton gradient across the membrane. However, archaeal flagella are notably different in composition and development. The two types of flagella evolved from different ancestors. The bacterial flagellum shares a common ancestor with the type III secretion system, while archaeal flagella appear to have evolved from bacterial type IV pili. In contrast to the bacterial flagellum, which is hollow and is assembled by subunits moving up the central pore to the tip of the flagella, archaeal flagella are synthesized by adding subunits at the base.

Membranes

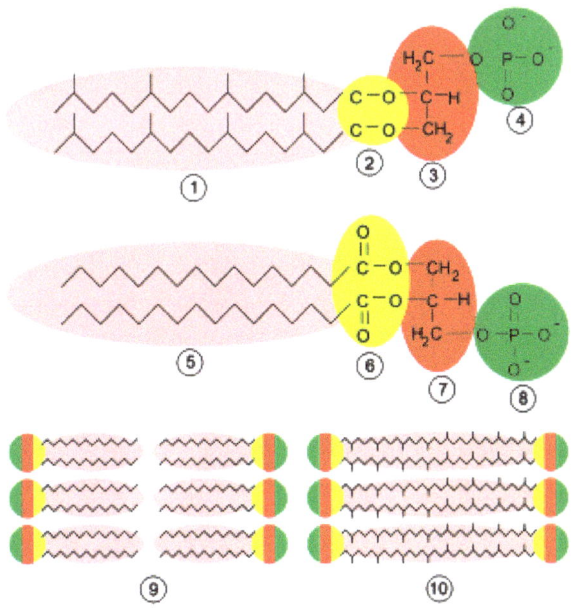

Membrane structures. Top, an archaeal phospholipid: 1, isoprene chains; 2, ether linkages; 3, L-glycerol moiety; 4, phosphate group. Middle, a bacterial or eukaryotic phospholipid: 5, fatty acid chains; 6, ester linkages; 7, D-glycerol moiety; 8, phosphate group. Bottom: 9, lipid bilayer of bacteria and eukaryotes; 10, lipid monolayer of some archaea.

Archaeal membranes are made of molecules that differ strongly from those in other life forms, showing that archaea are related only distantly to bacteria and eukaryotes. In all organisms, cell membranes are made of molecules known as phospholipids. These molecules possess both a polar part that dissolves in water (the phosphate "head"), and a "greasy" non-polar part that does not (the lipid tail). These dissimilar parts are connected by a glycerol moiety. In water, phospholipids cluster, with the heads facing the water and the tails facing away from it. The major structure in cell membranes is a double layer of these phospholipids, which is called a lipid bilayer.

These phospholipids are unusual in four ways:

- Bacteria and eukaryotes have membranes composed mainly of glycerol-ester lipids, whereas archaea have membranes composed of glycerol-ether lipids. The difference is the type of bond that joins the lipids to the glycerol moiety; the two types are shown in yellow in the figure at the right. In ester lipids this is an ester bond, whereas in ether lipids this is an ether bond. Ether bonds are chemically more resistant than ester bonds. This stability might help archaea to survive extreme temperatures and very acidic or alkaline environments. Bacteria and eukaryotes do contain some ether lipids, but in contrast to archaea these lipids are not a major part of their membranes.
- The stereochemistry of the glycerol moiety is the reverse of that found in other organisms. The glycerol moiety can occur in two forms that are mirror images of one another, called the right-handed and left-handed forms; in chemistry these are called *enantiomers*. Just as a right hand does not fit easily into a left-handed glove, a right-handed phospholipid generally cannot be used or made by enzymes adapted for the left-handed form. This suggests that archaea use entirely different enzymes for synthesizing phospholipids than do bacteria and eukaryotes. Such enzymes developed very early in life's history, suggesting an early split from the other two domains.
- Archaeal lipid tails are chemically different from other organisms. Archaeal lipids are based upon the isoprenoid sidechain and are long chains with multiple side-branches and sometimes even cyclopropane or cyclohexane rings. This is in contrast to the fatty acids found in other organisms' membranes, which have straight chains with no branches or rings. Although isoprenoids play an important role in the biochemistry of many organisms, only the archaea use them to make phospholipids. These branched chains may help prevent archaeal membranes from leaking at high temperatures.
- In some archaea, the lipid bilayer is replaced by a monolayer. In effect, the archaea fuse the tails of two independent phospholipid molecules into a single molecule with two polar heads (a bolaamphiphile); this fusion may make their membranes more rigid and better able to resist harsh environments. For example, the lipids in *Ferroplasma* are of this type, which is thought to aid this organism's survival in its highly acidic habitat.

Metabolism

Archaea exhibit a great variety of chemical reactions in their metabolism and use many sources of energy. These reactions are classified into nutritional groups, depending on energy and carbon sources. Some archaea obtain energy from inorganic compounds such as sulfur or ammonia (they are lithotrophs). These include nitrifiers, methanogens and anaerobic methane oxidisers. In these reactions one compound passes electrons to another (in a redox reaction), releasing energy to fuel the cell's activities. One compound acts as an electron donor and one as an electron acceptor. The energy released generates adenosine triphosphate (ATP) through chemiosmosis, in the same basic process that happens in the mitochondrion of eukaryotic cells.

Other groups of archaea use sunlight as a source of energy (they are phototrophs). However, oxygen–generating photosynthesis does not occur in any of these organisms. Many basic metabolic pathways are shared between all forms of life; for example, archaea use a modified form of glycolysis (the Entner–Doudoroff pathway) and either a complete or partial citric acid cycle. These similarities to other organisms probably reflect both early origins in the history of life and their high level of efficiency.

Nutritional types in archaeal metabolism

Nutritional type	Source of energy	Source of carbon	Examples
Phototrophs	Sunlight	Organic compounds	Halobacterium
Lithotrophs	Inorganic compounds	Organic compounds or carbon fixation	Ferroglobus, Methanobacteria or Pyrolobus
Organotrophs	Organic compounds	Organic compounds or carbon fixation	Pyrococcus, Sulfolobus or Methanosarcinales

Some Euryarchaeota are methanogens living in anaerobic environments, such as swamps. This form of metabolism evolved early, and it is even possible that the first free-living organism was a methanogen. A common reaction involves the use of carbon dioxide as an electron acceptor to oxidize hydrogen. Methanogenesis involves a range of coenzymes that are unique to these archaea, such as coenzyme M and methanofuran. Other organic compounds such as alcohols, acetic acid or formic acid are used as alternative electron acceptors by methanogens. These reactions are common in gut-dwelling archaea. Acetic acid is also broken down into methane and carbon dioxide directly, by acetotrophic archaea. These acetotrophs are archaea in the order Methanosarcinales, and are a major part of the communities of microorganisms that produce biogas.

Other archaea use CO2 in the atmosphere as a source of carbon, in a process called carbon fixation (they are autotrophs). This process involves either a highly modified form of the Calvin cycle or a recently discovered metabolic pathway called the 3-hydroxypropionate/4-hydroxybutyrate cycle. The Crenarchaeota also use the reverse Krebs cycle while the Euryarchaeota also use the reductive acetyl-CoA pathway. Carbon–fixation is powered by inorganic energy sources. No known archaea carry out photosynthesis. Archaeal energy sources are extremely diverse, and range from the oxidation of ammonia by the Nitrosopumilales to the oxidation of hydrogen sulfide or elemental sulfur by species of Sulfolobus, using either oxygen or metal ions as electron acceptors.

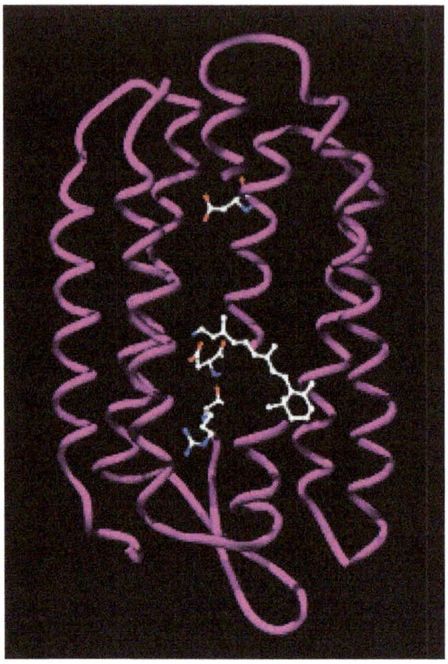

Bacteriorhodopsin from *Halobacterium salinarum*. The retinol cofactor and residues involved in proton transfer are shown as ball-and-stick models.

Phototrophic archaea use light to produce chemical energy in the form of ATP. In the Halobacteria, light-activated ion pumps like bacteriorhodopsin and halorhodopsin generate ion gradients by pumping ions out of the cell across the plasma membrane. The energy stored in these electrochemical gradients is then converted into ATP by ATP synthase. This process is a form of photophosphorylation. The ability of these light-driven pumps to move ions across membranes depends on light-driven changes in the structure of a retinol cofactor buried in the center of the protein.

Genetics

Archaea usually have a single circular chromosome, the size of which may be as great as 5,751,492 base pairs in Methanosarcina acetivorans, the largest known archaeal genome. The tiny 490,885 base-pair genome of Nanoarchaeum equitans is one-tenth of this size and the smallest archaeal genome known; it is estimated to contain only 537 protein-encoding genes. Smaller independent pieces of DNA, called plasmids, are also found in archaea. Plasmids may be transferred between cells by physical contact, in a process that may be similar to bacterial conjugation.

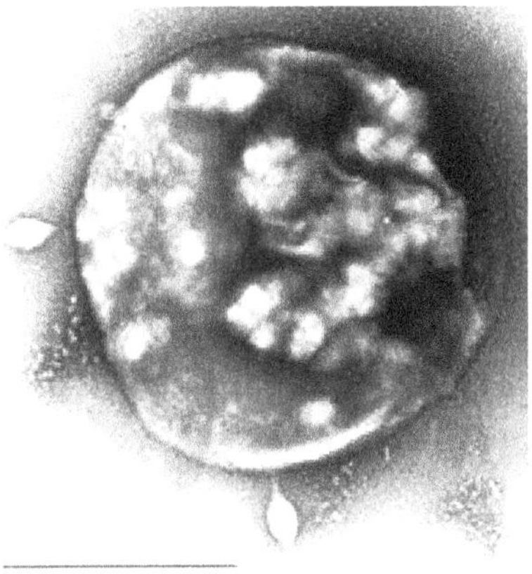

Sulfolobus infected with the DNA virus STSV1. Bar is 1 micrometer.

Archaea can be infected by double-stranded DNA viruses that are unrelated to any other form of virus and have a variety of unusual shapes, including bottles, hooked rods, or teardrops. These viruses have been studied in most detail in thermophilics, particularly the orders Sulfolobales and Thermoproteales. Two groups of single-stranded DNA viruses that infect archaea have been recently isolated. One group is exemplified by the Halorubrum pleomorphic virus 1 ("Pleolipoviridae") infecting halophilic archaea and the other one by the Aeropyrum coil-shaped virus ("Spiraviridae") infecting a hyperthermophilic (optimal growth at 90–95 °C) host. Notably, the latter virus has the largest currently reported ssDNA genome. Defenses against these viruses may involve RNA interference from repetitive DNA sequences that are related to the genes of the viruses.

Archaea are genetically distinct from bacteria and eukaryotes, with up to 15% of the proteins encoded by any one archaeal genome being unique to the domain, although most of these unique genes have no known function. Of the remainder of the unique proteins that have an identified function, most belong to the Euryarchaea and are involved in methanogenesis. The proteins that archaea, bacteria and eukaryotes share form a common core of cell function, relating mostly to transcription, translation, and nucleotide metabolism. Other characteristic archaeal features are the organization of genes of related function—such as enzymes that catalyze steps in the same metabolic pathway into novel operons, and large differences in tRNA genes and their aminoacyl tRNA synthetases.

Transcription in archaea more closely resembles eukaryotic than bacterial transcription, with the archaeal RNA polymerase being very close to its equivalent in eukaryotes; while archaeal translation shows signs of both bacterial and eukaryal equivalents. Although archaea only have one type of RNA polymerase, its structure and function in transcription seems to be close to that of the eukaryotic RNA polymerase II, with similar protein assemblies (the general transcription factors) directing the binding of the RNA polymerase to a gene's promoter. However, other archaeal transcription factors are closer to those found in bacteria. Post-transcriptional modification is simpler than in eukaryotes, since most archaeal genes lack introns, although there are many introns in their transfer RNA and ribosomal RNA genes, and introns may occur in a few protein-encoding genes.

Gene Transfer and Genetic Exchange

Halobacterium volcanii, an extreme halophilic archaeon, forms cytoplasmic bridges between cells that appear to be used for transfer of DNA from one cell to another in either direction.

When the hyperthermophilic archaea Sulfolobus solfataricus and Sulfolobus acidocaldarius are exposed to the DNA damaging agents UV irradiation, bleomycin or mitomycin C, species-specific cellular aggregation is induced. Aggregation in S. solfataricus could not be induced by other physical stressors, such as pH or temperature shift, suggesting that aggregation is induced specifically by DNA damage. Ajon et al.showed that UV-induced cellular aggregation mediates chromosomal marker exchange with high frequency in S. acidocaldarius. Recombination rates exceeded those of uninduced cultures by up to three orders of magnitude. Frols et al. and Ajon et al. hypothesized that cellular aggregation enhances species specific DNA transfer between Sulfolobus cells in order to provide increased repair of damaged DNA by means of homologous recombination. This response may be a primitive form of sexual interaction similar to the more well-studied bacterial transformation systems that are also associated with species specific DNA transfer between cells leading to homologous recombinational repair of DNA damage.

Reproduction

Archaea reproduce asexually by binary or multiple fission, fragmentation, or budding; meiosis does not occur, so if a species of archaea exists in more than one form, all have the same genetic material. Cell division is controlled in a cell cycle; after the cell's chromosome is replicated and the two daughter chromosomes separate, the cell divides. In the genus *Sulfolobus*, the cycle has characteristics that are similar to both bacterial and eukaryotic systems. The chromosomes replicate from multiple starting-points (origins of replication) using DNA polymerases that resemble the equivalent eukaryotic enzymes. In euryarchaea the cell division protein FtsZ, which forms a contracting ring around the cell, and the components of the septum that is constructed across the center of the cell, are similar to their bacterial equivalents. In cren- and thaumarchaea, however, the cell division machinery Cdv fulfills a similar role. This machinery is related to the eukaryotic ESCRT-III machinery which, while best known for its role in cell sorting, also has been seen to fulfill a role in separation between divided cell, suggesting an ancestral role in cell division.

Both bacteria and eukaryotes, but not archaea, make spores. Some species of Haloarchaea undergo phenotypic switching and grow as several different cell types, including thick-walled structures that are resistant to osmotic shock and allow the archaea to survive in water at low salt concentrations, but these are not reproductive structures and may instead help them reach new habitats.

Ecology

Habitats

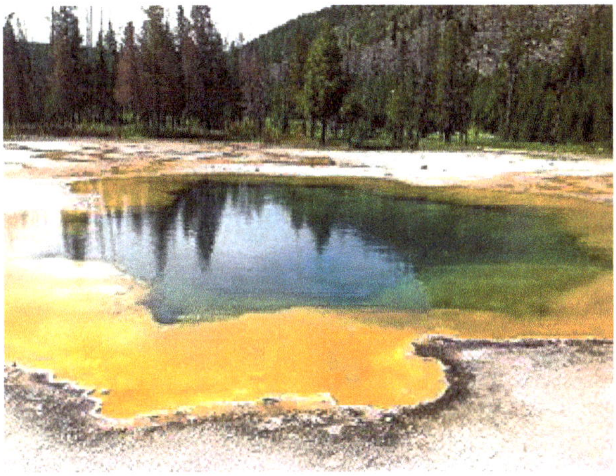

Archaea that grow in the hot water of the Morning Glory Hot Spring in Yellowstone National Park produce a bright colour

Archaea exist in a broad range of habitats, and as a major part of global ecosystems, may represent about 20% of microbial cells in the oceans. The first-discovered archaeans were extremophiles. Indeed, some archaea survive high temperatures, often above 100 °C (212 °F), as found in geysers, black smokers, and oil wells. Other common habitats include very cold habitats and highly saline, acidic, or alkaline water. However, archaea include mesophiles that grow in mild conditions, in swamps and marshland, sewage, the oceans, the intestinal tract of animals, and soils.

Extremophile archaea are members of four main physiological groups. These are the halophiles, thermophiles, alkaliphiles, and acidophiles. These groups are not comprehensive or phylum-specific, nor are they mutually exclusive, since some archaea belong to several groups. Nonetheless, they are a useful starting point for classification. Halophiles, including the genus Halobacterium, live in extremely saline environments such as salt lakes and outnumber their bacterial counterparts at salinities greater than 20–25%. Thermophiles grow best at temperatures above 45 °C (113 °F), in places such as hot springs; hyperthermophilic archaea grow optimally at temperatures greater than 80 °C (176 °F). The archaeal Methanopyrus kandleri Strain 116 can even reproduce at 122 °C (252 °F), the highest recorded temperature of any organism.

Other archaea exist in very acidic or alkaline conditions. For example, one of the most extreme archaean acidophiles is Picrophilus torridus, which grows at pH 0, which is equivalent to thriving in 1.2 molar sulfuric acid.

This resistance to extreme environments has made archaea the focus of speculation about the possible properties of extraterrestrial life. Some extremophile habitats are not dissimilar to those on Mars, leading to the suggestion that viable microbes could be transferred between planets in meteorites.

Recently, several studies have shown that archaea exist not only in mesophilic and thermophilic environments but are also present, sometimes in high numbers, at low temperatures as well. For example, archaea are common in cold oceanic environments such as polar seas. Even more significant are the large numbers of archaea found throughout the world's oceans in non-extreme habitats among the plankton community (as part of the picoplankton). Although these archaea can be present in extremely high numbers (up to 40% of the microbial biomass), almost none of these species have been isolated and studied in pure culture. Consequently, our understanding of the role of archaea in ocean ecology is rudimentary, so their full influence on global biogeochemical cycles remains largely unexplored. Some marine Crenarchaeota are capable of nitrification, suggesting these organisms may affect the oceanic nitrogen cycle, although these oceanic Crenarchaeota may also use other sources of energy. Vast numbers of archaea are also found in the sediments that cover the sea floor, with these organisms making up the majority of living cells at depths over 1 meter below the ocean bottom.

Role in Chemical Cycling

Archaea recycle elements such as carbon, nitrogen and sulfur through their various habitats. Although these activities are vital for normal ecosystem function, archaea can also contribute to human-made changes, and even cause pollution.

Archaea carry out many steps in the nitrogen cycle. This includes both reactions that remove nitrogen from ecosystems (such as nitrate-based respiration and denitrification) as well as processes that introduce nitrogen (such as nitrate assimilation and nitrogen fixation). Researchers recently discovered archaeal involvement in ammonia oxidation reactions. These reactions are particularly important in the oceans. The archaea also appear crucial for ammonia oxidation in soils. They produce nitrite, which other microbes then oxidize to nitrate. Plants and other organisms consume the latter.

In the sulfur cycle, archaea that grow by oxidizing sulfur compounds release this element from rocks, making it available to other organisms. However, the archaea that do this, such as Sulfolobus, produce sulfuric acid as a waste product, and the growth of these organisms in abandoned mines can contribute to acid mine drainage and other environmental damage.

In the carbon cycle, methanogen archaea remove hydrogen and play an important role in the decay of organic matter by the populations of microorganisms that act as decomposers in anaerobic ecosystems, such as sediments, marshes and sewage-treatment works. Global methane levels in 2011 had increased by a factor of 2.5 since pre-industrial times: from 722 ppb to 1800 ppb, the highest value in at least 800,000 years. Methane has an anthropogenic global warming potential (AGWP) of 29, which means that it's 29 times stronger in heat-trapping than carbon dioxide is, over a 100-year time scale.

Interactions with Other Organisms

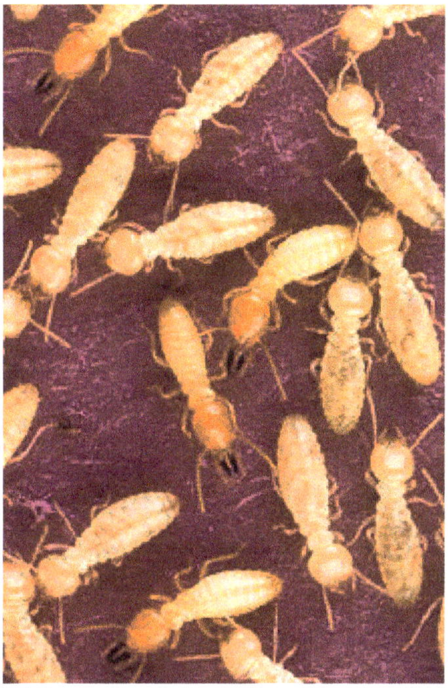

Methanogenic archaea form a symbiosis with termites.

The well-characterized interactions between archaea and other organisms are either mutual or commensal. There are no clear examples of known archaeal pathogens or parasites. However, some species of methanogens have been suggested to be involved in infections in the mouth, and Nanoarchaeum equitans may be a parasite of another species of archaea, since it only survives and reproduces within the cells of the Crenarchaeon Ignicoccus hospitalis, and appears to offer no benefit to its host. In contrast, Archaeal Richmond Mine Acidophilic Nanoorganisms (ARMAN) occasionally connect with other archaeal cells in acid mine drainage biofilms. The nature of this relationship is unknown. However, it is distinct from that of Nanarchaeaum–Ignicoccus in that the ultrasmall ARMAN cells are usually seen independent of the Thermoplasmatales cells.

Mutualism

One well-understood example of mutualism is the interaction between protozoa and methanogenic archaea in the digestive tracts of animals that digest cellulose, such as ruminants and termites. In these anaerobic environments, protozoa break down plant cellulose to obtain energy. This process releases hydrogen as a waste product, but high levels of hydrogen reduce energy production. When methanogens convert hydrogen to methane, protozoa benefit from more energy.

In anaerobic protozoa, such as Plagiopyla frontata, archaea reside inside the protozoa and consume hydrogen produced in their hydrogenosomes. Archaea also associate with larger organisms. For example, the marine archaean Cenarchaeum symbiosum lives within (is an endosymbiont of) the sponge Axinella mexicana.

Commensalism

Archaea can also be commensals, benefiting from an association without helping or harming the other organism. For example, the methanogen Methanobrevibacter smithii is by far the most common archaean in the human flora, making up about one in ten of all the prokaryotes in the human gut. In termites and in humans, these methanogens may in fact be mutualists, interacting with other microbes in the gut to aid digestion. Archaean communities also associate with a range of other organisms, such as on the surface of corals, and in the region of soil that surrounds plant roots (the rhizosphere).

Significance in Technology and Industry

Extremophile archaea, particularly those resistant either to heat or to extremes of acidity and alkalinity, are a source of enzymes that function under these harsh conditions. These enzymes have found many uses. For example, thermostable DNA polymerases, such as the Pfu DNA polymerase from Pyrococcus furiosus, revolutionized molecular biology by allowing the polymerase chain reaction to be used in research as a simple and rapid technique for cloning DNA. In industry, amylases, galactosidases and pullulanases in other species of Pyrococcus that function at over 100 °C (212 °F) allow food processing at high temperatures, such as the production of low lactose milk and whey. Enzymes from these thermophilic archaea also tend to be very stable in organic solvents, allowing their use in environmentally friendly processes in green chemistry that synthesize organic compounds. This stability makes them easier to use in structural biology. Consequently, the counterparts of bacterial or eukaryotic enzymes from extremophile archaea are often used in structural studies.

In contrast to the range of applications of archaean enzymes, the use of the organisms themselves in biotechnology is less developed. Methanogenic archaea are a vital part of sewage treatment, since they are part of the community of microorganisms that carry out anaerobic digestion and produce biogas. In mineral processing, acidophilic archaea display promise for the extraction of metals from ores, including gold, cobalt and copper.

Archaea host a new class of potentially useful antibiotics. A few of these archaeocins have been characterized, but hundreds more are believed to exist, especially within Haloarchaea and Sulfolobus. These compounds differ in structure from bacterial antibiotics, so they may have novel modes of action. In addition, they may allow the creation of new selectable markers for use in archaeal molecular biology.

REFERENCES

1. “Etymology of the word “bacteria””. Online Etymology dictionary. Archived from the original on 18 November 2006. Retrieved 2006-11-23.
2. “International Bacteriological Code of Nomenclature”. J. Bacteriol. 55 (3): 287–306. March 1948. PMC 518444Freely accessible. PMID 16561459.

3. Hierarchical classification of Prokaryotes entry in LPSN [Euzéby, J.P. (1997). "List of Bacterial Names with Standing in Nomenclature: a folder available on the Internet". Int J Syst Bacteriol. 47 (2): 590–2. doi:10.1099/00207713-47-2-590. ISSN 0020-7713. PMID 9103655.]
4. 1897, System der Bakterien. Gustav Fischer, Jena
5. 1925, Bergey's Manual of Determinative Bacteriology, Baltimore : Williams & Wilkins Co. (with many subsequent editions)
6. Achtman, M.; Zurth, K.; Morelli, G.; Torrea, G.; Guiyoule, A.; Carniel, E. (1999). "Yersinia pestis, the cause of plague, is a recently emerged clone of Yersinia pseudotuberculosis". Proceedings of the National Academy of Sciences of the United States of America. 96 (24): 14043–14048. Bibcode:1999PNAS...9614043A. doi:10.1073/pnas.96.24.14043. PMC 24187Freely accessible. PMID 10570195.
7. app. 9 of BC http://www.ncbi.nlm.nih.gov/books/NBK8808/
8. Balch, W.; Magrum, L.; Fox, G.; Wolfe, R.; Woese, C. (1977). "An ancient divergence among the bacteria". Journal of Molecular Evolution. 9 (4): 305–311. doi:10.1007/BF01796092. PMID 408502.
9. Bavykin, S. G.; Lysov, Y. P.; Zakhariev, V.; Kelly, J. J.; Jackman, J.; Stahl, D. A.; Cherni, A. (2004). "Use of 16S rRNA, 23S rRNA, and gyrB Gene Sequence Analysis to Determine Phylogenetic Relationships of Bacillus cereus Group Microorganisms". Journal of Clinical Microbiology. 42 (8): 3711–30. doi:10.1128/JCM.42.8.3711-3730.2004. PMC 497648Freely accessible. PMID 15297521.
10. Bisset, 1962, Bacteria, 2nd ed., Livingston, London
11. Buchanan RE (March 1917). "Studies in the Nomenclature and Classification of the Bacteria: II. The Primary Subdivisions of the Schizomycetes". J. Bacteriol. 2 (2): 155–64. PMC 378699Freely accessible. PMID 16558735.
12. Buchanan, R E J Bacteriol. 1916 Nov;1(6):591-6.ISSN 0021-9193 PMCID 378679
13. C. Jeffrey. 1989. Biological Nomenclature, 3rd ed. Edward Arnold, London, 86 pp.
14. C. Michael Hogan. 2010. Virus. Encyclopedia of Earth. Editors: Cutler Cleveland and Sidney Draggan
15. C. Von Nägeli (1857). R. Caspary, ed. "Bericht über die Verhandlungen der 33. Versammlung deutscher Naturforscher und Aerzte, gehalten in Bonn von 18 bis 24 September 1857" [Report on the negotiations on 33 Meeting of German Natural Scientists and Physicians, held in Bonn, 18 to 24 September 1857]. Botanische Zeitung. 15: 749–776. <https://archive.org/stream/botanischezeitun15mohl#page/372/mode/2up>
16. Cavalier-Smith, T (2002). "The neomuran origin of archaebacteria, the negibacterial root of the universal tree and bacterial megaclassification". International Journal of Systematic and Evolutionary Microbiology. 52 (Pt 1): 7–76. doi:10.1099/00207713-52-1-7. PMID 11837318.
17. Cavalier-Smith, T. (1998). "A revised six-kingdom system of life". Biological Reviews. 73 (03): 203–66. doi:10.1111/j.1469-185X.1998.tb00030.x. PMID 9809012.

18. Cavalier-Smith, T. (2006). "Rooting the tree of life by transition analyses". Biology Direct. 1: 19. doi:10.1186/1745-6150-1-19. PMC 1586193Freely accessible. PMID 16834776.
19. Chatton, É. (1925). "Pansporella perplexa. Réflexions sur la biologie et la phylogénie des protozoaires". Annales des Sciences Naturelles - Zoologie et Biologie Animale. 10-VII: 1–84.
20. Ciccarelli FD, Doerks T, von Mering C, Creevey CJ, Snel B, Bork P (2006). "Toward automatic reconstruction of a highly resolved tree of life". Science. 311 (5765): 1283–7. Bibcode:2006Sci...311.1283C. doi:10.1126/science.1123061. PMID 16513982.
21. Classification entry in LPSN [Euzéby, J.P. (1997). "List of Bacterial Names with Standing in Nomenclature: a folder available on the Internet". Int J Syst Bacteriol. 47 (2): 590–2. doi:10.1099/00207713-47-2-590. ISSN 0020-7713. PMID 9103655.]
22. Classification of Phyla entry in LPSN [Euzéby, J.P. (1997). "List of Bacterial Names with Standing in Nomenclature: a folder available on the Internet". Int J Syst Bacteriol. 47 (2): 590–2. doi:10.1099/00207713-47-2-590. ISSN 0020-7713. PMID 9103655.]
23. COHN, FERDINAND 1872 a Organismen in der Pockenlymphe. Virchow's Archiv, 55, 229-238. p. 237
24. COHN, FERDINAND 1872 b Untersuchungen ilber Bakterien. Beitrage zur Biologie der Pflanzen, 1 (Heft 1), 127-224. p. 136
25. Cohn, Ferdinand 1875, Untersuchungen uber Bakterien, II. Beitrage zur Biologie der Pfanzen 1: 141-207
26. Cole, J. R.; Wang, Q.; Cardenas, E.; Fish, J.; Chai, B.; Farris, R. J.; Kulam-Syed-Mohideen, A. S.; McGarrell, D. M.; Marsh, T.; Garrity, G. M.; Tiedje, J. M. (2009). "The Ribosomal Database Project: Improved alignments and new tools for rRNA analysis". Nucleic Acids Research. 37 (Database issue): D141–D145. doi:10.1093/nar/gkn879. PMC 2686447Freely accessible. PMID 19004872.
27. Copeland, H. (1938). "The kingdoms of organisms". Quarterly Review of Biology. 13: 383–420. doi:10.1086/394568.
28. DETONI, J. B., AND TREVISAN, V. 1889 Schizomycetaceae, in Saccardo's Sylloge Fungorum, 8, 923-1087. p. 923
29. É. Chatton (1925). "Pansporella perplexa. Réflexions sur la biologie et la phylogénie des protozoaires". Ann. Sci. Nat. Zool. 10-VII: 1–84.
30. EHRENBERG (C.G.): Beiträge zur Kenntnis der Organization der Infusorien und ihrer geographischen Verbreitung besonders in Sibirien. Abhandlungen der Koniglichen Akademie der Wissenschaften zu Berlin, 1832, 1830, 1-88.
31. EHRENBERG (C.G.): Dritter Beitrag zur Erkenntniss grosser Organisation in der Richtung des kleinsten Raumes. Physikalische Abhandlungen der Koeniglichen Akademie der Wissenschaften zu Berlin aus den Jahren 1833-1835, 1835, pp. 143-336.

32. EHRENBERG (C.G.): Dritter Beitrag zur Erkenntniss grosser Organisation in der Richtung des kleinsten Raumes. Abhandlungen der Preussischen Akademie der Wissenschaften (Berlin) aus den Jahre 1833-1835, pp. 143-336.
33. Erwin F. Smith Nomenclature and Classification in Bacteria in Relation to Plant Diseases vol. 1 (1905)
34. Farrand, S.; Van Berkum, P.; Oger, P. (2003). "Agrobacterium is a definable genus of the family Rhizobiaceae". International Journal of Systematic and Evolutionary Microbiology. 53 (Pt 5): 1681–1687. doi:10.1099/ijs.0.02445-0. PMID 13130068.
35. Fournier, G. P.; Gogarten, J. P. (2010). "Rooting the Ribosomal Tree of Life". Molecular Biology and Evolution. 27 (8): 1792–1801. doi:10.1093/molbev/msq057. PMID 20194428.
36. Fournier, G. P.; Gogarten, J. P. (2010). "Rooting the Ribosomal Tree of Life". Molecular Biology and Evolution. 27 (8): 1792–1801. doi:10.1093/molbev/msq057. PMID 20194428.
37. Francolini, C.; Egeth, H. (1979). "Perceptual selectivity is task dependent: The pop-out effect poops out". Perception & psychophysics. 25 (2): 99–110. doi:10.3758/bf03198793. PMID 432104.
38. ftp://ftp.ncbi.nih.gov/pub/taxonomy/
39. George M. Garrity: Bergey's manual of systematic bacteriology. 2. Auflage. Springer, New York, 2005, Volume 2: The Proteobacteria, Part B: The Gammaproteobacteria
40. Gevers, D.; Cohan, F. M.; Lawrence, J. G.; Spratt, B. G.; Coenye, T.; Feil, E. J.; Stackebrandt, E.; Van De Peer, Y. V.; Vandamme, P.; Thompson, F. L.; Swings, J. (2005). "Opinion: Re-evaluating prokaryotic species". Nature Reviews Microbiology. 3 (9): 733–739. doi:10.1038/nrmicro1236. PMID 16138101.
41. GIBBONS N.E.; MURRAY R.G.E. (1978). "Proposals concerning the higher taxa of bacteria". International Journal of Systematic Bacteriology. 28: 1–6. doi:10.1099/00207713-28-1-1.
42. Gribaldo S, Brochier-Armanet C (2006). "The origin and evolution of Archaea: a state of the art". Philosophical Transactions of the Royal Society B. 361 (1470): 1007–22. doi:10.1098/rstb.2006.1841. PMC 1578729Freely accessible. PMID 16754611.
43. Gupta RS (2000). "The natural evolutionary relationships among prokaryotes". Crit. Rev. Microbiol. 26 (2): 111–31. doi:10.1080/10408410091154219. PMID 10890353.
44. Gupta, R. S. (1998). "Life's third domain (Archaea): An established fact or an endangered paradigm?". Theoretical population biology. 54 (2): 91–104. doi:10.1006/tpbi.1998.1376. PMID 9733652.
45. Gupta, R. S. (1998). "Protein phylogenies and signature sequences: A reappraisal of evolutionary relationships among archaebacteria, eubacteria, and eukaryotes". Microbiology and molecular biology reviews : MMBR. 62 (4): 1435–1491. PMC

98952Freely accessible. PMID 9841678.

46. Gupta, R. S. (2000). "The Natural Evolutionary Relationships among Prokaryotes". Critical Reviews in Microbiology. 26 (2): 111–131. doi:10.1080/10408410091154219. PMID 10890353.
47. Haeckel, E. (1866). Generelle Morphologie der Organismen. Reimer, Berlin.
48. Haeckel, Ernst (1867). Generelle Morphologie der Organismen. Reimer, Berlin. ISBN 1-144-00186-2.
49. Help! Latin! How to avoid the most common mistakes while giving Latin names to newly discovered prokaryotes. Microbiología (Sociedad Española de Microbiología), 1996, 12, 473-475. http://www.bacterio.cict.fr/trueper.html
50. Holland L. (22 May 1990). "Woese,Carl in the forefront of bacterial evolution revolution". Scientist. 4 (10).
51. Hori, H.; Osawa, S. (1987). "Origin and evolution of organisms as deduced from 5S ribosomal RNA sequences". Molecular Biology and Evolution. 4 (5): 445–472. PMID 2452957.
52. http://www.bacterio.net/-number.html
53. Introductory entry in LPSN [Euzéby, J.P. (1997). "List of Bacterial Names with Standing in Nomenclature: a folder available on the Internet". Int J Syst Bacteriol. 47 (2): 590–2. doi:10.1099/00207713-47-2-590. ISSN 0020-7713. PMID 9103655.]
54. Lake, J. (2009). "Evidence for an early prokaryotic endosymbiosis". Nature. 460 (7258): 967–971. Bibcode:2009Natur.460..967L. doi:10.1038/nature08183. PMID 19693078.
55. Lake, J. A. (1986). "An alternative to archaebacterial dogma". Nature. 319 (6055): 626. Bibcode:1986Natur.319..626L. doi:10.1038/319626b0.
56. Lake, J. A.; Henderson, E.; Clark, M. W.; Scheinman, A.; Oakes, M. I. (1986). "Mapping evolution with three dimensional ribosome structure". Systematic and Applied Microbiology. 7: 131–136. doi:10.1016/S0723-2020(86)80135-7.
57. Lake, J.; Servin, J.; Herbold, C.; Skophammer, R. (2008). "Evidence for a New Root of the Tree of Life". Systematic Biology. 57 (6): 835–843. doi:10.1080/10635150802555933. PMID 19085327.
58. Lake, JA; Henderson, E; Oakes, M; Clark, MW (1984). "Eocytes: A new ribosome structure indicates a kingdom with a close relationship to eukaryotes". Proceedings of the National Academy of Sciences of the United States of America. 81 (12): 3786–3790. Bibcode:1984PNAS...81.3786L. doi:10.1073/pnas.81.12.3786. PMC 345305Freely accessible. PMID 6587394.
59. Lan, R; Reeves, PR (2002). "Escherichia coli in disguise: molecular origins of Shigella". Microbes and infection / Institut Pasteur. 4 (11): 1125–32. doi:10.1016/S1286-4579(02)01637-4. PMID 12361912.
60. Lapage, S.; Sneath, P.; Lessel, E.; Skerman, V.; Seeliger, H.; Clark, W. (1992). International Code of Nomenclature of Bacteria: Bacteriological Code, 1990 Revision. Washington, D.C.: ASM Press. PMID 21089234.

61. Linnaeus, C. (1735). Systemae Naturae, sive regna tria naturae, systematics proposita per classes, ordines, genera & species.
62. Linnaeus, Carl (1735). Systemae Naturae, sive regna tria naturae, systematics proposita per classes, ordines, genera & species.
63. Madigan, Michael (2009). Brock Biology of Microorganisms. San Francisco: Pearson/Benjamin Cummings. ISBN 0-13-232460-1.
64. minimal standards entry in LPSN [Euzéby, J.P. (1997). "List of Bacterial Names with Standing in Nomenclature: a folder available on the Internet". Int J Syst Bacteriol. 47 (2): 590–2. doi:10.1099/00207713-47-2-590. ISSN 0020-7713. PMID 9103655.]
65. MURRAY (R.G.E.): The higher taxa, or, a place for everything...? In: N.R. KRIEG and J.G. HOLT (ed.) Bergey's Manual of Systematic Bacteriology, vol. 1, The Williams & Wilkins Co., Baltimore, 1984, p. 31-34
66. Murray, R. G. E. 1984. The higher taxa, or, a place for everything . . .?, p. 33. In N. R. Krieg and J. G. Holt (ed.), Bergey's manual of systematic bacteriology, vol. 1. The Williams & Wilkins Co., Baltimore.
67. Olsen, G.; Larsen, N.; Woese, C. (1991). "The ribosomal RNA database project". Nucleic Acids Research. 19 Suppl: 2017–2021. doi:10.1093/nar/19.suppl.2017. PMC 331344Freely accessible. PMID 2041798.
68. Orla-Jensen, 1909, Die Hauptlinien des naturalischen Bakteriensystems nebst einer Ubersicht der Garungsphenomene. Zentr. Bakt. Parasitenk., II, 22: 305-346
69. Pace, N. R. (2009). "Mapping the Tree of Life: Progress and Prospects". Microbiology and Molecular Biology Reviews. 73 (4): 565–576. doi:10.1128/MMBR.00033-09. PMC 2786576Freely accessible. PMID 19946133.
70. PACINI (F.): Osservazione microscopiche e deduzioni patologiche sul cholera asiatico. Gazette Medicale de Italiana Toscano Firenze, 1854, 6, 405-412.
71. Palleroni, N. J. (2010). "The Pseudomonas Story". Environmental Microbiology. 12 (6): 1377–1383. doi:10.1111/j.1462-2920.2009.02041.x. PMID 20553550.
72. Porter JR (1976). "Antony van Leeuwenhoek: tercentenary of his discovery of bacteria". Bacteriological Reviews. 40 (2): 260–9. PMC 413956Freely accessible. PMID 786250.
73. Pot, B., Gillis, M., and De Ley, J., The genus Aquaspirillum. In: Balows, A., Trüper, H.G., Dworkin, M., Harder, W., Schleifer, K.-H. (Eds.). The prokaryotes, 2nd ed, vol. 3. Springer-Verlag. New York. 1991
74. Prévot, A.R. 1958. Manuel de classification et détermination des bactéries anaérobies. Masson, Paris
75. Prévot, A.R. Bactéries in Précis de Botanique, 1963, Masson, Paris
76. Protomonas entry in LPSN [Euzéby, J.P. (1997). "List of Bacterial Names with Standing in Nomenclature: a folder available on the Internet". Int J Syst Bacteriol. 47 (2): 590–2. doi:10.1099/00207713-47-2-590. ISSN 0020-7713. PMID 9103655.]
77. Pruesse, E.; Quast, C.; Knittel, K.; Fuchs, B. M.; Ludwig, W.; Peplies, J.;

Glockner, F. O. (2007). "SILVA: A comprehensive online resource for quality checked and aligned ribosomal RNA sequence data compatible with ARB". Nucleic Acids Research. 35 (21): 7188–7196. doi:10.1093/nar/gkm864. PMC 2175337Freely accessible. PMID 17947321.

78. R. E. BUCHANAN, Taxonomy, Annu. Rev. Microbiol. 1955.9:1-20. http://www.annualreviews.org/doi/pdf/10.1146/annurev.mi.09.100155.000245

79. Rediers, H; Vanderleyden, J; De Mot, R (2004). "Azotobacter vinelandii: a Pseudomonas in disguise?". Microbiology (Reading, England). 150 (Pt 5): 1117–9. doi:10.1099/mic.0.27096-0. PMID 15133068.

80. Salmonella entry in LPSN [Euzéby, J.P. (1997). "List of Bacterial Names with Standing in Nomenclature: a folder available on the Internet". Int J Syst Bacteriol. 47 (2): 590–2. doi:10.1099/00207713-47-2-590. ISSN 0020-7713. PMID 9103655.]

81. SCHROETER (J.). In: F. COHN (ed.), Kryptogamenflora von Schlesien. Band 3, Heft 3, Pilze. J.U. Kern's Verlag, Breslau, 1885-1889, pp. 1-814.

82. Skophammer, R. G.; Servin, J. A.; Herbold, C. W.; Lake, J. A. (2007). "Evidence for a Gram-positive, Eubacterial Root of the Tree of Life". Molecular Biology and Evolution. 24 (8): 1761–1768. doi:10.1093/molbev/msm096. PMID 17513883.

83. STACKEBRANDT, E.; RAINEY; WARD-RAINEY, N.L. (1997). "Proposal for a new hierarchic classification system, Actinobacteria classis nov". Int. J. Syst. Bacteriol. 47: 479–491. doi:10.1099/00207713-47-2-479.

84. Stackebrandt, E; Goebel, B.M. (1994). "Taxonomic note: a place for DNA–DNA reassociation and 16S rDNA sequence analysis in the present species definition in bacteriology". Int. J. Syst. Bacteriol. 44: 846–849. doi:10.1099/00207713-44-4-846.

85. Staley, J. (1997). "Biodiversity: Are microbial species threatened?". Current opinion in biotechnology. 8 (3): 340–345. doi:10.1016/s0958-1669(97)80014-6. PMID 9206017.

86. Staley, J. T. (2006). "The bacterial species dilemma and the genomic-phylogenetic species concept". Philosophical Transactions of the Royal Society B: Biological Sciences. 361 (1475): 1899–1909. doi:10.1098/rstb.2006.1914. PMC 1857736Freely accessible. PMID 17062409.

87. Stanier and van Neil,1941, The main outlines of bacterial classification. J Bacteriol 42: 437- 466

88. Valas, R. E.; Bourne, P. E. (2011). "The origin of a derived superkingdom: How a gram-positive bacterium crossed the desert to become an archaeon". Biology Direct. 6: 16. doi:10.1186/1745-6150-6-16. PMC 3056875Freely accessible. PMID 21356104.

89. van Leeuwenhoek A (1684). "An abstract of a letter from Mr. Anthony Leevvenhoek at Delft, dated Sep. 17, 1683, Containing Some Microscopical Observations, about Animals in the Scurf of the Teeth, the Substance Call'd Worms in the Nose, the Cuticula Consisting of Scales". Philosophical Transactions

(1683–1775). 14 (155–166): 568–574. doi:10.1098/rstl.1684.0030. Retrieved 2007-08-19.

90. van Leeuwenhoek A (1700). "Part of a Letter from Mr Antony van Leeuwenhoek, concerning the Worms in Sheeps Livers, Gnats, and Animalcula in the Excrements of Frogs". Philosophical Transactions (1683–1775). 22 (260–276): 509–518. doi:10.1098/rstl.1700.0013. Retrieved 2007-08-19.
91. van Leeuwenhoek A (1702). "Part of a Letter from Mr Antony van Leeuwenhoek, F. R. S. concerning Green Weeds Growing in Water, and Some Animalcula Found about Them". Philosophical Transactions (1683–1775). 23 (277–288): 1304–11. doi:10.1098/rstl.1702.0042. Retrieved 2007-08-19.
92. Vuillemin. 1913. Genera Schizomycetum. Annales Mycologici. 11,512-527.
93. Ward, B. B. (2002). "How many species of prokaryotes are there?". Proceedings of the National Academy of Sciences. 99 (16): 10234–10236. Bibcode:2002PNAS...9910234W. doi:10.1073/pnas.162359199.
94. Wayne, L. (1988). "International Committee on Systematic Bacteriology: Announcement of the report of the ad hoc Committee on Reconciliation of Approaches to Bacterial Systematics". Zentralblatt für Bakteriologie, Mikrobiologie, und Hygiene. Series A, Medical microbiology, infectious diseases, virology, parasitology. 268 (4): 433–434. doi:10.1016/s0176-6724(88)80120-2. PMID 3213314.
95. Whittaker, R. H. (January 1969). "New concepts of kingdoms of organisms". Science. 163 (3863): 150–60. Bibcode:1969Sci...163..150W. doi:10.1126/science.163.3863.150. PMID 5762760.
96. Woese C (1998). "The universal ancestor". Proceedings of the National Academy of Sciences of the United States of America. 95 (12): 6854–9. Bibcode:1998PNAS...95.6854W. doi:10.1073/pnas.95.12.6854. PMC 22660Freely accessible. PMID 9618502.
97. Woese CR (1 March 1994). "There must be a prokaryote somewhere: microbiology's search for itself". Microbiol. Rev. 58 (1): 1–9. PMC 372949Freely accessible. PMID 8177167.
98. Woese CR, Gupta R (1981). "Are archaebacteria merely derived 'prokaryotes'?". Nature. 289 (5793): 95–6. Bibcode:1981Natur.289...95W. doi:10.1038/289095a0. PMID 6161309.
99. Woese, C. R. (1987). "Bacterial evolution". Microbiological reviews. 51 (2): 221–271. PMC 373105Freely accessible. PMID 2439888.
100. Woese, C. R.; Kandler, O.; Wheelis, M. L. (1990). "Towards a natural system of organisms: proposal for the domains Archaea, Bacteria, and Eucarya". Proceedings of the National Academy of Sciences. 87 (12): 4576–4579. Bibcode:1990PNAS...87.4576W. doi:10.1073/pnas.87.12.4576. PMC 54159Freely accessible. PMID 2112744.
101. Woese, C.; Kandler, O.; Wheelis, M. (1990). "Towards a natural system of organisms: proposal for the domains Archaea, Bacteria, and Eucarya.". Proceedings of the National Academy of Sciences of the United States of America. 87 (12):

4576–9. Bibcode:1990PNAS...87.4576W. doi:10.1073/pnas.87.12.4576. PMC 54159Freely accessible. PMID 2112744.

102. Xu, D; Côté, JC (2003). "Phylogenetic relationships between Bacillus species and related genera inferred from comparison of 3' end 16S rDNA and 5' end 16S-23S ITS nucleotide sequences". International Journal of Systematic and Evolutionary Microbiology. 53 (Pt 3): 695–704. doi:10.1099/ijs.0.02346-0. PMID 12807189.
103. Young, J. M.; Park, D. -C. (2007). "Probable synonymy of the nitrogen-fixing genus Azotobacter and the genus Pseudomonas". International Journal of Systematic and Evolutionary Microbiology. 57 (12): 2894–2901. doi:10.1099/ijs.0.64969-0. PMID 18048745.
104. Young, J.; Kuykendall, L.; Martínez-Romero, E.; Kerr, A.; Sawada, H. (2001). "A revision of Rhizobium Frank 1889, with an emended description of the genus, and the inclusion of all species of Agrobacterium Conn 1942 and Allorhizobium undicola de Lajudie et al. 1998 as new combinations: Rhizobium radiobacter, R. Rhizogenes, R. Rubi, R. Undicola and R. Vitis". International Journal of Systematic and Evolutionary Microbiology. 51 (Pt 1): 89–103. doi:10.1099/00207713-51-1-89. PMID 11211278.
105. Young, J.; Kuykendall, L.; Martínez-Romero, E.; Kerr, A.; Sawada, H. (2003). "Classification and nomenclature of Agrobacterium and Rhizobium". International Journal of Systematic and Evolutionary Microbiology. 53 (Pt 5): 1689–1695. doi:10.1099/ijs.0.02762-0. PMID 13130069.

CHAPTER 4

Bacterial Cell Structure

Chapter Contents

- **Introduction**
- **Cell Morphology**

Procaryotic structural components consist of macromolecules such as DNA, RNA, proteins, polysaccharides, phospholipids, or some combination thereof. The macromolecules are made up of primary subunits such as nucleotides, amino acids and sugars (Table 1). It is the sequence in which the subunits are put together in the macromolecule, called the primary structure that determines many of the properties that the macromolecule will have.

INTRODUCTION

Bacteria, despite their simplicity, contain a well-developed cell structure which is responsible for some of their unique biological structures and pathogenicity. Many structural features are unique to bacteria and are not found among archaea or eukaryotes. Because of the simplicity of bacteria relative to larger organisms and the ease with which they can be manipulated experimentally, the cell structure of bacteria has been well studied, revealing many biochemical principles that have been subsequently applied to other organisms.

CELL MORPHOLOGY

Perhaps the most elemental structural property of bacteria is their morphology (shape). Typical examples include:

- coccus (spherical)
- bacillus (rod-like)
- spiral (DNA-like)
- filamentous (elongated)

Cell shape is generally characteristic of a given bacterial species, but can vary depending on growth conditions. Some bacteria have complex life cycles involving the production of stalks and appendages (e.g. Caulobacter) and some produce elaborate structures bearing reproductive spores (e.g. Myxococcus, Streptomyces). Bacteria generally form distinctive cell morphologies when examined by light microscopy and distinct colony morphologies when grown on Petri plates.

Perhaps the most obvious structural characteristic of bacteria is (with some exceptions) their small size. For example, Escherichia coli cells, an "average" sized bacterium, are about 2 µm (micrometres) long and 0.5 µm in diameter, with a cell volume of 0.6 - 0.7 µm3. This corresponds to a wet mass of about 1 picogram (pg), assuming that the cell consists mostly of water. The dry mass of a single cell can be estimated as 23% of the wet mass, amounting to 0.2 pg. About half of the dry mass of a bacterial cell consists of carbon, and also about half of it can be attributed to proteins. Therefore, a typical fully grown 1-liter culture of Escherichia coli (at an optical density of 1.0, corresponding to ca. 109cells/ml) yields about 1 g wet cell mass. Small size is extremely important because it allows for a large surface area-to-volume ratio which allows for rapid uptake and intracellular distribution of nutrients and excretion of wastes. At low surface area-to-volume ratios the diffusion of nutrients and waste products across the bacterial cell membrane limits the rate at which microbial metabolism can occur, making the cell less evolutionarily fit. The reason for the existence of large cells is unknown, although it is speculated that the increased cell volume is used primarily for storage of excess nutriets.

Cell Wall

The cell envelope is composed of the plasma membrane and cell wall. As in other organisms, the bacterial cell wall provides structural integrity to the cell. In prokaryotes, the primary function of the cell wall is to protect the cell from internal turgor pressure caused by the much higher concentrations of proteins and other molecules inside the cell compared to its external environment. The bacterial cell wall differs from that of all other organisms by the presence of peptidoglycan which is located immediately outside of the cytoplasmic membrane. Peptidoglycan is made up of a polysaccharide backbone consisting of alternating N-Acetylmuramic acid (NAM) and N-acetylglucosamine (NAG) residues in equal amounts. Peptidoglycan is responsible for the rigidity of the bacterial cell wall and for the determination of cell shape. It is relatively porous and is not considered to be a permeability barrier for small substrates. While all bacterial cell walls (with a few exceptions e.g. extracellular parasites such as Mycoplasma) contain peptidoglycan, not all cell walls have the same overall structures. Since the cell wall is required for bacterial survival, but is absent in some eukaryotes, several antibiotics (notably the penicillins and cephalosporins) stop bacterial infections by interfering with cell wall synthesis, while having no effects on human cells which have no cell wall only a cell membrane. There are two main types of bacterial cell walls, those of gram-positive bacteria and those of gram-negative bacteria, which are differentiated by their Gram staining characteristics. For both these types of bacteria, particles of approximately 2 nm can pass through the peptidoglycan. If the bacterial cell wall is entirely removed, it is called a protoplast while if it's partially removed, it is called a spheroplast. β-Lactam antibiotics such as penicillin inhibit the formation of peptidoglycan cross-links in the bacterial cell wall. The enzyme lysozyme, found in human tears, also digests the cell wall of bacteria and is the body›s main defense against eye infections.

The Gram-Positive Cell Wall

Gram-positive cell walls are thick and the peptidoglycan (also known as murein) layer constitutes almost 95% of the cell wall in some gram-positive bacteria and as little as 5-10% of the cell wall in gram-negative bacteria. The gram-positive bacteria take up the crystal violet dye and are stained purple. The cell wall of some gram-positive bacteria can be completely dissolved by lysozymes which attacks the bonds between GA and MA. In other gram-positive bacteria, such as Staphylococcus aureus, the walls are resistant to the action of lysozymes. They have O-acetyl groups on carbon-6 of some MA residues. The matrix substances in the walls of gram-positive bacteria may be polysaccharides or teichoic acids. The latter are very widespread, but have been found only in gram-positive bacteria. There are two main types of teichoic acid: ribitol teichoic acids and glycerol teichoic acids. The latter one is more widespread. These acids are polymers of ribitol phosphate and glycerol phosphate, respectively, and only located on the surface of many gram-positive bacteria. However, the exact function of teichoic acid is debated and not fully understood. A major component of the gram-positive cell wall is lipoteichoic acid. One of its purposes is providing an antigenic function. The lipid element is to be found in the membrane where its adhesive properties assist in its anchoring to the membrane.

The Gram-Negative Cell Wall

Gram-negative cell walls are thin and unlike the gram-positive cell walls, they contain a thin peptidoglycan layer adjacent to the cytoplasmic membrane. Gram-negative bacteria is stained as pink colour. The chemical structure of the outer membrane›s lipopolysaccharides is often unique to specific bacterial sub-species and is responsible for many of the antigenic properties of these strains. Lipopolysaccharides, also called endotoxins, are composed of polysaccharides and lipid A which are responsible for much of the toxicity of gram-negative bacteria.

Plasma Membrane

The plasma membrane or bacterial cytoplasmic membrane is composed of a phospholipid bilayer and thus has all of the general functions of a cell membrane such as acting as a permeability barrier for most molecules and serving as the location for the transport of molecules into the cell. In addition to these functions, prokaryotic membranes also function in energy conservation as the location about which a proton motive force is generated. Unlike eukaryotes, bacterial membranes (with some exceptions e.g. Mycoplasma and methanotrophs) generally do not contain sterols. However, many microbes do contain structurally related compounds called hopanoids which likely fulfill the same function. Unlike eukaryotes, bacteria can have a wide variety of fatty acids within their membranes. Along with typical saturated and unsaturated fatty acids, bacteria can contain fatty acids with additional methyl, hydroxy or even cyclic groups. The relative proportions of these fatty acids can be modulated by the bacterium to maintain the optimum fluidity of the membrane (e.g. following temperature change).

As a phospholipid bilayer, the lipid portion of the outer membrane is impermeable to charged molecules. However, channels called porins are present in the outer membrane that allow for passive transport of many ions, sugars and amino acids across the outer membrane. These molecules are therefore present in the periplasm, the region between the cytoplasmic and outer membranes. The periplasm contains the peptidoglycan layer and many proteins responsible for substrate binding or hydrolysis and reception of extracellular signals. The periplasm is thought to exist in a gel-like state rather than a liquid due to the high concentration of proteins and peptidoglycan found within it. Because of its location between the cytoplasmic and outer membranes, signals received and substrates bound are available to be transported across the cytoplasmic membrane using transport and signalling proteins imbedded there.

Extracellular (external) Structures

Fimbriae and Pili

Fimbriae (sometimes called “attachment pili») are protein tubes that extend out from the outer membrane in many members of the Proteobacteria. They are generally short in length and present in high numbers about the entire bacterial cell surface. Fimbriae usually function to facilitate the attachment of a bacterium to a surface (e.g. to form a biofilm) or to other cells (e.g. animal cells during pathogenesis). A few organisms (e.g. Myxococcus) use fimbriae for motility to facilitate the assembly of multicellular structures such as fruiting bodies. Pili are similar in structure to fimbriae but are much longer and present on the bacterial cell in low numbers. Pili are involved in the process of bacterial conjugation where they are called conjugation pili or “sex pili». Type IV pili (non-sex pili) also aid bacteria in gripping surfaces.Pili are absent in gram-positive bacteria and present in gram-negative bacteria.

S-layers

An S-layer (surface layer) is a cell surface protein layer found in many different bacteria and in some archaea, where it serves as the cell wall. All S-layers are made up of a two-dimensional array of proteins and have a crystalline appearance, the symmetry of which differs between species. The exact function of S-layers is unknown, but it has been suggested that they act as a partial permeability barrier for large substrates. For example, an S-layer could conceivably keep extracellular proteins near the cell membrane by preventing their diffusion away from the cell. In some pathogenic species, an S-layer may help to facilitate survival within the host by conferring protection against host defence mechanisms.

Glycocalyx

Many bacteria secrete extracellular polymers outside of their cell walls called glycocalyx. These polymers are usually composed of polysaccharides and sometimes protein. Capsules are relatively impermeable structures that cannot be stained with dyes such as India ink. They are structures that help protect bacteria from phagocytosis and desiccation. Slime layer is involved in attachment of bacteria to other cells or inanimate surfaces to form biofilms. Slime layers can also be used as a food reserve for the cell.

Flagella

Perhaps the most recognizable extracellular bacterial cell structures are flagella. Flagella are whip-like structures protruding from the bacterial cell wall and are responsible for bacterial motility (i.e. movement). The arrangement of flagella about the bacterial cell is unique to the species observed. Common forms include:

- Monotrichous - Single flagellum
- Lophotrichous - A tuft of flagella found at one of the cell pole
- Amphitrichous - Single flagellum found at each of two opposite poles
- Peritrichous - Multiple flagella found at several locations about the cell

The bacterial flagellum consists of three basic components: a whip-like filament, a motor complex, and a hook that connects them. The filament is approximately 20 nm in diameter and consists of several protofilaments, each made up of thousands of flagellin subunits. The bundle is held together by a cap and may or may not be encapsulated. The motor complex consists of a series of rings anchoring the flagellum in the inner and outer membranes, followed by a proton-driven motor that drives rotational movement in the filament.

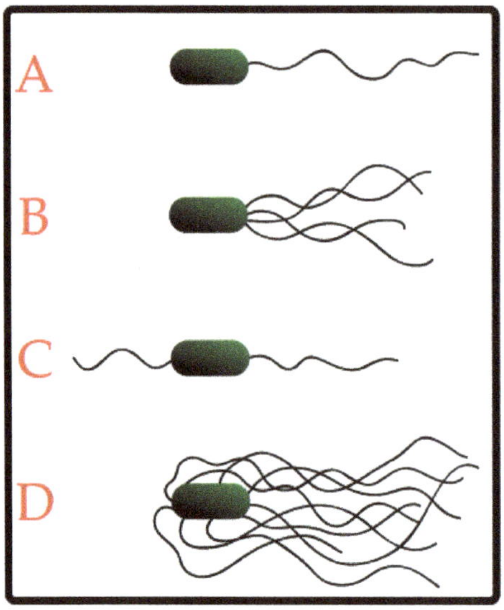

A-Monotrichous; B-Lophotrichous; C-Amphitrichous; D-Peritrichous;

Intracellular (internal) Structures

In comparison to eukaryotes, the intracellular features of the bacterial cell are extremely simple. Bacteria do not contain organelles in the same sense as eukaryotes. Instead, the chromosome and perhaps ribosomes are the only easily observable intracellular structures found in all bacteria. They do exist, however, specialized groups of bacteria that contain more complex intracellular structures, some of which are discussed below.

The Bacterial DNA and Plasmids

Unlike eukaryotes, the bacterial DNA is not enclosed inside of a membrane-bound nucleus but instead resides inside the bacterial cytoplasm. This means that the transfer of cellular information through the processes of translation, transcription and DNA replication all occur within the same compartment and can interact with other cytoplasmic structures, most notably ribosomes. The bacterial DNA is not packaged using histones to form chromatin as in eukaryotes but instead exists as a highly compact supercoiled structure, the precise nature of which remains unclear. Most bacterial DNA are circular although some examples of linear DNA exist (e.g. Borrelia burgdorferi). Along with chromosomal DNA, most bacteria also contain small independent pieces of DNA called plasmids that often encode for traits that are advantageous but not essential to their bacterial host. Plasmids can be easily gained or lost by a bacterium and can be transferred between bacteria as a form of horizontal gene transfer. So plasmids can be described as an extra chromosomal DNA in a bacterial cell.

Ribosomes and other Multiprotein Complexes

In most bacteria the most numerous intracellular structure is the ribosome, the site of protein synthesis in all living organisms. All prokaryotes have 70S (where S=Svedberg units) ribosomes while eukaryotes contain larger 80S ribosomes in their cytosol. The 70S ribosome is made up of a 50S and 30S subunits. The 50S subunit contains the 23S and 5S rRNA while the 30S subunit contains the 16S rRNA. These rRNA molecules differ in size in eukaryotes and are complexed with a large number of ribosomal proteins, the number and type of which can vary slightly between organisms. While the ribosome is the most commonly observed intracellular multiprotein complex in bacteria other large complexes do occur and can sometimes be seen using microscopy.

Intracellular Membranes

While not typical of all bacteria some microbes contain intracellular membranes in addition to (or as extensions of) their cytoplasmic membranes. An early idea was that bacteria might contain membrane folds termed mesosomes, but these were later shown to be artifacts produced by the chemicals used to prepare the cells for electron microscopy. Examples of bacteria containing intracellular membranes are phototrophs, nitrifying bacteria and methane-oxidising bacteria. Intracellular membranes are also found in bacteria belonging to the poorly studied Planctomycetes group, although these membranes more closely resemble organellar membranes in eukaryotes and are currently of unknown function.Chromatophores are intracellular membranes found in phototrophic bacteria. Used primarily for photosynthesis, they contain bacteriochlorophyll pigments and carotenoids.

Cytoskeleton

The prokaryotic cytoskeleton is the collective name for all structural filaments in prokaryotes. It was once thought that prokaryotic cells did not possess cytoskeletons, but recent advances in visualization technology and structure determination have shown that filaments indeed exist in these cells. In fact, homologues for all major cytoskeletal proteins in eukaryotes have been found in prokaryotes. Cytoskeletal elements play essential roles in cell division, protection, shape determination, and polarity determination in various prokaryotes.

Nutrient Storage Structures

Most bacteria do not live in environments that contain large amounts of nutrients at all times. To accommodate these transient levels of nutrients bacteria contain several different methods of nutrient storage in times of plenty for use in times of want. For example, many bacteria store excess carbon in the form of polyhydroxyalkanoates or glycogen. Some microbes store soluble nutrients such as nitrate in vacuoles. Sulfur is most often stored as elemental (S0) granules which can be deposited either intra- or extracellularly. Sulfur granules are especially common in bacteria that use hydrogen sulfide as an electron source. Most of the above-mentioned examples can be viewed using a microscope and are surrounded by a thin nonunit membrane to separate them from the cytoplasm.

Inclusions

Inclusions are considered to be nonliving components of the cell that do not possess metabolic activity and are not bounded by membranes. The most common inclusions are glycogen, lipid droplets, crystals, and pigments. Volutin granules are cytoplasmic inclusions of complexed inorganic polyphosphate. These granules are called metachromatic granules due to their displaying the metachromatic effect; they appear red or blue when stained with the blue dyes methylene blue or toluidine blue.

Gas Vacuoles

Gas vacuoles are membrane-bound, spindle-shaped vesicles, found in some planktonic bacteria and Cyanobacteria, that provides buoyancy to these cells by decreasing their overall cell density. Positive buoyancy is needed to keep the cells in the upper reaches of the water column, so that they can continue to perform photosynthesis. They are made up of a shell of protein that has a highly hydrophobic inner surface, making it impermeable to water (and stopping water vapour from condensing inside) but permeable to most gases. Because the gas vesicle is a hollow cylinder, it is liable to collapse when the surrounding pressure increases. Natural selection has fine tuned the structure of the gas vesicle to maximise its resistance to buckling, including an external strengthening protein, GvpC, rather like the green thread in a braided hosepipe. There is a simple relationship between the diameter of the gas vesicle and pressure at which it will collapse - the wider the gas vesicle the weaker it becomes. However, wider gas vesicles are more efficient, providing more buoyancy per unit of protein than narrow gas vesicles. Different species produce gas vesicle of different diameter, allowing them to colonise different depths of the water column (fast growing, highly competitive species with wide gas vesicles in the top most layers; slow growing, dark-adapted, species with strong narrow gas vesicles in the deeper layers). The diameter of the gas vesicle will also help determine which species survive in different bodies of water. Deep lakes that experience winter mixing expose the cells to the hydrostatic pressure generated by the full water column. This will select for species with narrower, stronger gas vesicles.

The cell achieves its height in the water column by synthesising gas vesicles. As the cell rises up, it is able to increase its carbohydrate load through increased photosynthesis. Too high and the cell will suffer photobleaching and possible death, however, the carbohydrate produced during photosynthesis increases the cell›s density, causing it to sink. The daily cycle of carbohydrate build-up from photosynthesis and carbohydrate catabolism during dark hours is enough to fine-tune the cell's position in the water column, bring it up toward the surface when its carbohydrate levels are low and it needs to photosynthesis, and allowing it to sink away from the harmful UV radiation when the cell's carbohydrate levels have been replenished. An extreme excess of carbohydrate causes a significant change in the internal pressure of the cell, which causes the gas vesicles to buckle and collapse and the cell to sink out.

Microcompartments

Bacterial microcompartments are widespread, membrane-bound organelles that are made of a protein shell that surrounds and encloses various enzymes. provide a further level of organization; they are compartments within bacteria that are surrounded by polyhedral protein shells, rather than by lipid membranes. These «polyhedral organelles» localize and compartmentalize bacterial metabolism, a function performed by the membrane-bound organelles in eukaryotes.

Carboxysomes

Carboxysomes are bacterial microcompartments found in many autotrophic bacteria such as Cyanobacteria, Knallgasbacteria, Nitroso- and Nitrobacteria. They are proteinaceous structures resembling phage heads in their morphology and contain the enzymes of carbon dioxide fixation in these organisms (especially ribulose bisphosphate carboxylase/oxygenase, RuBisCO, and carbonic anhydrase). It is thought that the high local concentration of the enzymes along with the fast conversion of bicarbonate to carbon dioxide by carbonic anhydrase allows faster and more efficient carbon dioxide fixation than possible inside the cytoplasm. Similar structures are known to harbor the coenzyme B12-containing glycerol dehydratase, the key enzyme of glycerol fermentation to 1,3-propanediol, in some Enterobacteriaceae (e. g. Salmonella).

Magnetosomes

Magnetosomes are bacterial microcompartments found in magnetotactic bacteria that allow them to sense and align themselves along a magnetic field (magnetotaxis). The ecological role of magnetotaxis is unknown but is thought to be involved in the determination of optimal oxygen concentrations. Magnetosomes are composed of the mineral magnetite or greigite and are surrounded by a lipid bilayer membrane. The morphology of magnetosomes is species-specific.

Endospores

Perhaps the best known bacterial adaptation to stress is the formation of endospores. Endospores are bacterial survival structures that are highly resistant to many different types of chemical and environmental stresses and therefore enable the survival of bacteria in environments that would be lethal for these cells in their normal vegetative form. It has been proposed that endospore formation has allowed for the survival of some bacteria for hundreds of millions of years (e.g. in salt crystals) although these publications have been questioned. Endospore formation is limited to several genera of gram-positive bacteria such as Bacillus and Clostridium. It differs from reproductive spores in that only one spore is formed per cell resulting in no net gain in cell number upon endospore germination. The location of an endospore within a cell is species-specific and can be used to determine the identity of a bacterium. Dipicolinic acid is a chemical compound which composes 5% to 15% of the dry weight of bacterial spores and is implicated in being responsible for the heat resistance of endospores. Archeologists have found viable endospores taken from the intestines of Egyptian mummies and also from sediment of over seven thousand years old taken from Minnesota's Elk Lake.

REFERENCES

1. Goldstein E, Drlica K (1984). "Regulation of bacterial DNA supercoiling: plasmid linking numbers very with growth temperature" (PDF). Proceedings of the National Academy of Sciences of the United States of America. 81: 4046–4050. doi:10.1073/pnas.81.13.4046. PMC 345365Freely accessible. PMID 6377307.
2. Ryter A (1988). "Contribution of new cryomethods to a better knowledge of bacterial anatomy". Ann. Inst. Pasteur Microbiol. 139 (1): 33–44. doi:10.1016/0769-2609(88)90095-6. PMID 3289587.
3. Fuerst J (2005). "Intracellular compartmentation in planctomycetes". Annu Rev Microbiol. 59: 299–328. doi:10.1146/annurev.micro.59.030804.121258. PMID 15910279.
4. Gitai Z (2005). "The new bacterial cell biology: moving parts and subcellular architecture". Cell. 120 (5): 577–86. doi:10.1016/j.cell.2005.02.026. PMID 15766522.
5. Shih YL, Rothfield L (2006). "The bacterial cytoskeleton". Microbiol. Mol. Biol. Rev. 70 (3): 729–54. doi:10.1128/MMBR.00017-06. PMC 1594594Freely accessible. PMID 16959967.
6. Cannon GC, Bradburne CE, Aldrich HC, Baker SH, Heinhorst S, Shively JM (2001). "Microcompartments in prokaryotes: carboxysomes and related polyhedra". Appl. Environ. Microbiol. 67 (12): 5351–61. doi:10.1128/AEM.67.12.5351-5361.2001. PMC 93316Freely accessible. PMID 11722879.
7. Capaldo-Kimball F (1 April 1971). "Involvement of Recombination Genes in Growth and Viability of Escherichia coli K-12". J. Bacteriol. 106 (1): 204–212. PMC 248663Freely accessible. PMID 4928007.
8. Kubitschek HE (1 January 1993). "Cell volume increase in Escherichia coli after shifts to richer media". J. Bacteriol. 172 (1): 94–101. PMC 208405Freely accessible. PMID 2403552.
9. Cano RJ, Borucki MK (May 1995). "Revival and identification of bacterial spores in 25- to 40-million-year-old Dominican amber". Science. 268 (5213): 1060–4. doi:10.1126/science.7538699. PMID 7538699.
10. Fischman J (May 1995). "Have 25-million-year-old bacteria returned to life?". Science. 268 (5213): 977. doi:10.1126/science.7754393. PMID 7754393.
11. Demchick, P; Koch, AL (1 February 1996). "The permeability of the wall fabric of Escherichia coli and Bacillus subtilis". J. Bacteriol. 178 (3): 768–73. PMC 177723Freely accessible. PMID 8550511.
12. Vreeland RH, Rosenzweig WD, Powers DW (October 2000). "Isolation of a 250 million-year-old halotolerant bacterium from a primary salt crystal". Nature. 407 (6806): 897–900. doi:10.1038/35038060. PMID 11057666.
13. Parkes RJ (October 2000). "A case of bacterial immortality?". Nature. 407 (6806): 844–5. doi:10.1038/35038181. PMID 11057647.

14. Badger MR, Price GD (February 2003). "CO2 concentrating mechanisms in cyanobacteria: molecular components, their diversity and evolution". J. Exp. Bot. 54 (383): 609–22. doi:10.1093/jxb/erg076. PMID 12554704.

CHAPTER 5

Bacterial Genetics

Chapter Contents

- **Introduction**
- **Microbial Genetics**
- **Catabolite Repression**

Bacterial genetics is the study of the mechanisms of heritable information in bacteria, their chromosomes, plasmids, transposons and phages. Techniques that have enabled this discipline are culture in defined media, replica plating, mutagenesis, transformation, conjugation and transduction.

INTRODUCTION

Bacterial genetics is the subfield of genetics devoted to the study of bacteria. Bacterial genetics are subtly different from eukaryotic genetics, however bacteria still serve as a good model for animal genetic studies. One of the major distinctions between bacterial and eukaryotic genetics stems from the bacteria's lack of membrane-bound organelles (this is true of all prokaryotes. While it is a fact that there are prokaryotic organelles, they are never bound by a lipid membrane, but by a shell of proteins), necessitating protein synthesis occur in the cytoplasm.

Like other organisms, bacteria also breed true and maintain their characteristics from generation to generation, yet at same time, exhibit variations in particular properties in a small proportion of their progeny. Though heritability and variations in bacteria had been noticed from the early days of bacteriology, it was not realised then that bacteria too obey the laws of genetics. Even the existence of a bacterial nucleus was a subject of controversy. The differences in morphology and other properties were attributed by Nageli in 1877, to bacterial pleomorphism, which postulated the existence of a single, a few species of bacteria, which possessed a protein capacity for a variation. With the development and application of precise methods of pure culture, it became apparent that different types of bacteria retained constant form and function through successive generations. This led to the concept of monomorphism.

Transformation

Transformation in bacteria was first observed in 1928 by F. Grffith and later (in 1944) examined at the molecular level by O. Avery and his colleagues who used the process to demonstrate that DNA was the genetic material of bacteria. In transformation, a cell takes up extraneous DNA found in the environment and incorporates it into its genome (genetic material) through recombination. Not all bacteria are competent to be transformed, and not all extracellular DNA is competent to transform. To be competent to transform, the extracellular DNA must be double-stranded and relatively large. To be competent to be transformed, a cell must have the surface protein Competent Factor›, which binds to the extracellular DNA in an energy requiring reaction. However bacteria that are not naturally competent can be treated in such a way to make them competent, usually by treatment with calcium chloride, which make them more permiable

Bacterial Conjugation

Bacterial conjugation is the transfer of genetic material (plasmid) between bacterial cells by direct cell-to-cell contact or by a bridge-like connection between two cells. Discovered in 1946 by Joshua Lederberg and Edward Tatum, conjugation is a mechanism of horizontal gene transfer as are transformation and transduction although these two other mechanisms do not involve cell-to-cell contact.

Bacterial conjugation is often regarded as the bacterial equivalent of sexual reproduction or mating since it involves the exchange of genetic material. During conjugation the donor cell provides a conjugative or mobilizable genetic element that is most often a plasmid or transposon. Most conjugative plasmids have systems ensuring that the recipient cell does not already contain a similar element.

The genetic information transferred is often beneficial to the recipient. Benefits may include antibiotic resistance, xenobiotic tolerance or the ability to use new metabolites. Such beneficial plasmids may be considered bacterial endosymbionts. Other elements, however, may be viewed as bacterial parasites and conjugation as a mechanism evolved by them to allow for their spread.

MICROBIAL GENETICS

Microbial genetics is a subject area within microbiology and genetic engineering. It studies the genetics of very small (micro) organisms; bacteria, archaea, viruses and some protozoa and fungi. This involves the study of the genotype of microbial species and also the expression system in the form of phenotypes.

Since the discovery of microorganisms by two Fellows of The Royal Society, Robert Hooke and Antoni van Leeuwenhoek during the period 1665-1885 they have been used to study many processes and have had applications in various areas of study in genetics. For example: Microorganisms› rapid growth rates and short generation times are used by scientists to study evolution. Microbial genetics also has applications in being able to study processes and pathways that are similar to those found in humans such as drug metabolism.

Microorganisms whose study is encompassed by Microbial Genetics

Bacteria

Bacteria have been on this planet for approximately 3.5 billion years, and are classified by their shape.Bacterial genetics studies the mechanisms of their heritable information, their chromosomes, plasmids, transposons, and phages.

Gene transfer systems that have been extensively studied in bacteria include genetic transformation, conjugation and transduction. Natural transformation is a bacterial adaptation for DNA transfer between two cells through the intervening medium. The uptake of donor DNA and its recombinational incorporation into the recipient chromosome depends on the expression of numerous bacterial genes whose products direct this process. In general, transformation is a complex, energy-requiring developmental process that appears to be an adaptation for repairing DNA damage.

Bacterial conjugation is the transfer of genetic material between bacterial cells by direct cell-to-cell contact or by a bridge-like connection between two cells. Bacterial conjugation has been extensively studied in Escherichia coli, but also occurs in other bacteria such as Mycobacterium smegmatis. Conjugation requires stable and extended contact between a donor and a recipient strain, is DNase resistant, and the transferred DNA is incorporated into the recipient chromosome by homologous recombination. E. coli conjugation is mediated by expression of plasmid genes, whereas mycobacterial conjugation is mediated by genes on the bacterial chromosome.

Transduction is the process by which foreign DNA is introduced into a cell by a virus or viral vector. Transduction is a common tool used by molecular biologists to stably introduce a foreign gene into a host cell›s genome.

Archaea

Archaea is a domain of organisms that are prokaryotic, single-celled, and are thought to have developed 4 billion years ago. They share a common ancestor with bacteria, but are more closely related to eukaryotes in comparison to bacteria. Some Archaea are able to survive extreme environments, which leads to many applications in the field of genetics. One of such applications is the use of archaeal enzymes, which would be better able to survive harsh conditions in vitro.

Gene transfer and genetic exchange have been studied in the halophilic archaeon Halobacterium volcanii and the hyperthermophilic archaeons Sulfolobus solfataricus and Sulfolobus acidocaldarius. H. volcani forms cytoplasmic bridges between cells that appear to be used for transfer of DNA from one cell to another in either direction. When S. solfataricus and S. acidocaldarius are exposed to DNA damaging agents, species-specific cellular aggregation is induced. Cellular aggregation mediates chromosomal marker exchange and genetic recombination with high frequency. Cellular aggregation is thought to enhance species specific DNA transfer between Sulfolobus cells in order to provide increased repair of damaged DNA by means of homologous recombination.

Fungi

Fungi can be both multicellular and unicellular organisms, and are distinguished from other microbes by the way they obtain nutrients. Fungi secrete enzymes into their surroundings, to break down organic matter. Fungal genetics uses yeast, and filamentous fungi as model organisms for eukaryotic genetic research, including cell cycle regulation, chromatin structure and gene regulation.

Studies of the fungus Neurospora crassa have contributed substantially to understanding how genes work. N. crassa is a type of red bread mold of the phylum Ascomycota. It is used as a model organism because it is easy to grow and has a haploid life cycle that makes genetic analysis simple since recessive traits will show up in the offspring. Analysis of genetic recombination is facilitated by the ordered arrangement of the products of meiosis in ascospores. In its natural environment, N. crassa lives mainly in tropical and sub-tropical regions. It often can be found growing on dead plant matter after fires.

Neurospora was used by Edward Tatum and George Beadle in their experiments for which they won the Nobel Prize in Physiology or Medicine in 1958. The results of these experiments led directly to the one gene-one enzyme hypothesis that specific genes code for specific proteins. This concept proved to be the opening gun in what became molecular genetics and all the developments that have followed from that.

Saccharomyces cerevisiae is a yeast of the phylum Ascomycota. During vegetative growth that ordinarily occurs when nutrients are abundant, S. cerevisiae reproduces by mitosis as diploid cells. However, when starved, these cells undergo meiosis to form haploid spores. Mating occurs when haploid cells of opposite mating types MATa and MATα come into contact. Ruderfer et al. pointed out that, in nature, such contacts are frequent between closely related yeast cells for two reasons. The first is that cells of opposite mating type are present together in the same acus, the sac that contains the cells directly produced by a single meiosis, and these cells can mate with each other. The second reason is that haploid cells of one mating type, upon cell division, often produce cells of the opposite mating type. An analysis of the ancestry of natural S. cerevisiae strains concluded that outcrossing occurs very infrequently (only about once every 50,000 cell divisions). The relative rarity in nature of meiotic events that result from outcrossing suggests that the possible long-term benefits of outcrossing (e.g. generation of diversity) are unlikely to be sufficient for generally maintaining sex from one generation to the next. Rather, a short term benefit, such as meiotic recombinational repair of DNA damages caused by stressful conditions (such as starvation) may be the key to the maintenance of sex in S. cerevisiae.

Candida albicans is a diploid fungus that grows both as a yeast and as a filament. C. albicans is the most common fungal pathogen in humans. It causes both debilitating mucosal infections and potentially life-threatening systemic infections. C. albicans has maintained an elaborate, but largely hidden, mating apparatus. Johnson suggested that mating strategies may allow C. albicans to survive in the hostile environment of a mammalian host.

Among the 250 known species of aspergilli, about 33% have an identified sexual state. Among those Aspergillus species that exhibit a sexual cycle the overwhelming majority in nature are homothallic (self-fertilizing). Selfing in the homothallic fungus Aspergillus nidulans involves activation of the same mating pathways characteristic of sex in outcrossing species, i.e. self-fertilization does not bypass required pathways for outcrossing sex but instead requires activation of these pathways within a single individual. Fusion of haploid nuclei occurs within reproductive structures termed cleistothecia, in which the diploid zygote undergoes meiotic divisions to yield haploid ascospores.

Protozoa

Protozoa are unicellular organisms, which have nuclei, and ultramicroscopic cellular bodies within their cytoplasm. One particular aspect of protozoa that are of interest to human geneticists are their flagella, which are very similar to human sperm flagella.

Studies of Paramecia have contributed to our understanding of the function of meiosis. Like all ciliates, Paramecia have a polyploid macronucleus, and one or more diploid micronuclei. The macronucleus controls non-reproductive cell functions, expressing the genes needed for daily functioning. The micronucleus is the generative, or germline nucleus, containing the genetic material that is passed along from one generation to the next.

In the asexual fission phase of growth, during which cell divisions occur by mitosis rather than meiosis, clonal aging occurs leading to a gradual loss of vitality. In some species, such as the well studied Paramecium tetraurelia, the asexual line of clonally aging paramecia loses vitality and expires after about 200 fissions if the cells fail to undergo meiosis followed by either autogamy (self-fertilizaion) or conjugation (outcrossing) (see aging in Paramecium). DNA damage increases dramatically during successive clonal cell divisions and is a likely cause of clonal aging in P. tetraurelia.

When clonally aged P. tetraurelia are stimulated to undergo meiosis in association with either autogamy or conjugation, the progeny are rejuvenated, and are able to have many more mitotic binary fission divisions. During either of these processes the micronuclei of the cell(s) undergo meiosis, the old macronucleus disintegrates and a new macronucleus is formed by replication of the micronuclear DNA that had recently undergone meiosis. There is apparently little, if any, DNA damage in the new macronucleus, suggesting that rejuvenation is associated with the repair of these damages in the micronucleus during meiosis.

Viruses

Viruses are capsid-encoding organisms composed of proteins and nucleic acids that can self-assemble after replication in a host cell using the host›s replication machinery. There is a disagreement in science about whether viruses are living due to their lack of ribosomes.

Comprehending the viral genome is important not only for studies in genetics but also for understanding their pathogenic properties.

Many types of virus are capable of genetic recombination. When two or more individual viruses of the same type infect a cell, their genomes may recombine with each other to produce recombinant virus progeny. Both DNA and RNA viruses can undergo recombination. When two or more viruses, each containing lethal genomic damage infect the same host cell, the virus genomes often can pair with each other and undergo homologous recombinational repair to produce viable progeny. This process is known as multiplicity reactivation. Enzymes employed in multiplicity reactivation are functionally homologous to enzymes employed in bacterial and eukaryotic recombinational repair. Multiplicity reactivation has been found to occur with pathogenic viruses including influenza virus, HIV-1, adenovirus simian virus 40, vaccinia virus, reovirus, poliovirus and herpes simplex virus as well as numerous bacteriophages.

Applications of Microbial Genetics

Microbes are ideally suited for biochemical and genetics studies and have made huge contributions to these fields of science such as the demonstration that DNA is the genetic material, that the gene has a simple linear structure, that the genetic code is a triplet code, and that gene expression is regulated by specific genetic processes. Jacques Monod and François Jacob used Escherichia coli, a type of bacteria, in order to develop the operon model of gene expression, which lay down the basis of gene expression and regulation. Furthermore the hereditary processes of single-celled eukaryotic microorganisms are similar to those in multi-cellular organisms allowing researchers to gather information on this process as well. Another bacterium which has greatly contributed to the field of genetics is Thermus aquaticus, which is a bacterium that tolerates high temperatures. From this microbe scientists isolated the enzyme Taq polymerase, which is now used in the powerful experimental technique, Polymerase chain reaction(PCR). Additionally the development of recombinant DNA technology through the use of bacteria has led to the birth of modern genetic engineering and biotechnology.

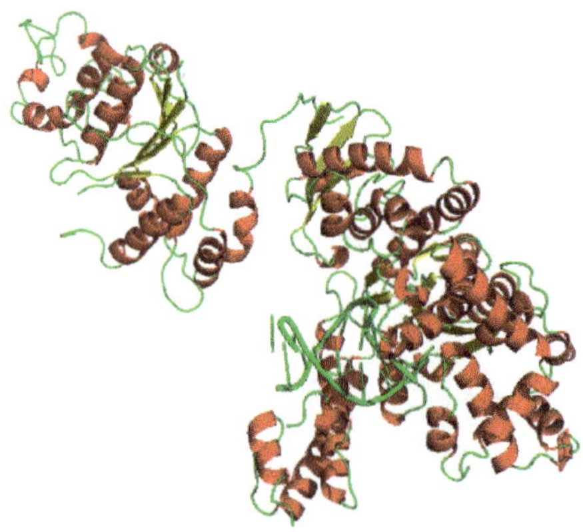

Taq polymerase which is used in Polymerase Chain Reaction(PCR)

Using microbes, protocols were developed to insert genes into bacterial plasmids, taking advantage of their fast reproduction, to make biofactories for the gene of interest. Such genetically engineered bacteria can produce pharmaceuticals such as insulin, human growth hormone, interferons and blood clotting factors. Microbes synthesize a variety of enzymes for industrial applications, such as fermented foods, laboratory test reagents, dairy products (such as renin), and even in clothing (such as Trichoderma fungus whose enzyme is used to give jeans a stone washed appearance).

LAC OPERON

The lac operon (lactose operon) is an operon required for the transport and metabolism of lactose in Escherichia coli and many other enteric bacteria. Although glucose is the preferred carbon source for most bacteria, the lac operon allows for the effective digestion of lactose when glucose is not available. Gene regulation of the lac operon was the first genetic regulatory mechanism to be understood clearly, so it has become a foremost example of prokaryotic gene regulation. It is often discussed in introductory molecular and cellular biology classes for this reason.

Bacterial operons are polycistronic transcripts that are able to produce multiple proteins from one mRNA transcript. In this case, when lactose is required as a sugar source for the bacterium, the three genes of the lac operon can be expressed and their subsequent proteins translated: lacZ, lacY, and lacA. The gene product of lacZ is β-galactosidase which cleaves lactose, a disaccharide, into glucose and galactose. lacY encodes Beta-galactoside permease, a protein which becomes embedded in the cytoplasmic membrane to enable transport of lactose into the cell. Finally, lacA encodes β-galactoside transacetylase.

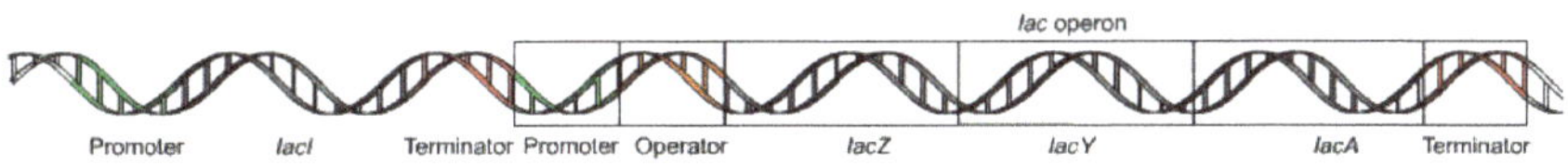

It would be wasteful to produce the enzymes when there is no lactose available or if there is a more preferable energy source available, such as glucose. The lac operon uses a two-part control mechanism to ensure that the cell expends energy producing the enzymes encoded by the lac operon only when necessary. In the absence of lactose, the lac repressor halts production of the enzymes encoded by the lac operon. In the presence of glucose, the catabolite activator protein (CAP), required for production of the enzymes, remains inactive, and EIIAGlc shuts down lactose permease to prevent transport of lactose into the cell. This dual control mechanism causes the sequential utilization of glucose and lactose in two distinct growth phases, known as diauxie.

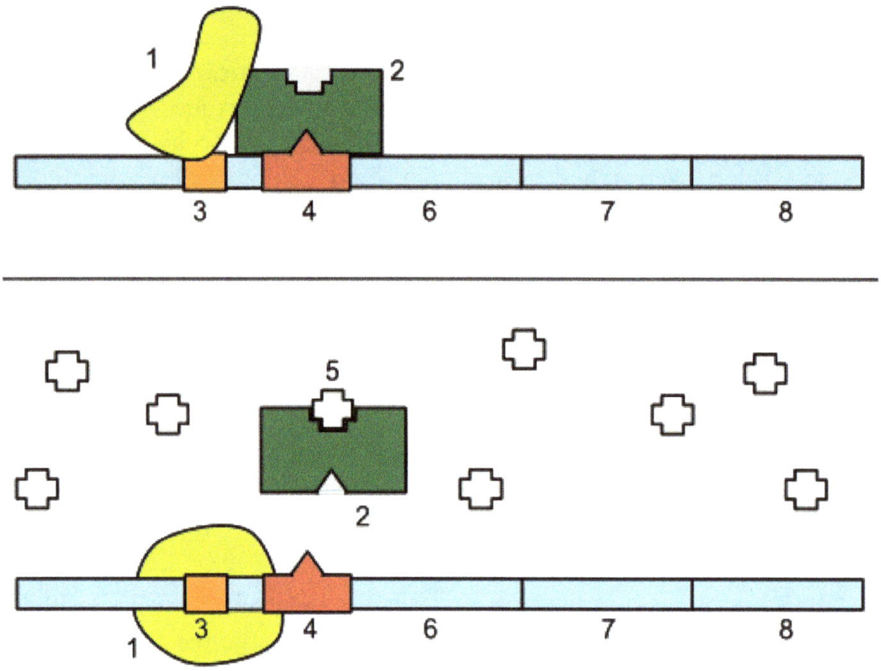

The lac operon. Top:Repressed, Bottom:Active.

1: RNA Polymerase, 2: Repressor, 3: Promoter, 4: Operator, 5: Lactose, 6: lacZ, 7: lacY, 8: lacA.

Structure of the lac operon

- The *lac* operon consists of three structural genes, and a promoter, a terminator, regulator, and an operator. The three structural genes are: *lacZ*, *lacY*, and *lacA*.

  lacZ encodes β-galactosidase (LacZ), an intracellular enzyme that cleaves the disaccharide lactose into glucose and galactose.

  lacY encodes Beta-galactoside permease (LacY), a transmembrane symporter that pumps β-galactosides including lactose into the cell using a proton gradient in the same direction.

  lacA encodes β-galactoside transacetylase (LacA), an enzyme that transfers an acetyl group from acetyl-CoA to β-galactosides.

Only lacZ and lacY appear to be necessary for lactose catabolism.

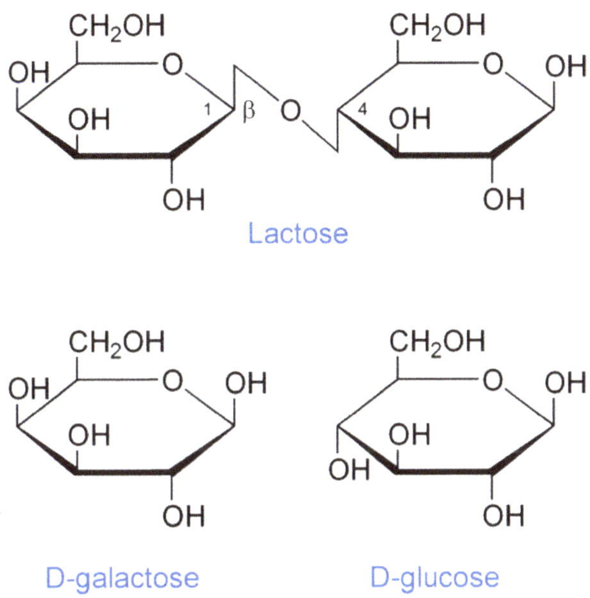

Structure of lactose and the products of its cleavage.

Genetic Nomenclature

Three-letter abbreviations are used to describe phenotypes in bacteria including *E. coli*.

Examples include:

- Lac (the ability to use lactose),
- His (the ability to synthesize the amino acid histidine)
- Mot (swimming motility)
- Sm^R (resistance to the antibiotic streptomycin)

In the case of Lac, wild type cells are Lac+ and are able to use lactose as a carbon and energy source, while Lac− mutant derivatives cannot use lactose. The same three letters are typically used (lower-case, italicized) to label the genes involved in a particular phenotype, where each different gene is additionally distinguished by an extra letter. The lac genes encoding enzymes are lacZ, lacY, and lacA. The fourth lac gene is lacI, encoding the lactose repressor—"I" stands for inducibility.

One may distinguish between structural genes encoding enzymes, and regulatory genes encoding proteins that affect gene expression. Current usage expands the phenotypic nomenclature to apply to proteins: thus, LacZ is the protein product of the lacZ gene, β-galactosidase. Various short sequences that are not genes also affect gene expression, including the lac promoter, lac p, and the lac operator, lac o. Although it is not strictly standard usage, mutations affecting lac o are referred to as lac oc, for historical reasons.

Regulation

Specific control of the lac genes depends on the availability of the substrate lactose to the bacterium. The proteins are not produced by the bacterium when lactose is unavailable as a carbon source. The lac genes are organized into an operon; that is, they are oriented in the same direction immediately adjacent on the chromosome and are co-transcribed into a single polycistronic mRNA molecule. Transcription of all genes starts with the binding of the enzyme RNA polymerase (RNAP), a DNA-binding protein, which binds to a specific DNA binding site, the promoter, immediately upstream of the genes. Binding of RNA polymerase to the promoter is aided by the cAMP-bound catabolite activator protein (CAP, also known as the cAMP receptor protein). However, the lacI gene (regulatory gene for lac operon) produces a protein that blocks RNAP from binding to the promoter of the operon. This protein can only be removed when allolactose binds to it, and inactivates it. The protein that is formed by the lacI gene is known as the lac repressor. The type of regulation that the lac operon undergoes is referred to as negative inducible, meaning that the gene is turned off by the regulatory factor (lac repressor) unless some molecule (lactose) is added. Because of the presence of the lac repressor protein, genetic engineers who replace the lacZ gene with another gene will have to grow the experimental bacteria on agar with lactose available on it. If they do not, the gene they are trying to express will not be expressed as the repressor protein is still blocking RNAP from binding to the promoter and transcribing the gene. Once the repressor is removed, RNAP then proceeds to transcribe all three genes (lacZYA) into mRNA. Each of the three genes on the mRNA strand has its own Shine-Dalgarno sequence, so the genes are independently translated. The DNA sequence of the E. coli lac operon, the lacZYA mRNA, and the lacI genes are available from GenBank (view).

The first control mechanism is the regulatory response to lactose, which uses an intracellular regulatory protein called the lactose repressor to hinder production of β-galactosidase in the absence of lactose. The lacI gene coding for the repressor lies nearby the lac operon and is always expressed (constitutive). If lactose is missing from the growth medium, the repressor binds very tightly to a short DNA sequence just downstream of the promoter near the beginning of lacZ called the lac operator. The repressor binding to the operator interferes with binding of RNAP to the promoter, and therefore mRNA encoding LacZ and LacY is only made at very low levels. When cells are grown in the presence of lactose, however, a lactose metabolite called allolactose, made from lactose by the product of the lacZ gene, binds to the repressor, causing an allosteric shift. Thus altered, the repressor is unable to bind to the operator, allowing RNAP to transcribe the lac genes and thereby leading to higher levels of the encoded proteins.

The second control mechanism is a response to glucose, which uses the catabolite activator protein (CAP) homodimer to greatly increase production of β-galactosidase in the absence of glucose. Cyclic adenosine monophosphate (cAMP) is a signal molecule whose prevalence is inversely proportional to that of glucose. It binds to the CAP, which in turn allows the CAP to bind to the CAP binding site (a 16 bp DNA sequence upstream of the promoter on the left in the diagram below, about 60 bp upstream of the transcription start site), which assists the RNAP in binding to the DNA. In the absence of glucose, the cAMP concentration is high and binding of CAP-cAMP to the DNA significantly increases the production of β-galactosidase, enabling the cell to hydrolyse lactose and release galactose and glucose.

More recently inducer exclusion was shown to block expression of the lac operon when glucose is present. Glucose is transported into the cell by the PEP-dependent phosphotransferase system. The phosphate group of phosphoenolpyruvate is transferred via a phosphorylation cascade consisting of the general PTS (phosphotransferase system) proteins HPr and EIA and the glucose-specific PTS proteins EIIAGlc and EIIBGlc, the cytoplasmic domain of the EII glucose transporter. Transport of glucose is accompanied by its phosphorylation by EIIBGlc, draining the phosphate group from the other PTS proteins, including EIIAGlc. The unphosphorylated form of EIIAGlc binds to the lac permease and prevents it from bringing lactose into the cell. Therefore, if both glucose and lactose are present, the transport of glucose blocks the transport of the inducer of the lac operon.

Repressor Structure

The lac repressor is a four-part protein, a tetramer, with identical subunits. Each subunit contains a helix-turn-helix (HTH) motif capable of binding to DNA. The operator site where repressor binds is a DNA sequence with inverted repeat symmetry. The two DNA half-sites of the operator together bind to two of the subunits of the repressor. Although the other two subunits of repressor are not doing anything in this model, this property was not understood for many years.

Eventually it was discovered that two additional operators are involved in lac regulation. One (O3) lies about -90 bp upstream of O1 in the end of the lacI gene, and the other (O2) is about +410 bp downstream of O1 in the early part of lacZ. These two sites were not found in the early work because they have redundant functions and individual mutations do not affect repression very much. Single mutations to either O2 or O3 have only 2 to 3-fold effects. However, their importance is demonstrated by the fact that a double mutant defective in both O2 and O3 is dramatically de-repressed (by about 70-fold).

In the current model, lac repressor is bound simultaneously to both the main operator O1 and to either O2 or O3. The intervening DNA loops out from the complex. The redundant nature of the two minor operators suggests that it is not a specific looped complex that is important. One idea is that the system works through tethering; if bound repressor releases from O1momentarily, binding to a minor operator keeps it in the vicinity, so that it may rebind quickly. This would increase the affinity of repressor for O1.

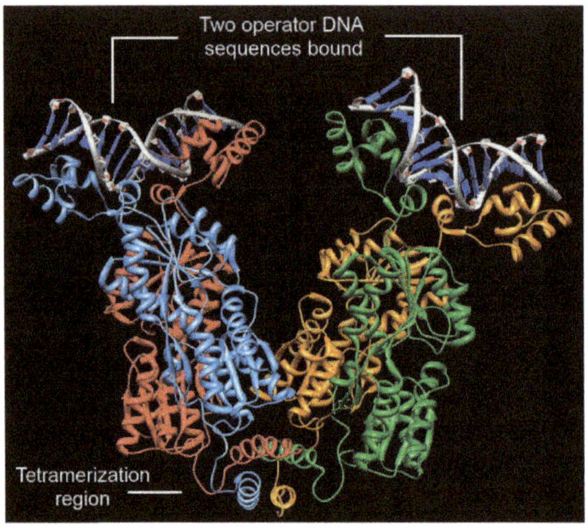

Tetrameric LacI binds two operator sequences and induces DNA looping. Two dimeric LacI functional subunits (red+blue and green+orange) each bind a DNA operator sequence (labeled). These two functional subunits are coupled at the tetramerization region (labeled); thus, tetrameric LacI binds two operator sequences. This allows tetrameric LacI to induce DNA looping.

Mechanism of induction

The repressor is an allosteric protein, i.e. it can assume either one of two slightly different shapes, which are in equilibrium with each other. In one form the repressor will bind to the operator DNA with high specificity, and in the other form it has lost its specificity. According to the classical model of induction, binding of the inducer, either allolactose or IPTG, to the repressor affects the distribution of repressor between the two shapes. Thus, repressor with inducer bound is stabilized in the non-DNA-binding conformation. However, this simple model cannot be the whole story, because repressor is bound quite stably to DNA, yet it is released rapidly by addition of inducer. Therefore, it seems clear that inducer can also bind to the repressor when the repressor is already bound to DNA. It is still not entirely known what the exact mechanism of binding is.

Role of Non-Specific Binding

Non-specific binding of the repressor to DNA plays a crucial role in the repression and induction of the Lac-operon. The specific binding site for the Lac-repressor protein is the operator. The non-specific interaction is mediated mainly by charge-charge interactions while binding to the operator is reinforced by hydrophobic interactions. Additionally, there is an abundance of non-specific DNA sequences to which the repressor can bind. Essentially, any sequence that is not the operator, is considered non-specific. Studies have shown, that without the presence of non-specific binding, induction (or unrepression) of the Lac-operon could not occur even with saturated levels of inducer. It had been demonstrated that, without non-specific binding, the basal level of induction is ten thousand times smaller than observed normally. This is because the non-specific DNA acts as sort of a "sink" for the repressor proteins, distracting them from the operator.

The non-specific sequences decrease the amount of available repressor in the cell. This in turn reduces the amount of inducer required to unrepress the system.

Lactose Analogs

A number of lactose derivatives or analogs have been described that are useful for work with the lac operon. These compounds are mainly substituted galactosides, where the glucose moiety of lactose is replaced by another chemical group.

- Isopropyl-β-D-thiogalactoside (IPTG) is frequently used as an inducer of the *lac* operon for physiological work.IPTG binds to repressor and inactivates it, but is not a substrate for β-galactosidase. One advantage of IPTG for *in vivo* studies is that since it cannot be metabolized by *E. coli* its concentration remains constant and the rate of expression of *lac p/o*-controlled genes, is not a variable in the experiment. IPTG intake is dependent on the action of lactose permease in *P. fluorescens*, but not in *E. coli*.

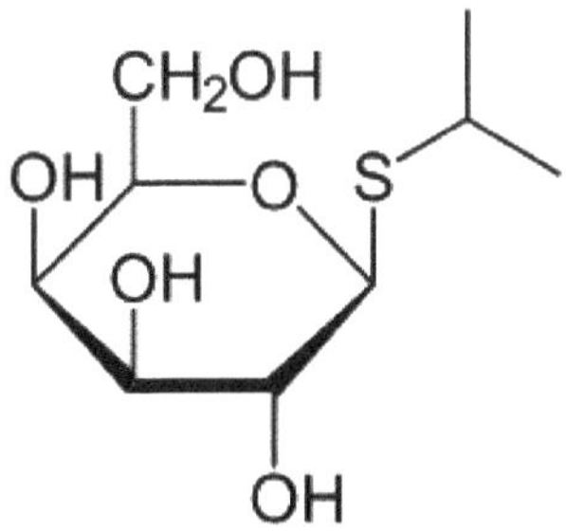

- Phenyl-β-D-galactose (phenyl-Gal) is a substrate for β-galactosidase, but does not inactivate repressor and so is not an inducer. Since wild type cells produce very little β-galactosidase, they cannot grow on phenyl-Gal as a carbon and energy source. Mutants lacking represso r are able to grow on phenyl-Gal. Thus, minimal medium containing only phenyl-Gal as a source of carbon and energy is selective for repressor mutants and operator mutants. If 10^8 cells of a wild type strain are plated on agar plates containing phenyl-Gal, the rare colonies which grow are mainly spontaneous mutants affecting the repressor. The relative distribution of repressor and operator mutants is affected by the target size. Since the *lacI gene* encoding repressor is about 50 times larger than the operator, repressor mutants predominate in the selection.

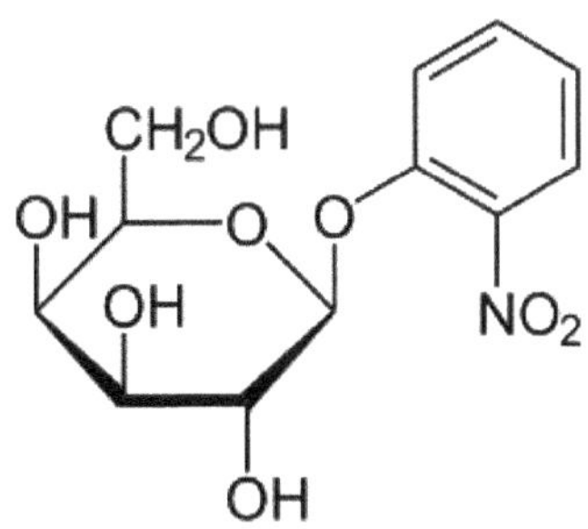

- Other compounds serve as colorful indicators of β-galactosidase activity.
    - ONPG is cleaved to produce the intensely yellow compound, orthonitrophenol, and is commonly used as a substrate for assay of β-galactosidase *in vitro*.
    - Colonies that produce β-galactosidase are turned blue by X-gal (5-bromo-4-chloro-3-indolyl-β-D-galactoside).

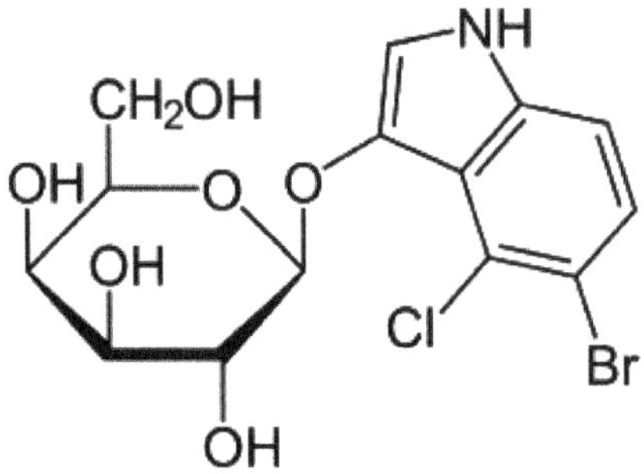

- Allolactose is an isomer of lactose and is the inducer of the lac operon. Lactose is galactose-(β1->4)-glucose, whereas allolactose is galactose-(β1->6)-glucose. Lactose is converted to allolactose by β-galactosidase in an alternative reaction to the hydrolytic one. A physiological experiment which demonstrates the role of LacZ in production of the «true» inducer in *E. coli* cells is the observation that a null mutant of *lacZ* can still produce LacY permease when grown with IPTG but not when grown with lactose. The explanation is that processing of lactose to allolactose (catalyzed by β-galactosidase) is needed to produce the inducer inside the cell.

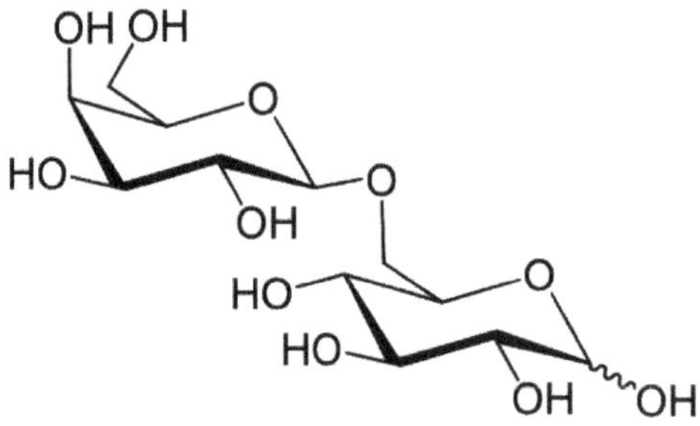

Development of the Classic Model

The experimental microorganism used by François Jacob and Jacques Monod was the common laboratory bacterium, E. coli, but many of the basic regulatory concepts that were discovered by Jacob and Monod are fundamental to cellular regulation in all organisms. The key idea is that proteins are not synthesized when they are not needed--- E. coli conserves cellular resources and energy by not making the three Lac proteins when there is no need to metabolize lactose, such as when other sugars like glucose are available. The following section discusses how E. coli controls certain genes in response to metabolic needs.

During World War II, Monod was testing the effects of combinations of sugars as nutrient sources for E. coli and B. subtilis. Monod was following up on similar studies that had been conducted by other scientists with bacteria and yeast. He found that bacteria grown with two different sugars often displayed two phases of growth. For example, if glucose and lactose were both provided, glucose was metabolized first (growth phase I, see Figure 2) and then lactose (growth phase II). Lactose was not metabolized during the first part of the diauxic growth curve because β-galactosidase was not made when both glucose and lactose were present in the medium. Monod named this phenomenon diauxie.

Monod then focused his attention on the induction of β-galactosidase formation that occurred when lactose was the sole sugar in the culture medium.

Classification of Regulatory Mutants

A conceptual breakthrough of Jacob and Monod was to recognize the distinction between regulatory substances and sites where they act to change gene expression. A former soldier, Jacob used the analogy of a bomber that would release its lethal cargo upon receipt of a special radio transmission or signal. A working system requires both a ground transmitter and a receiver in the airplane. Now, suppose that the usual transmitter is broken. This system can be made to work by introduction of a second, functional transmitter. In contrast, he said, consider a bomber with a defective receiver. The behavior of this bomber cannot be changed by introduction of a second, functional aeroplane.

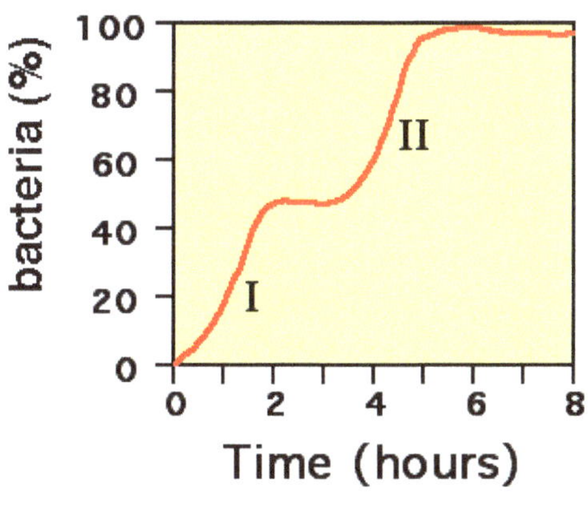

Figure 2: Monod's "bi-phasic" growth curve

To analyze regulatory mutants of the lac operon, Jacob developed a system by which a second copy of the lac genes (lacI with its promoter, and lacZYA with promoter and operator) could be introduced into a single cell. A culture of such bacteria, which are diploid for the lac genes but otherwise normal, is then tested for the regulatory phenotype. In particular, it is determined whether LacZ and LacY are made even in the absence of IPTG (due to the lactose repressor produced by the mutant gene being non-functional). This experiment, in which genes or gene clusters are tested pairwise, is called a complementation test.

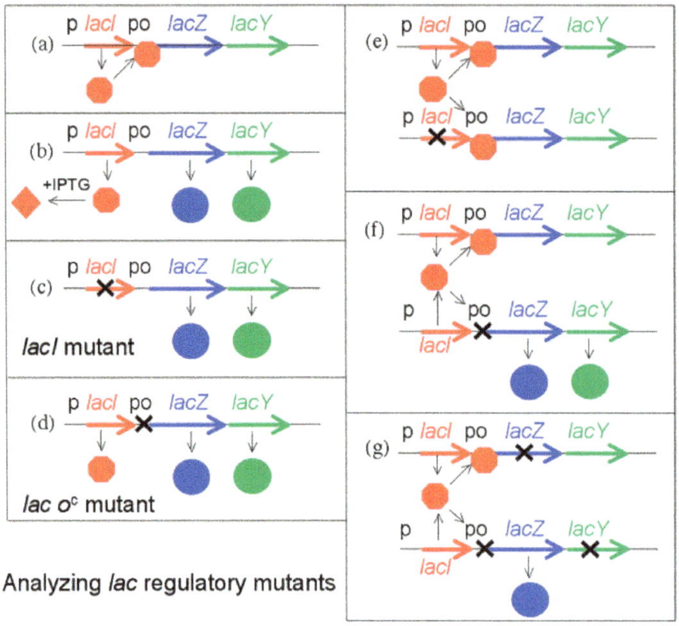

Analyzing *lac* regulatory mutants

This test is illustrated in the figure (lacA is omitted for simplicity). First, certain haploid states are shown (i.e. the cell carries only a single copy of the lac genes). Panel (a) shows repression, (b) shows induction by IPTG, and (c) and (d) show the effect of a mutation to the lacI gene or to the operator, respectively. In panel (e) the complementation test for repressor is shown. If one copy of the lac genes carries a mutation in lacI, but the second copy is wild type for lacI, the resulting phenotype is normal---but lacZ is expressed when exposed to inducer IPTG. Mutations affecting repressor are said to be recessive to wild type (and that wild type is dominant), and this is explained by the fact that repressor is a small protein which can diffuse in the cell. The copy of the lac operon adjacent to the defective lacI gene is effectively shut off by protein produced from the second copy of lacI.

If the same experiment is carried out using an operator mutation, a different result is obtained (panel (f)). The phenotype of a cell carrying one mutant and one wild type operator site is that LacZ and LacY are produced even in the absence of the inducer IPTG; because the damaged operator site, does not permit binding of the repressor to inhibit transcription of the structural genes. The operator mutation is dominant. When the operator site where repressor must bind is damaged by mutation, the presence of a second functional site in the same cell makes no difference to expression of genes controlled by the mutant site.

A more sophisticated version of this experiment uses marked operons to distinguish between the two copies of the lac genes and show that the unregulated structural gene(s) is(are) the one(s) next to the mutant operator (panel (g). For example, suppose that one copy is marked by a mutation inactivating lacZ so that it can only produce the LacY protein, while the second copy carries a mutation affecting lacY and can only produce LacZ. In this version, only the copy of the lac operon that is adjacent to the mutant operator is expressed without IPTG. We say that the operator mutation is cis-dominant, it is dominant to wild type but affects only the copy of the operon which is immediately adjacent to it.

This explanation is misleading in an important sense, because it proceeds from a description of the experiment and then explains the results in terms of a model. But in fact, it is often true that the model comes first, and an experiment is fashioned specifically to test the model. Jacob and Monod first imagined that there must be a site in DNA with the properties of the operator, and then designed their complementation tests to show this.

The dominance of operator mutants also suggests a procedure to select them specifically. If regulatory mutants are selected from a culture of wild type using phenyl-Gal, as described above, operator mutations are rare compared to repressor mutants because the target-size is so small. But if instead we start with a strain which carries two copies of the whole lac region (that is diploid for lac), the repressor mutations (which still occur) are not recovered because complementation by the second, wild type lacI gene confers a wild type phenotype. In contrast, mutation of one copy of the operator confers a mutant phenotype because it is dominant to the second, wild type copy.

Regulation by cyclic AMP

Explanation of diauxie depended on the characterization of additional mutations affecting the lac genes other than those explained by the classical model. Two other genes, cya and crp, subsequently were identified that mapped far from lac, and that, when mutated, result in a decreased level of expression in the presence of IPTG and even in strains of the bacterium lacking the repressor or operator. The discovery of cAMP in E. coli led to the demonstration that mutants defective the cya gene but not the crp gene could be restored to full activity by the addition of cAMP to the medium.

The cya gene encodes adenylate cyclase, which produces cAMP. In a cya mutant, the absence of cAMP makes the expression of the lacZYA genes more than ten times lower than normal. Addition of cAMP corrects the low Lac expression characteristic of cya mutants. The second gene, crp, encodes a protein called catabolite activator protein (CAP) or cAMP receptor protein (CRP).

However the lactose metabolism enzymes are made in small quantities in the presence of both glucose and lactose (sometimes called leaky expression) due to the fact that the LacI repressor rapidly associates/dissociates from the DNA rather than tightly binding to it, which can allow time for RNAP to bind and transcribe mRNAs of lacZYA. Leaky expression is necessary in order to allow for metabolism of some lactose after the glucose source is expended, but before lac expression is fully activated.

In summary:

- When lactose is absent then there is very little Lac enzyme production (the operator has Lac repressor bound to it).
- When lactose is present but a preferred carbon source (like glucose) is also present then a small amount of enzyme is produced (Lac repressor is not bound to the operator).
- When glucose is absent, CAP-cAMP binds to a specific DNA site upstream of the promoter and makes a direct protein-protein interaction with RNAP that

facilitates the binding of RNAP to the promoter.

The delay between growth phases reflects the time needed to produce sufficient quantities of lactose-metabolizing enzymes. First, the CAP regulatory protein has to assemble on the lac promoter, resulting in an increase in the production of lac mRNA. More available copies of the lac mRNA results in the production (see translation) of significantly more copies of LacZ (β-galactosidase, for lactose metabolism) and LacY (lactose permease to transport lactose into the cell). After a delay needed to increase the level of the lactose metabolizing enzymes, the bacteria enter into a new rapid phase of cell growth.

The *lac* Operon and its Control Elements

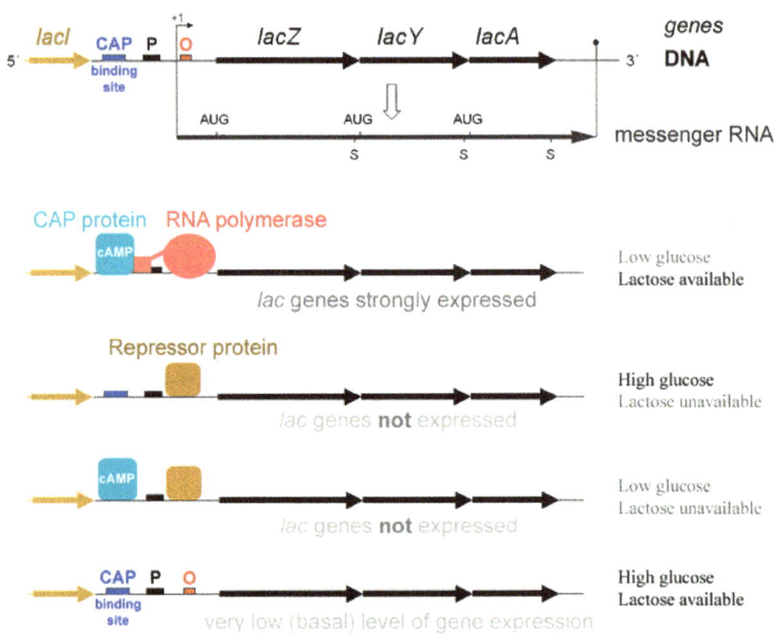

lac operon in detail

Two puzzles of catabolite repression relate to how cAMP levels are coupled to the presence of glucose, and secondly, why the cells should even bother. After lactose is cleaved it actually forms glucose and galactose (easily converted to glucose). In metabolic terms, lactose is just as good a carbon and energy source as glucose. The cAMP level is related not to intracellular glucose concentration but to the rate of glucose transport, which influences the activity of adenylate cyclase. (In addition, glucose transport also leads to direct inhibition of the lactose permease.) As to why E. coli works this way, one can only speculate. All enteric bacteria ferment glucose, which suggests they encounter it frequently. It is possible that a small difference in efficiency of transport or metabolism of glucose v. lactose makes it advantageous for cells to regulate the lac operon in this way.

Use in Molecular Biology

The lac gene and its derivatives are amenable to use as a reporter gene in a number of bacterial-based selection techniques such as two hybrid analysis, in which the successful binding of a transcriptional activator to a specific promoter sequence must be determined. In LB plates containing X-gal, the colour change from white colonies to a shade of blue corresponds to about 20-100 β-galactosidase units, while tetrazolium lactose and MacConkey lactose media have a range of 100-1000 units, being most sensitive in the high and low parts of this range respectively.Since MacConkey lactose and tetrazolium lactose media both rely on the products of lactose breakdown, they require the presence of both lacZ and lacY genes. The many lac fusion techniques which include only the lacZ gene are thus suited to X-gal plates or ONPG liquid broths.

CATABOLITE REPRESSION

Carbon catabolite repression, or simply catabolite repression, is an important part of global control system of various bacteria and other micro-organisms. Catabolite repression allows micro-organisms to adapt quickly to a preferred (rapidly metabolisable) carbon and energy source first. This is usually achieved through inhibition of synthesis of enzymes involved in catabolism of carbon sources other than the preferred one. The catabolite repression was first shown to be initiated by glucose and therefore sometimes referred to as the glucose effect. However, the term «glucose effect» is actually a misnomer since other carbon sources are known to induce catabolite repression.

Escherichia coli

Catabolite repression was extensively studied in Escherichia coli. E. coli grows faster on glucose than on any other carbon source. For example, if E. coli is placed on an agar plate containing only glucose and lactose, the bacteria will use glucose first and lactose second. When glucose is available in the environment, the synthesis of β-galactosidase is under repression due to the effect of catabolite repression caused by glucose. The catabolite repression in this case is achieved through the utilization of phosphotransferase system.

An important enzyme from the phosphotranferase system called Enzyme II A (EIIA) plays a central role in this mechanism. There are different catabolite-specific EIIA in a single cell, even though different bacterial groups have specificities to different sets of catabolites. In enteric bacteria one of the EIIA enzymes in their set is specific for glucose transport only. When glucose levels are high inside the bacteria, EIIA mostly exists in its unphosphorylated form. This leads to inhibition of adenylyl cyclase and lactose permease, therefore cAMP levels are low and lactose can not be transported inside the bacteria.

Once the glucose is all used up, the second preferred carbon source (i.e. lactose) has to be used by bacteria. Absence of glucose will «turn off» catabolite repression. When glucose levels are low the phosphorylated form of EIIA accumulates and consequently activates the enzyme adenylyl cyclase, which will produce high levels of cAMP. cAMP binds to catabolite activator protein (CAP) and together they will bind to a promoter sequence on the lac operon. However, this is not enough for the lactose genes to be transcribed. Lactose must be present inside the cell to remove the lactose repressor from the operator sequence (transcriptional regulation). When these two conditions are satisfied, it means for the bacteria that glucose is absent and lactose is available. Next, bacteria start to transcribe the lac operon and produce β-galactosidase enzymes for lactose metabolism. The example above is a simplification of a complex process. Catabolite repression is considered to be a part of global control system and therefore it affects more genes rather than just lactose gene transcription.

Bacillus Subtilis

Gram positive bacteria such as Bacillus subtilis have a cAMP-independent catabolite repression mechanism controlled by catabolite control protein A (CcpA). In this alternative pathway CcpA negatively represses other sugar operons so they are off in the presence of glucose. It works by the fact that Hpr is phosphorylated by a specific mechanism, when glucose enters through the cell membrane protein EIIC, and when Hpr is phosphoralated it can then allow CcpA to block transcription of the alternative sugar pathway operons at their respective cre sequence binding sites. Note that E. coli has a similar cAMP-independent catabolite repression mechanism that utilizes a protein called catabolite repressor activator (Cra).

REFERENCES

1. "Archaea". Microbe WORLD. Microbe WORLD. Retrieved 8 November 2015.
2. "Bacterial genetics". Nature. Macmillan Publishers Limmited. Retrieved 8 November 2015.
3. "Fungal Genetics". Nature.com. Macmillan Publishers Limited. Retrieved 9 November 2015.
4. "Induction of the lac operon in E. coli" (PDF). SAPS. Retrieved 29 June 2016.
5. "Microbial genetics". Nature. Nature Publishing Group, A division of Macmillan Publishers Limmited. Retrieved 2015-09-24.
6. "Microbial Genetics". World Of Micorbiology and Immunology. 2003. Retrieved 9 November 2015.
7. "Milestone 2 - A visionary pair : Nature Milestones in gene expression". www.nature.com. Retrieved 2015-12-27.
8. "ONPG (β-Galactosidase) test". September 2000.
9. Ajon M, Fröls S, van Wolferen M, Stoecker K, Teichmann D, Driessen AJ, Grogan DW, Albers SV, Schleper C (2011). "UV-inducible DNA exchange in hyperthermophilic archaea mediated by type IV pili". Mol. Microbiol. 82 (4): 807–17. doi:10.1111/j.1365-2958.2011.07861.x. PMID 21999488.
10. Avery OT, MacLeod CM, McCarty M (1979). "Studies on the chemical nature of the substance inducing transformation of pneumococcal types. Inductions of transformation by a desoxyribonucleic acid fraction isolated from pneumococcus

type III". J. Exp. Med. 149 (2): 297–326. doi:10.1084/jem.149.2.297. PMC 2184805Freely accessible. PMID 33226.

11. Bainbridge, B.W. (1987). Genetics of microbes (2nd ed.). Glasgow: Blackie. ISBN 0-412-01281-2.
12. Beadle GW, Tatum EL (1941). "Genetic Control of Biochemical Reactions in Neurospora". Proc. Natl. Acad. Sci. U.S.A. 27 (11): 499–506. PMC 1078370Freely accessible. PMID 16588492.
13. Benzer S (1959). "On The Topology Of The Genetic Fine Structure". Proc. Natl. Acad. Sci. U.S.A. 45 (11): 1607–20. PMC 222769Freely accessible. PMID 16590553.
14. Bernstein C (1981). "Deoxyribonucleic acid repair in bacteriophage". Microbiol. Rev. 45 (1): 72–98. PMC 281499Freely accessible. PMID 6261109.
15. Bernstein H and Bernstein C (2013). Evolutionary Origin and Adaptive Function of Meiosis. In Meiosis: Bernstein C and Bernstein H, editors. ISBN 978-953-51-1197-9, InTech, http://www.intechopen.com/books/meiosis/evolutionary-origin-and-adaptive-function-of-meiosis
16. Birdsell JA, Wills C (2003). The evolutionary origin and maintenance of sexual recombination: A review of contemporary models. Evolutionary Biology Series >> Evolutionary Biology, Vol. 33 pp. 27-137. MacIntyre, Ross J.; Clegg, Michael, T (Eds.), Springer. Hardcover ISBN 978-0306472619, ISBN 0306472619 Softcover ISBN 978-1-4419-3385-0.
17. Busby S., Ebright RH. (2001). "Transcription activation by catabolite activator protein (CAP)". J. Mol. Biol. 293: 199–213. doi:10.1006/jmbi.1999.3161. PMID 10550204.
18. Chambers, Cecilia R.; Patrick, Wayne M. (2015). "Archaeal Nucleic Acid Ligases and Their Potential in Biotechnology". Archaea. 2015: 1–10. doi:10.1155/2015/170571.
19. Chen D, Bernstein C (1987). "Recombinational repair of hydrogen peroxide-induced damages in DNA of phage T4". Mutat. Res. 184 (2): 87–98. doi:10.1016/0167-8817(87)90064-2. PMID 3627145.
20. Chen I, Dubnau D (2004). "DNA uptake during bacterial transformation". Nat. Rev. Microbiol. 2 (3): 241–9. doi:10.1038/nrmicro844. PMID 15083159.
21. Crick Fh, Barnett L, Brenner S, Watts-Tobin Rj (1961). "General nature of the genetic code for proteins". Nature. 192: 1227–32. doi:10.1038/1921227a0. PMID 13882203.
22. Deutscher, Josef (April 2008). "The mechanisms of carbon catabolite repression in bacteria". Current Opinion in Microbiology. 11 (2): 87–93. doi:10.1016/j.mib.2008.02.007. ISSN 1369-5274. PMID 18359269.
23. Dyer PS, O'Gorman CM (2012). "Sexual development and cryptic sexuality in fungi: insights from Aspergillus species". FEMS Microbiol. Rev. 36 (1): 165–92. doi:10.1111/j.1574-6976.2011.00308.x. PMID 22091779.

24. Elvira Hörandl (2013). Meiosis and the Paradox of Sex in Nature, Meiosis, ISBN 978-953-51-1197-9, InTech, DOI: 10.5772/56542. Available from: http://www.intechopen.com/books/meiosis/meiosis-and-the-paradox-of-sex-in-nature
25. Fröls S, Ajon M, Wagner M, Teichmann D, Zolghadr B, Folea M, Boekema EJ, Driessen AJ, Schleper C, Albers SV (2008). "UV-inducible cellular aggregation of the hyperthermophilic archaeon Sulfolobus solfataricus is mediated by pili formation". Mol. Microbiol. 70 (4): 938–52. doi:10.1111/j.1365-2958.2008.06459.x. PMID 18990182.
26. Fröls S, White MF, Schleper C (2009). "Reactions to UV damage in the model archaeon Sulfolobus solfataricus". Biochem. Soc. Trans. 37 (Pt 1): 36–41. doi:10.1042/BST0370036. PMID 19143598.
27. Gest, Hau (22 May 2004). "The discovery of microorganisms by Robert Hooke and Antoni van Leeuwenhoek, Fellows of The Royal Society". The Royal Society. 58: 137–201. doi:10.1098/rsnr.2004.0055. PMID 15209075. Retrieved 2015-09-25.
28. Gilley D, Blackburn EH (1994). "Lack of telomere shortening during senescence in Paramecium". Proc. Natl. Acad. Sci. U.S.A. 91 (5): 1955–8. doi:10.1073/pnas.91.5.1955. PMC 43283Freely accessible. PMID 8127914.
29. Görke B, Stülke J (August 2008). "Carbon catabolite repression in bacteria: many ways to make the most out of nutrients". Nature Reviews. Microbiology. 6 (8): 613–24. doi:10.1038/nrmicro1932. PMID 18628769.
30. Gray TA, Krywy JA, Harold J, Palumbo MJ, Derbyshire KM (2013). "Distributive conjugal transfer in mycobacteria generates progeny with meiotic-like genome-wide mosaicism, allowing mapping of a mating identity locus". PLoS Biol. 11 (7): e1001602. doi:10.1371/journal.pbio.1001602. PMC 3706393Freely accessible. PMID 23874149.
31. Hansen LH, Knudsen S, Sørensen SJ (June 1998). "The effect of the lacY gene on the induction of IPTG inducible promoters, studied in Escherichia coli and Pseudomonas fluorescens". Curr. Microbiol. 36 (6): 341–7. doi:10.1007/s002849900320. PMID 9608745.
32. Hershey Ad, Chase M (1952). "Independent functions of viral protein and nucleic acid in growth of bacteriophage". J. Gen. Physiol. 36 (1): 39–56. doi:10.1085/jgp.36.1.39. PMC 2147348Freely accessible. PMID 12981234.
33. Herskowitz I (1988). "Life cycle of the budding yeast Saccharomyces cerevisiae". Microbiol. Rev. 52 (4): 536–53. PMC 373162Freely accessible. PMID 3070323.
34. Holmes GE, Holmes NR (1986). "Accumulation of DNA damages in aging Paramecium tetraurelia". Mol. Gen. Genet. 204 (1): 108–14. doi:10.1007/bf00330196. PMID 3091993.
35. Horowitz NH, Berg P, Singer M, Lederberg J, Susman M, Doebley J, Crow JF (2004). "A centennial: George W. Beadle, 1903-1989". Genetics. 166 (1): 1–10. doi:10.1534/genetics.166.1.1. PMC 1470705Freely accessible. PMID 15020400.
36. Jacob F, Monod J (1961). "Genetic regulatory mechanisms in the synthesis of proteins". J. Mol. Biol. 3: 318–56. PMID 13718526.

37. Jacob F.; Monod J (June 1961). "Genetic regulatory mechanisms in the synthesis of proteins". J Mol Biol. 3 (3): 318–56. doi:10.1016/S0022-2836(61)80072-7. PMID 13718526.

38. Johnsborg O, Eldholm V, Håvarstein LS (2007). "Natural genetic transformation: prevalence, mechanisms and function". Res. Microbiol. 158 (10): 767–78. doi:10.1016/j.resmic.2007.09.004. PMID 17997281.

39. Johnson A (2003). "The biology of mating in Candida albicans". Nat. Rev. Microbiol. 1 (2): 106–16. doi:10.1038/nrmicro752. PMID 15035040.

40. Joung J, Ramm E, Pabo C (2000). "A bacterial two-hybrid selection system for studying protein–DNA and protein–protein interactions". Proc Natl Acad Sci USA. 97 (13): 7382–7. doi:10.1073/pnas.110149297. PMC 16554Freely accessible. PMID 10852947.

41. Kennell, David; Riezman, Howard (July 1977). "Transcription and translation initiation frequencies of the Escherichia coli lac operon". Journal of Molecular Biology. 114 (1): 1–21. doi:10.1016/0022-2836(77)90279-0.

42. Madigan, M. T., J. M. Martinko, P. V. Dunlap, and D. P. Clark. Brock biology of microorganisms. 12th ed. San Francisco, CA: Pearson/Benjamin Cummings, 2009.

43. Malan, T. Philip; Kolb, Annie; Buc, Henri; McClure, William (December 1984). "Mechanism of CRP-cAMP Activation of lac Operon Transcription Initiation Activation of the P1 Promoter". J. Mol. Biol. 180: 881–909. doi:10.1016/0022-2836(84)90262-6. PMID 6098691.

44. McKnight, Steven L. (1992). Transcriptional Regulation. Cold Spring Harbor, NY: Cold Spring Harbor Laboratory Press. pp. 3–24. ISBN 0-87969-410-6.

45. Michod RE, Bernstein H, Nedelcu AM (2008). "Adaptive value of sex in microbial pathogens". Infect. Genet. Evol. 8 (3): 267–85. doi:10.1016/j.meegid.2008.01.002. PMID 18295550.

46. Michod RE, Bernstein H, Nedelcu AM (May 2008). "Adaptive value of sex in microbial pathogens". Infection, Genetics and Evolution. 8 (3): 267–85. doi:10.1016/j.meegid.2008.01.002. PMID 18295550.http://www.hummingbirds.arizona.edu/Faculty/Michod/Downloads/IGE%20review%20sex.pdf

47. Mortlock, Robert (2013). Microorganisms As Model Systems for Studying Evolution. Springer Verlag. p. 2. ISBN 978-1-4684-4846-7.

48. Muller-Hill, Benno (1996). The lac Operon, a Short History of a Genetic Paradigm. Berlin: Walter de Gruyter. pp. 7–10. ISBN 3-11-014830-7.

49. Murphy, Cormac D. (2 September 2014). "Drug metabolism in microorganisms". Biotechnology Letters. 37 (1): 19–28. doi:10.1007/s10529-014-1653-8.

50. Oehler, S.; Eismann, E. R.; Krämer, H.; Müller-Hill, B. (1990). "The three operators of the lac operon cooperate in repression". The EMBO Journal. 9 (4): 973–979. PMC 551766Freely accessible. PMID 2182324.

51. Paoletti M, Seymour FA, Alcocer MJ, Kaur N, Calvo AM, Archer DB, Dyer PS (2007). "Mating type and the genetic basis of self-fertility in the model fungus

Aspergillus nidulans". Curr. Biol. 17 (16): 1384–9. doi:10.1016/j.cub.2007.07.012. PMID 17669651.

52. Prescott DM (1994). "The DNA of ciliated protozoa". Microbiol. Rev. 58 (2): 233–67. PMC 372963Freely accessible. PMID 8078435.

53. Raoult, Didier; Forterre, Patrick (3 March 2008). "Redefining viruses: lessons from Mimivirus". Nature Reviews Microbiology. 6 (4): 315–319. doi:10.1038/nrmicro1858.

54. Rosenshine I, Tchelet R, Mevarech M (1989). "The mechanism of DNA transfer in the mating system of an archaebacterium". Science. 245 (4924): 1387–9. doi:10.1126/science.2818746. PMID 2818746.

55. Ruderfer DM, Pratt SC, Seidel HS, Kruglyak L (2006). "Population genomic analysis of outcrossing and recombination in yeast". Nat. Genet. 38 (9): 1077–81. doi:10.1038/ng1859. PMID 16892060.

56. Seiboth, Bernhard; Ivanova, Christa; Seidl-Seiboth, Verena (September 15, 2011). "Chapter 13: Trichoderma reesei: A Fungal Enzyme Producer for Cellulosic Biofuels". In Dos Santos Bernardes, Marco Aurélio. Biofuel Production-Recent Developments and Prospects. InTech. p. 321. doi:10.5772/16848. ISBN 978-953-307-478-8.

57. Seto, Donald (30 November 2010). "Viral Genomics and Bioinformatics". Viruses. 2 (12): 2587–2593. doi:10.3390/v2122587.

58. Smith-Sonneborn J (1979). "DNA repair and longevity assurance in Paramecium tetraurelia". Science. 203 (4385): 1115–7. doi:10.1126/science.424739. PMID 424739.

59. Terpe, Kay (1 November 2013). "Overview of thermostable DNA polymerases for classical PCR applications: from molecular and biochemical fundamentals to commercial systems". Applied Microbiology and Biotechnology. 97 (24): 10243–10254. doi:10.1007/s00253-013-5290-2

60. Vazquez A, Beg QK, Demenezes MA, et al. (2008). "Impact of the solvent capacity constraint on E. coli metabolism". BMC Syst Biol. 2: 7. doi:10.1186/1752-0509-2-7. PMC 2270259Freely accessible. PMID 18215292.

61. von Hippel, P.H.; Revzin, A.; Gross, C.A.; Wang, A.C. (December 1974). "Non-specific DNA binding of genome regulating proteins as a biological control mechanism: I. The lac operon: equilibrium aspects". PNAS. 71 (12): 4808–12. doi:10.1073/pnas.71.12.4808. PMC 433986Freely accessible. PMID 4612528.

62. Weeks, Benjamin S. (2012). Alcamo's microbes and society (3rd ed.). Sudbury, MA: Jones & Bartlett Learning. ISBN 978-0-7637-9064-6.

CHAPTER 6

Theory of Bacteriophage

Chapter Contents

- **Introduction**
- **Replication**
- **DNA Virus**
- **Phage Ecology**

Bacteriophage is a virus which infects bacteria.These are obligate intracellular parasites that multiply inside bacteria by making use of some or all of the host biosynthetic machinery. Like all viruses, phages are simple organisms that consist of a core of genetic material (nucleic acid) surrounded by a protein capsid. The nucleic acid may be either DNA or RNA and may be double-stranded or single-stranded.

INTRODUCTION

A bacteriophage is a virus that infects and replicates within a bacterium. The term is derived from bacteria and the Greek: φαγεῖν (phagein), "to devour". Bacteriophages are composed of proteins that encapsulate a DNA or RNA genome, and may have relatively simple or elaborate structures. Their genomes may encode as few as four genes, and as many as hundreds of genes. Phages replicate within the bacterium following the injection of their genome into its cytoplasm. Bacteriophages are among the most common and diverse entities in the biosphere.

Phages are widely distributed in locations populated by bacterial hosts, such as soil or the intestines of animals. One of the densest natural sources for phages and other viruses is sea water, where up to 9×10^8 virions per milliliter have been found in microbial mats at the surface, and up to 70% of marine bacteria may be infected by phages. They have been used for over 90 years as an alternative to antibiotics in the former Soviet Union and Central Europe, as well as in France. They are seen as a possible therapy against multi-drug-resistant strains of many bacteria (see phage therapy). Nevertheless, phages of Inoviridae have been shown to complicate biofilms involved in pneumonia and cystic fibrosis, shelter the bacteria from drugs meant to eradicate disease and promote persistent infection.

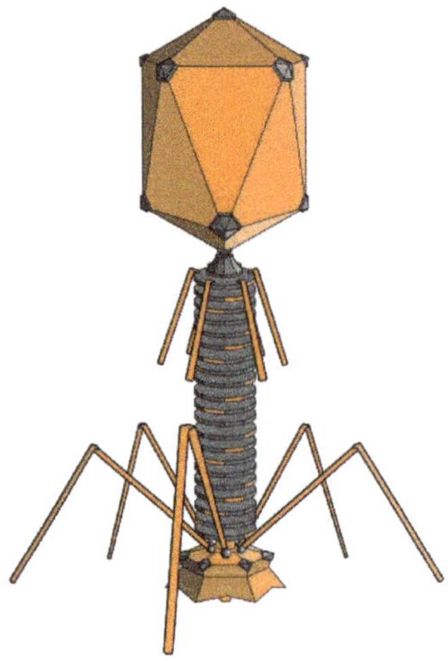

structure of a typical myovirus bacteriophage

Classification

Bacteriophages occur abundantly in the biosphere, with different virions, genomes, and lifestyles. Phages are classified by the International Committee on Taxonomy of Viruses (ICTV) according to morphology and nucleic acid.

Nineteen families are currently recognized by the ICTV that infect bacteria and archaea. Of these, only two families have RNA genomes, and only five families are enveloped. Of the viral families with DNA genomes, only two have single-stranded genomes. Eight of the viral families with DNA genomes have circular genomes while nine have linear genomes. Nine families infect bacteria only, nine infect archaea only, and one (Tectiviridae) infects both bacteria and archaea.

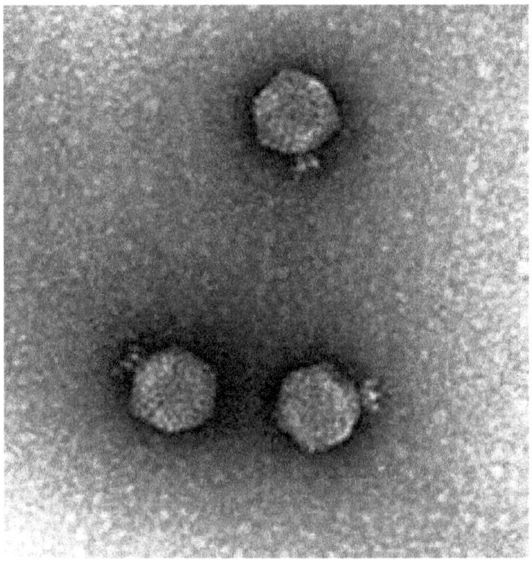

Bacteriophage P22, a member of the *Podoviridae* by morphology due to its short, non-contractile tail.

ICTV classification of prokaryotic (bacterial and archaeal) viruses

Order	Family	Morphology	Nucleic acid	Examples
Caudovirales	*Myoviridae*	Nonenveloped, contractile tail	Linear dsDNA	T4 phage, Mu, PBSX, P1Puna-like, P2, I3, Bcep 1, Bcep 43, Bcep 78
	Siphoviridae	Nonenveloped, noncontractile tail (long)	Linear dsDNA	λ phage, T5 phage, phi, C2, L5, HK97, N15
	Podoviridae	Nonenveloped, noncontractile tail (short)	Linear dsDNA	T7 phage, T3 phage, Φ29, P22, P37
Ligamenvirales	*Lipothrixviridae*	Enveloped, rod-shaped	Linear dsDNA	Acidianus filamentous virus 1
	Rudiviridae	Nonenveloped, rod-shaped	Linear dsDNA	Sulfolobus islandicus rod-shaped virus 1

Unassigned	*Ampullaviridae*	Enveloped, bottle-shaped	Linear dsDNA	
	Bicaudaviridae	Nonenveloped, lemon-shaped	Circular dsDNA	
	Clavaviridae	Nonenveloped, rod-shaped	Circular dsDNA	
	Corticoviridae	Nonenveloped, isometric	Circular dsDNA	
	Cystoviridae	Enveloped, spherical	Segmented dsRNA	
	Fuselloviridae	Nonenveloped, lemon-shaped	Circular dsDNA	
	Globuloviridae	Enveloped, isometric	Linear dsDNA	
	Guttaviridae	Nonenveloped, ovoid	Circular dsDNA	
	Inoviridae	Nonenveloped, filamentous	Circular ssDNA	M13
	Leviviridae	Nonenveloped, isometric	Linear ssRNA	MS2, Qβ
	Microviridae	Nonenveloped, isometric	Circular ssDNA	ΦX174
	Plasmaviridae	Enveloped, pleomorphic	Circular dsDNA	
	Tectiviridae	Nonenveloped, isometric	Linear dsDNA	

In 1896, Ernest Hanbury Hankin reported that something in the waters of the Ganges and Yamuna rivers in India had marked antibacterial action against cholera and could pass through a very fine porcelain filter. In 1915, British bacteriologist Frederick Twort, superintendent of the Brown Institution of London, discovered a small agent that infected and killed bacteria. He believed the agent must be one of the following:

- a stage in the life cycle of the bacteria;
- an enzyme produced by the bacteria themselves; or
- a virus that grew on and destroyed the bacteria

Twort›s work was interrupted by the onset of World War I and shortage of funding. Independently, French-Canadian microbiologist Félix d›Hérelle, working at the Pasteur Institute in Paris, announced on 3 September 1917, that he had discovered an invisible, antagonistic microbe of the dysentery bacillus". For d'Hérelle, there was no question as to the nature of his discovery: "In a flash I had understood: what caused my clear spots was in fact an invisible microbe … a virus parasitic on bacteria." D'Hérelle called the virus a bacteriophage or bacteria-eater (from the Greek phagein meaning to eat). He also recorded a dramatic account of a man suffering from dysentery who was restored to good health by the bacteriophages. It was D'Herelle who conducted much research into bacteriophages and introduced the concept of phage therapy.

In 1969, Max Delbrück, Alfred Hershey and Salvador Luria were awarded the Nobel Prize in Physiology and Medicine for their discoveries of the replication of viruses and their genetic structure.

Phage Therapy

Main article: Phage therapy

Phages were discovered to be antibacterial agents and were used in the former Soviet Republic of Georgia (pioneered there by Giorgi Eliava with help from the co-discoverer of bacteriophages, Felix d'Herelle) and the United States during the 1920s and 1930s for treating bacterial infections. They had widespread use, including treatment of soldiers in the Red Army. However, they were abandoned for general use in the West for several reasons:

- Medical trials were carried out, but a basic lack of understanding of phages made these invalid.
- Antibiotics were discovered and marketed widely. They were easier to make, store and to prescribe.
- Former Soviet research continued, but publications were mainly in Russian or Georgian languages and were unavailable internationally for many years.
- Clinical trials evaluating the antibacterial efficacy of bacteriophage preparations were conducted without proper controls and were methodologically incomplete preventing the formulation of important conclusions.

Their use has continued since the end of the Cold War in Georgia and elsewhere in Central and Eastern Europe. Globalyz Biotech is an international joint venture that commercializes bacteriophage treatment and its various applications across the globe. The company has successfully used bacteriophages in administering phage therapy to patients suffering from bacterial infections, including Staphylococcus (including MRSA), Streptococcus, Pseudomonas, Salmonella, skin and soft tissue, gastrointestinal, respiratory, and orthopedic infections. In 1923, the Eliava Institute was opened in Tbilisi, Georgia, to research this new science and put it into practice.

The first regulated, randomized, double-blind clinical trial was reported in the Journal of Wound Care in June 2009, which evaluated the safety and efficacy of a bacteriophage cocktail to treat infected venous leg ulcers in human patients. The FDA approved the study as a Phase I clinical trial. The study›s results demonstrated the safety of therapeutic application of bacteriophages but did not show efficacy. The authors explain that the use of certain chemicals that are part of standard wound care (e.g. lactoferrin or silver) may have interfered with bacteriophage viability. Another controlled clinical trial in Western Europe (treatment of ear infections caused by Pseudomonas aeruginosa) was reported shortly after in the journal Clinical Otolaryngology in August 2009. The study concludes that bacteriophage preparations were safe and effective for treatment of chronic ear infections in humans. Additionally, there have been numerous animal and other experimental clinical trials evaluating the efficacy of bacteriophages for various diseases, such as infected burns and wounds, and cystic fibrosis associated lung infections, among others. Meanwhile, bacteriophage researchers are developing engineered viruses to overcome antibiotic resistance, and engineering the phage genes responsible for coding enzymes which degrade the biofilm matrix, phage structural proteins and also enzymes responsible for lysis of bacterial cell wall.

D'Herelle "quickly learned that bacteriophages are found wherever bacteria thrive: in sewers, in rivers that catch waste runoff from pipes, and in the stools of convalescent patients." This includes rivers traditionally thought to have healing powers, including India's Ganges River.

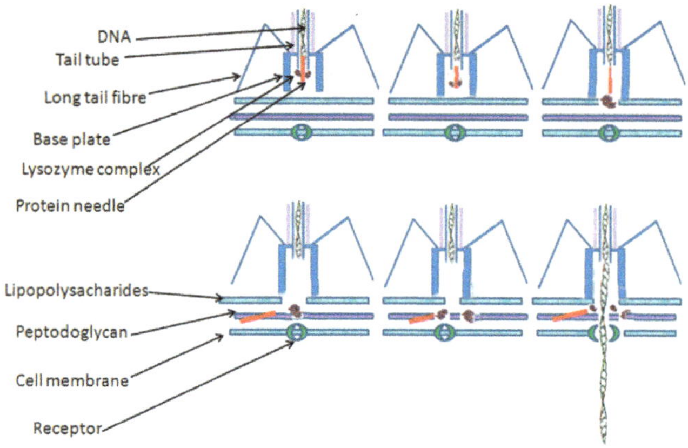

Diagram of the DNA injection process

REPLICATION

Bacteriophages may have a lytic cycle or a lysogenic cycle, and a few viruses are capable of carrying out both. With lytic phages such as the T4 phage, bacterial cells are broken open (lysed) and destroyed after immediate replication of the virion. As soon as the cell is destroyed, the phage progeny can find new hosts to infect. Lytic phages are more suitable for phage therapy. Some lytic phages undergo a phenomenon known as lysis inhibition, where completed phage progeny will not immediately lyse out of the cell if extracellular phage concentrations are high. This mechanism is not identical to that of temperate phage going dormant and is usually temporary.

In contrast, the lysogenic cycle does not result in immediate lysing of the host cell. Those phages able to undergo lysogeny are known as temperate phages. Their viral genome will integrate with host DNA and replicate along with it relatively harmlessly, or may even become established as a plasmid. The virus remains dormant until host conditions deteriorate, perhaps due to depletion of nutrients; then, the endogenous phages (known as prophages) become active. At this point they initiate the reproductive cycle, resulting in lysis of the host cell. As the lysogenic cycle allows the host cell to continue to survive and reproduce, the virus is replicated in all of the cell's offspring. An example of a bacteriophage known to follow the lysogenic cycle and the lytic cycle is the phage lambda of E. coli.

Sometimes prophages may provide benefits to the host bacterium while they are dormant by adding new functions to the bacterial genome in a phenomenon called lysogenic conversion. Examples are the conversion of harmless strains of Corynebacterium diphtheriae or Vibrio cholerae by bacteriophages to highly virulent ones, which cause Diphtheria or cholera, respectively. Strategies to combat certain bacterial infections by targeting these toxin-encoding prophages have been proposed.

Attachment and Penetration

To enter a host cell, bacteriophages attach to specific receptors on the surface of bacteria, including lipopolysaccharides, teichoic acids, proteins, or even flagella. This specificity means a bacteriophage can infect only certain bacteria bearing receptors to which they can bind, which in turn determines the phage's host range.

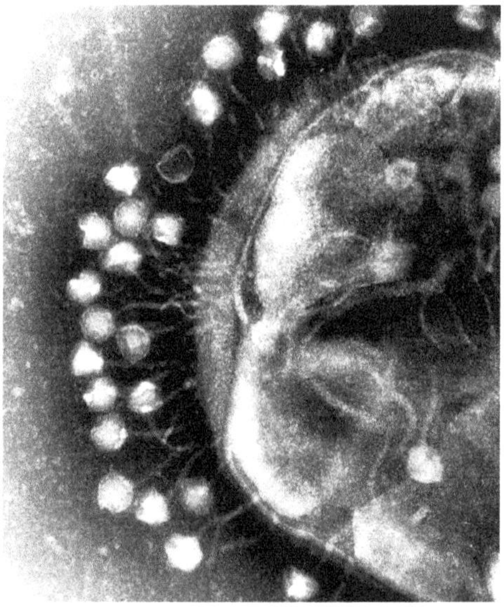

In this electron micrograph of bacteriophages attached to a bacterial cell, the viruses are the size and shape of coliphage T1.

Host growth conditions also influence the ability of the phage to attach and invade them. As phage virions do not move independently, they must rely on random encounters with the right receptors when in solution (blood, lymphatic circulation, irrigation, soil water, etc.).

Myovirus bacteriophages use a hypodermic syringe-like motion to inject their genetic material into the cell. After making contact with the appropriate receptor, the tail fibers flex to bring the base plate closer to the surface of the cell; this is known as reversible binding. Once attached completely, irreversible binding is initiated and the tail contracts, possibly with the help of ATP present in the tail, injecting genetic material through the bacterial membrane. Podoviruses lack an elongated tail sheath similar to that of a myovirus, so they instead use their small, tooth-like tail fibers enzymatically to degrade a portion of the cell membrane before inserting their genetic material.

Synthesis of Proteins and Nucleic Acid

Within minutes, bacterial ribosomes start translating viral mRNA into protein. For RNA-based phages, RNA replicase is synthesized early in the process. Proteins modify the bacterial RNA polymerase so it preferentially transcribes viral mRNA. The host's normal synthesis of proteins and nucleic acids is disrupted, and it is forced to manufacture viral products instead. These products go on to become part of new virions within the cell, helper proteins that help assemble the new virions, or proteins involved in cell lysis. Walter Fiers (University of Ghent, Belgium) was the first to establish the complete nucleotide sequence of a gene (1972) and of the viral genome of bacteriophage MS2 (1976).

Virion Assembly

In the case of the T4 phage, the construction of new virus particles involves the assistance of helper proteins. The base plates are assembled first, with the tails being built upon them afterward. The head capsids, constructed separately, will spontaneously assemble with the tails. The DNA is packed efficiently within the heads. The whole process takes about 15 minutes.

Release of Virions

Phages may be released via cell lysis, by extrusion, or, in a few cases, by budding. Lysis, by tailed phages, is achieved by an enzyme called endolysin, which attacks and breaks down the cell wall peptidoglycan. An altogether different phage type, the filamentous phages, make the host cell continually secrete new virus particles. Released virions are described as free, and, unless defective, are capable of infecting a new bacterium. Budding is associated with certain Mycoplasma phages. In contrast to virion release, phages displaying a lysogenic cycle do not kill the host but, rather, become long-term residents as prophage.

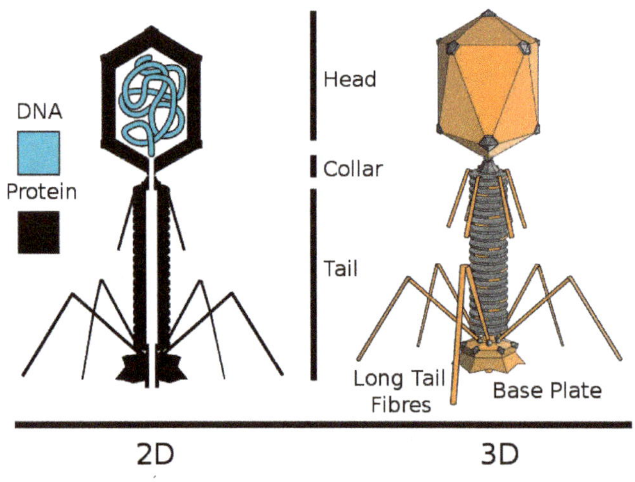

Diagram of a typical tailed bacteriophage structure

Genome Structure

Given the millions of different phages in the environment, phages genomes come in a variety of forms and sizes. RNA phage such as MS2 have the smallest genomes of only a few kilobases. However, some DNA phages such as T4 may have large genomes with hundreds of genes.

Bacteriophage genomes can be highly mosaic, i.e. the genome of many phage species appear to be composed of numerous individual modules. These modules may be found in other phage species in different arrangements. Mycobacteriophages – bacteriophages with mycobacterial hosts – have provided excellent examples of this mosaicism. In these mycobacteriophages, genetic assortment may be the result of repeated instances of site-specific recombination and illegitimate recombination (the result of phage genome acquisition of bacterial host genetic sequences). It should be noted, however, that evolutionary mechanisms shaping the genomes of bacterial viruses vary between different families and depend on the type of the nucleic acid, characteristics of the virion structure, as well as the mode of the viral life cycle.

Systems Biology

Phages often have dramatic effects on their hosts. As a consequence, the transcription pattern of the infected bacterium may change considerably. For instance, infection of Pseudomonas aeruginosa by the temperate phage PaP3 changed the expression of 38% (2160/5633) of its host's genes. Many of these effects are probably indirect, hence the challenge becomes to identify the direct interactions among bacteria and phage.

Several attempts have been made to map Protein–protein interactions among phage and their host. For instance, bacteriophage lambda was found to interact with its host E. coli by 31 interactions. However, a large-scale study revealed 62 interactions, most of which were new. Again, the significance of many of these interactions remains unclear, but these studies suggest that there are most likely several key interactions and many indirect interactions whose role remains uncharacterized.

In the Environment

Main article: Marine bacteriophage

Metagenomics has allowed the in-water detection of bacteriophages that was not possible previously.

Bacteriophages have also been used in hydrological tracing and modelling in river systems, especially where surface water and groundwater interactions occur. The use of phages is preferred to the more conventional dye marker because they are significantly less absorbed when passing through ground waters and they are readily detected at very low concentrations. Non-polluted water may contain ca. 2×10^{8} bacteriophages per mL.

Other Areas of Use

Since 2006, the United States Food and Drug Administration (FDA) and United States Department of Agriculture (USDA) have approved several bacteriophage products. LMP-102 (Intralytix) was approved for treating ready-to-eat (RTE) poultry and meat products. In that same year, the FDA approved LISTEX (developed and produced by Micreos) using bacteriophages on cheese to kill Listeria monocytogenes bacteria, giving them generally recognized as safe (GRAS) status. In July 2007, the same bacteriophage were approved for use on all food products. In 2011 USDA confirmed that LISTEX is a clean label processing aid and is included in USDA. Research in the field of food safety is continuing to see if lytic phages are a viable option to control other food-borne pathogens in various food products.

In 2011 the FDA cleared the first bacteriophage-based product for in vitro diagnostic use. The KeyPath MRSA/MSSA Blood Culture Test uses a cocktail of bacteriophage to detect Staphylococcus aureus in positive blood cultures and determine methicillin resistance or susceptibility. The test returns results in about 5 hours, compared to 2–3 days for standard microbial identification and susceptibility test methods. It was the first accelerated antibiotic susceptibility test approved by the FDA.

Government agencies in the West have for several years been looking to Georgia and the former Soviet Union for help with exploiting phages for counteracting bioweapons and toxins, such as anthrax and botulism. Developments are continuing among research groups in the US. Other uses include spray application in horticulture for protecting plants and vegetable produce from decay and the spread of bacterial disease. Other applications for bacteriophages are as biocides for environmental surfaces, e.g., in hospitals, and as preventative treatments for catheters and medical devices before use in clinical settings. The technology for phages to be applied to dry surfaces, e.g., uniforms, curtains, or even sutures for surgery now exists. Clinical trials reported in the Lancet show success in veterinary treatment of pet dogs with otitis.

Phage display is a different use of phages involving a library of phages with a variable peptide linked to a surface protein. Each phage's genome encodes the variant of the protein displayed on its surface (hence the name), providing a link between the peptide variant and its encoding gene. Variant phages from the library can be selected through their binding affinity to an immobilized molecule (e.g., botulism toxin) to neutralize it. The bound, selected phages can be multiplied by reinfecting a susceptible bacterial strain, thus allowing them to retrieve the peptides encoded in them for further study.

The SEPTIC bacterium sensing and identification method uses the ion emission and its dynamics during phage infection and offers high specificity and speed for detection.

Phage-ligand technology makes use of proteins, which are identified from bacteriophages, characterized and recombinantly expressed for various applications such as binding of bacteria and bacterial components (e.g. endotoxin) and lysis of bacteria.

Bacteriophages are also important model organisms for studying principles of evolution and ecology.

DNA VIRUS

A DNA virus is a virus that has DNA as its genetic material and replicates using a DNA-dependent DNA polymerase. The nucleic acid is usually double-stranded DNA (dsDNA) but may also be single-stranded DNA (ssDNA). DNA viruses belong to either Group I or Group II of the Baltimore classification system for viruses. Single-stranded DNA is usually expanded to double-stranded in infected cells. Although Group VII viruses such as hepatitis B contain a DNA genome, they are not considered DNA viruses according to the Baltimore classification, but rather reverse transcribing viruses because they replicate through an RNA intermediate. Notable diseases like smallpox, herpes, and chickenpox are caused by such DNA viruses.

Group I: dsDNA Viruses

Genome organization within this group varies considerably. Some have circular genomes (Baculoviridae, Papovaviridae and Polydnaviridae) while others have linear genomes (Adenoviridae, Herpesviridae and some phages). Some families have circularly permuted linear genomes (phage T4 and some Iridoviridae). Others have linear genomes with covalently closed ends (Poxviridae and Phycodnaviridae).

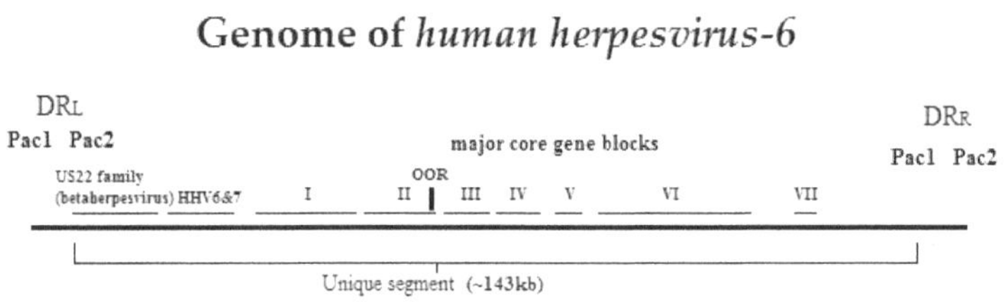

Genome of *human herpesvirus-6*, a member of the Herpesviridae family

A virus infecting archaea was first described in 1974. Several others have been described since: most have head-tail morphologies and linear double-stranded DNA genomes. Other morphologies have also been described: spindle shaped, rod shaped, filamentous, icosahedral and spherical. Additional morphological types may exist.

Orders within this group are defined on the basis of morphology rather than DNA sequence similarity. It is thought that morphology is more conserved in this group than sequence similarity or gene order which is extremely variable. Three orders and 31 families are currently recognised. A fourth order—Megavirales—for the nucleocytoplasmic large DNA viruses has been proposed. Four genera are recognised that have not yet been assigned a family. The species Sulfolobus turreted icosahedral virus is so unlike any previously described virus that it will almost certainly be placed in a new family on the next revision of viral families.

Fifteen families are enveloped. These include all three families in the order Herpesvirales and the following families: Ascoviridae, Ampullaviridae, Asfarviridae, Baculoviridae, Fuselloviridae, Globuloviridae, Guttaviridae, Hytrosaviridae, Iridoviridae, Lipothrixviridae, Nimaviridae and Poxviridae.

Bacteriophages (viruses infecting bacteria) belonging to the families Tectiviridae and Corticoviridae have a lipid bilayer membrane inside the icosahedral protein capsid and the membrane surrounds the genome. The crenarchaeal virus Sulfolobus turreted icosahedral virus has a similar structure.

The genomes in this group vary considerably from ~10 kilobases to over 2.5 megabases in length. The largest bacteriophage known is Klebsiella Phage vB_KleM-RaK2 which has a genome of 346 kilobases.

A recently proposed clade is the Megavirales which includes the nucleocytoplasmic large DNA viruses. This proposal has yet to be ratified by the ICTV.

The virophages are a group of viruses that infect other viruses. Their classification has yet to be decided. A family Lavidaviridae has been proposed.

Host Range

Species of the order Caudovirales and of the families Corticoviridae and Tectiviridae infect bacteria.

Species of the order Ligamenvirales and the families Ampullaviridae, Bicaudaviridae, Clavaviridae, Fuselloviridae, Globuloviridae, Guttaviridae and Turriviridae infect hyperthermophilic archaea species of the Crenarchaeota.

Species of the order Herpesvirales and of the families Adenoviridae, Asfarviridae, Iridoviridae, Papillomaviridae, Polyomaviridae and Poxviridae infect vertebrates.

Species of the families Ascovirus, Baculovirus, Hytrosaviridae, Iridoviridae and Polydnaviruses and of the genus Nudivirus infect insects.

Species of the family Mimiviridae and the species Marseillevirus, Megavirus, Mavirus virophage and Sputnik virophage infect protozoa.

Species of the family Nimaviridae infect crustaceans.

Species of the family Phycodnaviridae and the species Organic Lake virophage infect algae. These are the only known dsDNA viruses that infect plants.

Species of the family Plasmaviridae infect species of the class Mollicutes.

Species of the family Pandoraviridae infect amoebae.

Species of the genus Dinodnavirus infect dinoflagellates. These are the only known viruses that infect dinoflagellates.

Species of the genus Rhizidiovirus infect stramenopiles. These are the only known dsDNA viruses that infect stramenopiles.

Species of the genus Salterprovirus and Sphaerolipoviridae infect species of the Euryarchaeota.

Taxonomy

- Order *Caudovirales*
    - Family *Myoviridae*—includes Enterobacteria phage T4

- Family *Podoviridae*—includes Enterobacteria phage T7
- Family *Siphoviridae*—includes Enterobacteria phage λ

■ Order *Herpesvirales*
  - Family *Alloherpesviridae*
  - Family *Herpesviridae*—includes human herpesviruses, Varicella Zoster virus
  - Family *Malacoherpesviridae*

■ Order *Ligamenvirales*
  - Family *Lipothrixviridae*
  - Family *Rudiviridae*

■ Unassigned families
  - Family *Adenoviridae*—includes viruses which cause human adenovirus infection
  - Family *Ampullaviridae*
  - Family *Ascoviridae*
  - Family *Asfarviridae*—includes African swine fever virus
  - Family *Baculoviridae*
  - Family *Bicaudaviridae*
  - Family *Clavaviridae*
  - Family *Corticoviridae*
  - Family *Fuselloviridae*
  - Family *Globuloviridae*
  - Family *Guttaviridae*
  - Family *Hytrosaviridae*
  - Family *Iridoviridae*
  - Family *Marseilleviridae*
  - Family *Mimiviridae*
  - Family *Nudiviridae*
  - Family *Nimaviridae*
  - Family *Pandoraviridae*

- Family *Papillomaviridae*
- Family *Phycodnaviridae*
- Family *Plasmaviridae*
- Family *Polydnaviruses*
- Family *Polyomaviridae*—includes Simian virus 40, JC virus, BK virus
- Family *Poxviridae*—includes Cowpox virus, smallpox
- Family *Sphaerolipoviridae*
- Family *Tectiviridae*
- Family *Turriviridae*

■ Unassigned genera
- *Dinodnavirus*
- *Salterprovirus*
- *Rhizidiovirus*

■ Unassigned species
- *Abalone shriveling syndrome-associated virus*
- *Bandicoot papillomatosis carcinomatosis virus*
- *Cedratvirus*
- *Kaumoebavirus*
- *KIs-V*
- *Lentille virus*
- *Megavirus*
- *Mollivirus sibericum virus*
- *Phaeocystis globosa virus*
- *Pithovirus*

■ Virophages
- *Ace Lake Mavirus virophage*
- *Dishui Lake virophage 1*
- *Mavirus virophage*

- *Organic Lake virophage*
- *Phaeocystis globosa virus virophage*
- *Rio Negro virophage*
- *Sputnik virophage*
- *Sputnik virophage 2*
- *Yellowstone Lake virophage 1*
- *Yellowstone Lake virophage 2*
- *Yellowstone Lake virophage 3*
- *Yellowstone Lake virophage 4*
- *Yellowstone Lake virophage 5*
- *Yellowstone Lake virophage 6*
- *Yellowstone Lake virophage 7*
- *Zamilon virophage*
- *Zamilon virophage 2*

Pleolipoviruses

A group known as the pleolipoviruses, although having a similar genome organisation, differ in having either single or double stranded DNA genomes. Within the double stranded forms have runs of single stranded DNA. This group does not fit into the current classification system and a new taxon is required.

These viruses are nonlytic and form virions characterized by a lipid vesicle enclosing the genome. They do not have nucleoproteins. The lipids in the viral membrane are unselectively acquired from host cell membranes. The virions contain two to three major structural proteins, which either are embedded in the membrane or form spikes distributed randomly on the external membrane surface. This group includes the following viruses:

- Haloarcula hispanica pleomorphic virus 1
- Halogeometricum pleomorphic virus 1
- Halorubrum pleomorphic virus 1
- Halorubrum pleomorphic virus 2
- Halorubrum pleomorphic virus 3
- Halorubrum pleomorphic virus 6
- SNJ2

Group II: ssDNA Viruses

Although bacteriophages were first described in 1927, it was only in 1959 that Sinshemer working with phage Phi X 174 showed that they could possess single-stranded DNA genomes. Despite this discovery until relatively recently it was believed that the majority of DNA viruses belonged to the double-stranded clade. Recent work suggests that this may not be the case with single-stranded viruses forming the majority of viruses found in sea water, fresh water, sediment, terrestrial, extreme, metazoan-associated and marine microbial mats. Many of these environmental viruses belong to the family Microviridae. However, the vast majority has yet to be classified and assigned to genera and higher taxa. Because most of these viruses do not appear to be related or are only distantly related to known viruses additional taxa will be created for these.

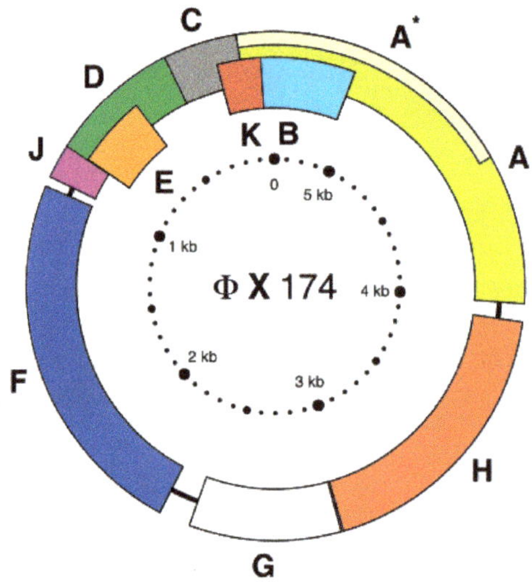

Genome of bacteriophage ΦX174, a single-stranded DNA virus

Taxonomy

Families in this group have been assigned on the basis of the nature of the genome (circular or linear) and the host range. Eleven families are currently recognised.

- Family *Anelloviridae*
- Family *Bacillariodnaviridae*
- Family *Bidnaviridae*
- Family *Circoviridae*
- Family *Geminiviridae*
- Family *Inoviridae*
- Family *Microviridae*

- Family *Nanoviridae*
- Family *Parvoviridae*
- Family *Spiraviridae*

Classification

A division of the circular single stranded viruses into four types has been proposed. This division seems likely reflects their phylogenetic relationships.

Type I genomes are characterized by a small circular DNA genome (approximately 2-kb), with the Rep protein and the major open reading frame (ORF) in opposite orientations. This type is characteristic of the circoviruses, geminiviruses and nanoviruses.

Type II genomes have the unique feature of two separate Rep ORFs.

Type III genomes contain two major ORFs in the same orientation. This arrangement is typical of the anelloviruses.

Type IV genomes have the largest genomes of nearly 4-kb, with up to eight ORFs. This type of genome is found in the Inoviridae and the Microviridae.

Given the variety of single stranded viruses that have been described this scheme—if it is accepted by the ICTV—will need to be extended.

Host Range

The families Bidnaviridae and Parvoviridae have linear genomes while the other families have circular genomes. The Bidnaviridae have a two part genome and infect invertebrates. The Inoviridae and Microviridae infect bacteria; the Anelloviridae and Circoviridae infect animals (mammals and birds respectively); and the Geminiviridae and Nanoviridae infect plants. In both the Geminiviridae and Nanoviridae the genome is composed of more than a single chromosome. The Bacillariodnaviridae infect diatoms and have a unique genome: the major chromosome is circular (~6 kilobases in length): the minor chromosome is linear (~1 kilobase in length) and complementary to part of the major chromosome. Members of the Spiraviridae infect archaea. Members of the Mycodnaviridae infect fungi.

Molecular Biology

All viruses in this group require formation of a replicative form—a double stranded DNA intermediate—for genome replication. This is normally created from the viral DNA with the assistance of the host's own DNA polymerase.

Recently classified Viruses

In the 9th edition of the viral taxonomy of the ICTV (published 2011) the Bombyx mori densovirus type 2 was placed in a new family—the Bidnaviridae on the basis of its genome structure and replication mechanism. This is currently the only member of this family but it seems likely that other species will be allocated to this family in the near future.

A new genus—Bufavirus—was proposed on the basis of the isolation of two new viruses from human stool. These viruses have since been renamed Primate protoparvovirus and been placed in the genus Protoparvovirus. Another member of this genus—megabat bufavius 1—has been reported from bats.

Gemycircularvirus

The following viruses have been placed in the proposed Gemycircularvirus genus of the family Microvirus subfamily Mycodnaviridae. This genus includes the species bovine stool associated circular virus and chimpanzee stool associated circular virus. The closest relations to this genus appear to be the Nanoviridae but further work will be needed to confirm this. Another isolate that appears to be related to these viruses has been isolated from pig faeces in New Zealand. This isolate also appears to be related to the pig stool-associated single-stranded DNA virus. This virus has two large open reading frames one encoding the capsid gene and the other the Rep gene. These are bidirectionally transcribed and separated by intergenic regions. The name Gemycircularvirus (Gemini-like myco-infecting circular virus) has been proposed for this group of viruses. Another virus of this group has been reported again from pigs. Some of this group of viruses may infect fungi. A virus from this group has been isolated from turkey faeces. Another ten viruses from this group have been isolated from pig faeces. Additional viruses from this group have been reported from dragonflies and damselflies. Viruses that appear to belong to this group have been isolated from other mammals including cows, rodents, bats, badgers and foxes. A isolate from this group has also been identified in a child with encephalitis. The genomes in this group have some similarity with the Sclerotinia sclerotiorum hypovirulence associated DNA virus 1 which infects fungi. Another virus from this group has been isolated from mosquitoes. Viruses from this group have also been isolaed from the blood of HIV+ve patients.Viruses in this group have also been isolated from other cases of encephalitis, diarrhoea and sewage. Isolates from this group have also been isolated from the cerebrospinal fluid and brains of patients with multiple sclerosis. Two additional viruses that may belong to this group are Ostrich faecal associated ssDNA virus and Rabbit faecal associated ssDNA virus. Three viruses in this group have been isolated from plants.Another virus has been isolated from birds. A single stranded DNA fungal virus—Sclerotinia sclerotiorum hypovirulence associated DNA virus 1—has been described. This virus appears to be related to the Geminiviridae but is distinct from them. It has also been placed in thc Gemycircularvirus group.

Unassigned Species

A number of additional single stranded DNA viruses have been described but are as yet unclassified.

Animal Viruses—Vertebrates

Among these are the parvovirus-like viruses. These have linear single-stranded DNA genomes but unlike the parvoviruses the genome is bipartate. This group includes the Bombyx mori densovirus type 2, Hepatopancreatic parvo-like virus and Lymphoidal parvo-like virus. A new family Bidensoviridae has been proposed for this group but this proposal has not been ratified by the ICTV to date. Their closest relations appear to be the Brevidensoviruses (family Parvoviridae).

Fur seal feces-associated circular DNA virus was isolate from the faeces of a fur seal (Arctocephalus forsteri) in New Zealand. The genome has 2 main open reading frames and is 2925 nucleotides in length. Another virus porcine stool associated virus 4 has been isolated that appears to be related to the fur seal virus.

Two viruses have been isolated from human faeces—circo-like virus-Brazil hs1 and hs2—with genome lengths of 2526 and 2533 nucleotides respectively. These viruses have four open reading frames. These viruses appear to be related to three viruses previously isolated from waste water, a bat and from a rodent.

This appears to belong to a novel group.

Two viruses have been described from the nesting material yellow crowned parakeet (*Cyanoramphus auriceps*)—Cyanoramphus nest-associated circular X virus (2308 nt) and Cyanoramphus nest-associated circular K virus (2087 nt) Both viruses have two bidirectional open reading frames. Within these are the rolling-circle replication motifs I, II, III and the helicase motifs Walker A and Walker B. There is also a conserved nonanucleotide motif required for rolling-circle replication. CynNCKV has some similarity to the picobiliphyte nano-like virus (Picobiliphyte M5584-5) and CynNCXV has some similarity to the rodent stool associated virus (RodSCV M-45).

Psittacine beak and feather disease virus is a single stranded circular molecule of 1993 nucleotide bases encoding seven open reading frames—three in the virion strand and four in the complementary strand. The open reading frames have some homology to porcine circovirus, subterranean clover stunt virus and faba bean necrotic yellows virus.

A virus with a circular genome—sea turtle tornovirus 1—has been isolated from a sea turtle with fibropapillomatosis. It is sufficiently unrelated to any other known virus that it may belong to a new family. The closest relations seem to be the *Gyrovirinae*. The proposed genus name for this virus is Tornovirus.

Animal Viruses—Invertebrates

A virus—Acheta domesticus volvovirus has been isolated from the house cricket (Acheta domesticus). The genome is circular, has four open reading frames and is 2,517 nucleotides in length. It appears to be unrelated to previously described species. The genus name Volvovirus has been proposed for these species. The genomes in this genus are ~2.5 nucleotides in length and encode 4 open reading frames.

Two new viruses have been isolated from the copepods Acartia tonsa and Labidocera aestiva—Acartia tonsa copepod circo-like virus and Labidocera aestiva copepod circo-like virus respectively. A virus has been isolated from the mud flat snail (Amphibola crenata). This virus has a single stranded circular genome of 2351 nucleotides that encoded 2 open reading frames that are oriented in opposite directions. The smaller open reading frame (874 nucleotides) encodes a protein with similarities to the Rep (replication) proteins of circoviruses and plasmids. The larger open reading frame (955 nucleotides) has no homology to any currently known protein.

An unusual—and as yet unnamed—virus has been isolated from the flatwom *Girardia tigrina*. Because of its genome organisation, this virus appears to belong to an entirely new family. It is the first virus to be isolated from a flatworm.

From the hepatopancreas of the shrimp (Farfantepenaeus duorarum) a circular single stranded DNA virus has been isolated. This virus does not appear to cause disease in the shrimp.

A circo-like virus has been isolated from the shrimp (*Penaeus monodon*). The 1,777-nucleotide genome is circular and single stranded. It has some similarity to the circoviruses and cycloviruses.

Ten new circular viruses have been isolated from dragonfly larvae. The genomes range from 1628 to 2668 nucleotides in length.

Ten viruses have been isolated from echinoderms. All appear to belong to as yet undescribed genera.

Fungal

Most known fungal viruses have either double stranded DNA or RNA genomes. A genus—Breviviridae—has been proposed for Sclerotinia sclerotiorum hypovirulence associated DNA virus 1 and a European badger fecal virus.

Plants

A virus—Cassava associated circular DNA virus—that has some similarity to Sclerotinia sclerotiorum hypovirulence associated DNA virus 1 has been isolated.

A circular single stranded DNA virus has been isolated from a grapevine. This species may be related to the family Geminiviridae but differs from this family in a number of important respects including genome size.

Grapevine red blotch associated virus and Grapevine cabernet franc associated virus are two single stranded DNA viruses associated with infections of grape vines.

A virus— Euphorbia caput medusae latent virus —is so divergent from the other members of the geminiviruses that a new genus has been proposed for it. The name of this new genus is proposed to be Capulavirus. Another virus in this genus is Alfalfa leaf curl virus.

Several viruses—baminivirus, nepavirus and niminivirus—related to geminvirus have also been reported.

A virus - Ancient caribou feces associated virus - has been cloned from 700-y-old caribou faeces.

Archaea

Although ~50 archaeal viruses are known, all but two have double stranded genomes. The first archaeal ssDNA virus to be isolated is the Halorubrum pleomorphic virus 1, which has a pleomorphic enveloped virion and a circular genome.

The second single stranded DNA virus infecting Archaea is Aeropyrum coil-shaped virus (ACV). The genome is circular and with 24,893 nucleotides is currently the largest known ssDNA genome. The viron is nonenveloped, hollow, cylindrical and formed from a coiling fiber. The morphology and the genome appear to be unique.

The new family Spiraviridae (from Latin spira, "a coil") has been created by the ICTV to accommodate ACV.

Marine and Other

Several hundred single stranded DNA viral genomes have been isolated from seawater. Their hosts have yet to be identified but are likely to be eukaryotic phytoplankton and zooplankton. They fall into at least 11 distinct groups that are unrelated to previously described viral families.

A virus—Boiling Springs Lake virus—appears to have evolved by a recombination event between a DNA virus (circovirus) and an RNA virus (tombusvirus). The genome is circular and encodes two proteins—a Rep protein and a capsid protein.

Further reports of viruses that appear to have evolved from recombination events between ssRNA and ssDNA viruses have been made.

A new virus has been isolated from the diatom *Chaetoceros setoensis*. It has a single stranded DNA genome and does not appear to be a member of any previously described group.

Satellite Viruses

Satellite viruses are small viruses with either RNA or DNA as their genomic material that require another virus to replicate. There are two types of DNA satellite viruses—the alphasatellites and the betasatellites—both of which are dependent on begomoviruses. At present satellite viruses are not classified into genera or higher taxa.

Alphasatellites are small circular single strand DNA viruses that require a begomovirus for transmission. Betasatellites are small linear single stranded DNA viruses that require a begomovirus to replicate.

Phylogenetic Relationships

Phylogenetic relationships between these families are difficult to determine. The genomes differ significantly in size and organisation. Most studies that have attempted to determine these relationships are based either on some of the more conserved proteins—DNA polymerase and others—or on common structural features. In general most of the proposed relationships are tentative and have not yet been used by the ICTV in their classification.

ds DNA viruses

Herpesviruses and caudoviruses

While determining the phylogenetic relations between the various known clades of viruses is difficult, on a number of grounds the herpesviruses and caudoviruses appear to be related. While the three families in the order Herpesvirales are clearly related on morphological grounds, it has proven difficult to determine the dates of divergence between them because of the lack of gene conservation. On morphological grounds they appear to be related to the bacteriophages—specifically the Caudoviruses.

The branching order among the herpesviruses suggests that Alloherpesviridae is the basal clade and that Herpesviridae and Malacoherpesviridae are sister clades. Given the phylogenetic distances between vertebrates and molluscs this suggests that herpesviruses were initially fish viruses and that they have evolved with their hosts to infect other vertebrates.

The vertebrate herpesviruses initially evolved ~400 million years ago and underwent subsequent evolution on the supercontinent Pangaea.The alphaherpesvirinae separated from the branch leading to the betaherpesvirinae and gammaherpesvirinae about 180 million years ago to 220 million years ago. The avian herpes viruses diverged from the branch leading to the mammalian species. The mammalian species divided into two branches—the Simplexvirus and Varicellovirus genera. This latter divergence appears to have occurred around the time of the mammalian radiation.

Several dsDNA bacteriophages and the herpesviruses encode a powerful ATP driven DNA translocating machine that encapsidates a viral genome into a preformed capsid shell or prohead. The critical components of the packaging machine are the packaging enzyme (terminase) which acts as the motor and the portal protein that forms the unique DNA entrance vertex of prohead. The terminase complex consists of a recognition subunit (small terminase) and an endonuclease/translocase subunit (large terminase) and cuts viral genome concatemers. It forms a motor complex containing five large terminase subunits. The terminase-viral DNA complex docks on the portal vertex. The pentameric motor processively translocates DNA until the head shell is full with one viral genome. The motor cuts the DNA again and dissociates from the full head, allowing head-finishing proteins to assemble on the portal, sealing the portal, and constructing a platform for tail attachment. Only a single gene encoding the putative ATPase subunit of the terminase (UL15) is conserved among all herpesviruses. To a lesser extent this gene is also found in T4-like bacteriophages suggesting a common ancestor for these two groups of viruses. Another paper has also suggested that herpesviruses originated among the bacteriophages.

A common origin for the herpesviruses and the caudoviruses has been suggested on the basis of parallels in their capsid assembly pathways and similarities between their portal complexes, through which DNA enters the capsid. These two groups of viruses share a distinctive 12-fold arrangement of subunits in the portal complex. A second paper has suggested an evolutionary relationship between these two groups of viruses.

It seems likely that the tailed viruses infecting the archaea are also related to the tailed viruses infecting bacteria.

Large DNA viruses

The family Ascoviridae appear to have evolved from the Iridoviridae. The family Polydnaviridae may have evolved from the Ascoviridae. Molecular evidence suggests that the Phycodnaviridae may have evolved from the family Iridoviridae. These four families (Ascoviridae, Iridoviridae, Phycodnaviridae and Polydnaviridae) may form a clade but more work is needed to confirm this. Based on the genome organisation and DNA replication mechanism it seems that phylogenetic relationships may exist between the rudiviruses (Rudiviridae) and the large eukaryal DNA viruses: the African swine fever virus (Asfarviridae), Chlorella viruses (Phycodnaviridae) and poxviruses (Poxviridae).

Based on the analysis of the DNA polymerase the genus Dinodnavirus may be a member of the family Asfarviridae. Further work on this virus will required before a final assignment can be made.

The nucleocytoplasmic large DNA virus group (Asfarviridae, Iridoviridae, Marseilleviridae, Mimiviridae, Phycodnaviridae and Poxviridae) along with three other families—Adenoviridae, Cortiviridae and Tectiviridae—and the phage Sulfolobus turreted icosahedral virus and the satellite virus Sputnik all possess double β-barrel major capsid proteins suggesting a common origin.

Some of the relations among the large viruses have been established. Mimiviruses are distantly related to Phycodnaviridae. Pandoraviruses share a common ancestor with Coccolithoviruses within the Phycodnaviridae family.

Pithoviruses are related to Iridoviridae and Marseilleviridae.

Other viruses

Based on the analysis of the coat protein, Sulfolobus turreted icosahedral virus may share a common ancestry with the Tectiviridae.

The families Adenoviridae and Tectiviridae appear to be related structurally.

Baculoviruses evolved from the nudiviruses 310 million years ago.

The Hytrosaviridae are related to the baculoviruses and to a lesser extent the nudiviruses suggesting they may have evolved from the baculoviruses.

The Nimaviridae may be related to nudiviruses and baculoviruses.

The Nudiviruses seem to be related to the polydnaviruses.

A protein common to the families Bicaudaviridae, Lipotrixviridae and Rudiviridae and the unclassified virus Sulfolobus turreted icosahedral virus is known suggesting a common origin.

Examination of the pol genes that encode the DNA dependent DNA polymerase in various groups of viruses suggests a number of possible evolutionary relationships. All know viral DNA polymerases belong to the DNA pol families A and B. All possess a 3'-5'-exonuclease domain with three sequence motifs Exo I, Exo II and Exo III. The families A and B are distinguishable with family A Pol sharing 9 distinct consensus sequences and only two of them are convincingly homologous to sequence motif B of family B. The putative sequence motifs A, B, and C of the polymerase domain are located near the C-terminus in family A Pol and more central in family B Pol.

Phylogenetic analysis of these genes places the adenoviruses (Adenoviridae), bacteriophages (Caudovirales) and the plant and fungal linear plasmids into a single clade. A second clade includes the alpha- and delta-like viral Pol from insect ascovirus

(Ascoviridae), mammalian herpesviruses (Herpesviridae), fish lymphocystis disease virus (Iridoviridae) and chlorella virus (Phycoviridae). The pol genes of the African swine fever virus (Asfarviridae), baculoviruses (Baculoviridae), fish herpesvirus (Herpesviridae), T-even bacteriophages (Myoviridae) and poxviruses (Poxviridae) were not clearly resolved. A second study showed that poxvirus, baculovirus and the animal herpesviruses form separate and distinct clades. Their relationship to the Asfarviridae and the Myoviridae was not examined and remains unclear. The polymerases from the archaea are similar to family B DNA Pols. The T4-like viruses infect both bacteria and archaea and their pol gene resembles that of eukaryotes. The DNA polymerase of mitochondria resembles that of the T odd phages (Myoviridae).

The virophage—Mavirus—may have evolved from a recombination between a transposon of the Polinton (Maverick) family and an unknown virus.

The polyoma and papillomaviruses appear to have evolved from single-stranded DNA viruses and ultimately from plasmids.

ss DNA Viruses

The evolutionary history of this group is currently poorly understood. An ancient origin for the single stranded circular DNA viruses has been proposed.

Capsid proteins of most icosahedral ssRNA and ssDNA viruses display the same structural fold, the eight-stranded beta-barrel, also known as the jelly-roll fold. On the other hand, the replication proteins of icosahedral ssDNA viruses belong to the superfamily of rolling-circle replication initiation proteins that are commonly found in prokaryotic plasmids. Based on these observations, it has been proposed that small DNA viruses have originated via recombination between RNA viruses and plasmids.

Circoviruses may have evolved from a nanovirus.

Given the similarities between the rep proteins of the alphasatellites and the nanoviruses, it is likely that the alphasatellites evolved from the nanoviruses. Further work in this area is needed to clarify this.

The geminiviruses may have evolved from phytoplasmal plasmids.

Based on the three-dimensional structure of the Rep proteins the geminiviruses and parvoviruses may be related.

The ancestor of the geminiviruses probably infected dicots.

The parvoviruses have frequently invaded the germ lines of diverse animal species including mammals, fishes, birds, tunicates, arthropods and flatworms. In particular they have been associated with the human genome for ~98 million years.

Members of the family Bidnaviridae have evolved from insect parvoviruses by replacing the typical replication-initiation endonuclease with a protein-primed family B DNA polymerase acquired from large DNA transposons of the Polinton/Maverick family. Some bidnavirus genes were also horizontally acquired from reoviruses (dsRNA genomes) and baculoviruses (dsDNA genomes).

Bacteriophage Evolution

Since 1959 ~6300 prokaryote viruses have been described morphologically, including ~6200 bacterial and ~100 archaeal viruses. Archaeal viruses belong to 15 families and infect members of 16 archaeal genera. These are nearly exclusively hyperthermophiles or extreme halophiles. Tailed archaeal viruses are found only in the Euryarchaeota, whereas most filamentous and pleomorphic archaeal viruses occur in the Crenarchaeota. Bacterial viruses belong to 10 families and infect members of 179 bacterial genera: most these are members of the Firmicutes and γ-proteobacteria.

The vast majority (96.3%) are tailed with and only 230 (3.7%) are polyhedral, filamentous or pleomorphic. The family Siphoviridae is the largest family (>3600 descriptions: 57.3%). The tailed phages appear to be monophyletic and are the oldest known virus group. They arose repeatedly in different hosts and there are at least 11 separate lines of descent.

All of the known temperate phages employ one of only three different systems for their lysogenic cycle: lambda-like integration/excision, Mu-like transposition or the plasmid-like partitioning of phage N15.

A putative course of evolution of these phages has been proposed by Ackermann.

Tailed phages originated in the early Precambrian, long before eukaryotes and their viruses. The ancestral tailed phage had an icosahedral head of about 60 nanometers in diameter and a long non contractile tail with sixfold symmetry. The capsid contained a single molecule of double stranded DNA of about 50 kilobases. The tail was probably provided with a fixation apparatus. The head and tail were held together by a connector. The viral particle contained no lipids, was heavier than its descendant viruses and had a high DNA content proportional to its capsid size (~50%). Most of the genome coded for structural proteins. Morphopoietic genes clustered at one end of the genome, with head genes preceding tail genes. Lytic enzymes were probably coded for. Part of the phage genome was nonessential and possibly bacterial.

The virus infected its host from the outside and injected its DNA. Replication involved transcription in several waves and formation of DNA concatemers.

New phages were released by burst of the infected cell after lysis of host membranes by a peptidoglycan hydrolase. Capsids were assembled from a starting point, the connector and around a scaffold. They underwent an elaborate maturation process involving protein cleavage and capsid expansion. Heads and tails were assembled separately and joined later. The DNA was cut to size and entered preformed capsids by a headful mechanism.

Subsequently the phages evolved contractile or short tails and elongated heads. Some viruses become temperate by acquiring an integrase-excisionase complex, plasmid parts or transposons.

NCLDVs

The asfarviruses, iridoviruses, mimiviruses, phycodnaviruses and poxviruses have been shown to belong to a single group,—the large nuclear and cytoplasmic DNA viruses. These are also abbreviated "NCLDV". This clade can be divided into two groups:

- the iridoviruses-phycodnaviruses-mimiviruses group. The phycodnaviruses and mimiviruses are sister clades.
- the poxvirus-asfarviruses group.

It is probable that these viruses evolved before the separation of eukaryoyes into the extant crown groups. The ancestral genome was complex with at least 41 genes including (1) the replication machinery (2) up to four RNA polymerase subunits (3) at least three transcription factors (4) capping and polyadenylation enzymes (5) the DNA packaging apparatus (6) and structural components of an icosahedral capsid and the viral membrane.

The evolution of this group of viruses appears to be complex with genes having been gained from multiple sources. It has been proposed that the ancestor of NCLDVs has evolved from large, virus-like DNA transposons of the Polinton/Maverick family. From Polinton/Maverick transposons NCLDVs might have inherited the key components required for virion morphogenesis, including the major and minor capsid proteins, maturation protease and genome packaging ATPase.

Another group of large viruses—the Pandoraviridae—has been described. Two species—Pandoravirus salinus and Pandoravirus dulcis—have been recognized. These were isolated from Chile and Australia respectively. These viruses are about one micrometer in diameter making them one of the largest viruses discovered so far. Their gene complement is larger than any other known virus to date. At present they appear to be unrelated to any other species of virus.

An even larger genus, Pithovirus, has since been discovered, measuring about 1.5 μm in length. Another virus - Cedratvirus - may be related this group.

PHAGE ECOLOGY

Bacteriophages (phages), potentially the most numerous organisms on Earth, are the viruses of bacteria (more generally, of prokaryotes). Phage ecology is the study of the interaction of bacteriophages with their environments.

Vastness of Phage Ecology

Phages are obligate intracellular parasites meaning that they are able to reproduce only while infecting bacteria. Phages therefore are found only within environments that contain bacteria. Most environments contain bacteria, including our own bodies (called normal flora). Often these bacteria are found in large numbers. As a consequence, phages are found almost everywhere.

As a rule of thumb, many phage biologists expect that phage population densities will exceed bacterial densities by a ratio of 10-to-1 or more (VBR or virus-to-bacterium ratio; see for a summary of actual data). As there exist estimates of bacterial numbers on Earth of approximately 1030,there consequently is an expectation that 1031 or more individual virus (mostly phage) particles exist , making phages the most numerous category of “organisms on our planet.

Bacteria (along with archaea) appear to be highly diverse and there possibly are millions of species. Phage-ecological interactions therefore are quantitatively vast: huge numbers of interactions. Phage-ecological interactions are also qualitatively diverse: There are huge numbers of environment types, bacterial-host types, and also individual phage types

Studying Phage Ecology

The study of phage ecology reflects established scientific disciplines in ecological studies in scope, the most obvious being general ecology. Accordingly, phage ecology is treated under the following heads— "organismal" ecology, population ecology, community ecology, and ecosystem ecology. Phage ecology also may be considered (though mostly less well formally explored) from perspectives of phage behavioral ecology, evolutionary ecology, functional ecology, landscape ecology, mathematical ecology, molecular ecology, physiological ecology (or ecophysiology), and spatial ecology. Phage ecology additionally draws (extensively) from microbiology, particularly in terms of environmental microbiology, but also from an enormous catalog (90 years) of study of phage and phage-bacterial interactions in terms of their physiology and, especially, their molecular biology.

Phage "Organismal" Ecology

Phage "organismal" ecology is primarily the study of the evolutionary ecological impact of phage growth parameters:

- latent period, plus
    - eclipse period (or simply eclipse)
    - rise period (or simply rise)
- burst size, plus
    - rate of intracellular phage-progeny maturation
- adsorption constant, plus
    - rates of virion diffusion
    - virion decay (inactivation) rates
- host range, plus
    - resistance to restriction
    - resistance to abortive infection
- various temperate-phage properties, including
    - rates of reduction to lysogeny
    - rates of lysogen induction
- the tendency of at least some phage to enter into (and then subsequently leave) a not very well understood state known (inconsistently) as pseudolysogeny

Another way of envisioning phage organismal ecology is that it is the study of phage adaptations that contribute to phage survival and transmission to new hosts or environments. Phage organismal ecology is the most closely aligned of phage ecology disciplines with the classical molecular and molecular genetic analyses of bacteriophage.

From the perspective of ecological subdisciplines, we can also consider phage behavioral ecology, functional ecology, and physiological ecology under the heading of phage organismal ecology. However, as noted, these subdisciplines are not as well developed as more general considerations of phage organismal ecology. Phage growth parameters often evolve over the course of phage experimental adaptation studies.

Historical Overview

In the mid 1910s, when phage were first discovered, the concept of phage was very much a whole-culture phenomenon (like much of microbiology), where various types of bacterial cultures (on solid media, in broth) were visibly cleared by phage action. Though from the start there was some sense, especially by Fėlix d›Hėrelle, that phage consisted of individual organisms, in fact it wasn›t until the late 1930s through the 1940s that phage were studied, with rigor, as individuals, e.g., by electron microscopy and single-step growth experiments. Note, though, that for practical reasons much of "organismal" phage study is of their properties in bulk culture (many phage) rather than the properties of individual phage virions or individual infections.

This somewhat whole-organismal view of phage biology saw its heyday during the 1940s and 1950s, before giving way to much more biochemical, molecular genetic, and molecular biological analyses of phage, as seen during the 1960s and onward. This shift, paralleled in much of the rest of microbiology , represented a retreat from a much more ecological view of phages (first as bacterial killers, and then as organisms unto themselves). However, the organismal view of phage biology lives on as a foundation of phage ecological understanding. Indeed, it represents a key thread that ties together the ecological thinking on phage ecology with the more "modern" considerations of phage as molecular model systems.

Methods

The basic experimental toolkit of phage "organismal" ecology consists of the single-step growth (or one-step growth;) experiment and the phage adsorption curve. Single-step growth is a means of determining the phage latent period (example), which is approximately equivalent (depending on how it is defined) to the phage period of infection. Single-step growth experiments also are employed to determine a phage›s burst size, which is the number of phage (on average) that are produced per phage-infected bacterium.

The adsorption curve is obtained by measuring the rate at which phage virion particles (see Virion#Structure) attach to bacteria. This is usually done by separating free phage from phage-infected bacteria in some manner so that either the loss of not currently infecting (free) phage or the gain of infected bacteria may be measured over time.

Phage Population Ecology

A population is a group of individuals which either do or can interbreed or, if incapable of interbreeding, then are recently derived from a single individual (a clonal population). Population ecology considers characteristics that are apparent in populations of individuals but either are not apparent or are much less apparent among individuals. These characteristics include so-called intraspecific interactions, that is between individuals making up the same population, and can include competition as well as cooperation. Competition can be either in terms of rates of population growth (as seen especially at lower population densities in resource-rich environments) or in terms of retention of population sizes (seen especially at higher population densities where individuals are directly competing over limited resources). Respectively, these are population-density independent and dependent effects.

Phage population ecology considers issues of rates of phage population growth, but also phage-phage interactions as can occur when two or more phage adsorb an individual bacterium.

Phage Community Ecology

A community consists of all of the biological individuals found within a given environment (more formally, within an ecosystem), particularly when more than one species is present. Community ecology studies those characteristics of communities that either are not apparent or which are much less apparent if a community consists of only a single population. Community ecology thus deals with interspecific interactions. Interspecific interactions, like intraspecific interactions, can range from cooperative to competitive but also to quite antagonistic (as are seen, for example, with predator-prey interactions). An important consequence of these interactions is coevolution.

Relationship with Bacteria

The interaction of phage with bacteria is the primary concern of phage community ecologists. Bacteria have developed mechanisms that prevent phage from having an effect on them, which has led to this evolutionary arms race between the phage and their host bacteria. Bacterial resistance to phage puts pressure on the phage to develop stronger effects on the bacteria. The Red Queen hypothesis describes this relationship, as the organisms must constantly adapt and evolve in order to survive. This relationship is important to understand as phage are now being used for more practical and medicinal purposes.

Bacteria have developed multiple defense mechanisms to fight off the effects of bacteriophage. In experimentation, amount of resistance can be determined by how much of a plate (generally agar with bacteria, infected with phage) ends up being clear. The clearer, the less resistant as more bacteria have been lysed. The most common of these defense mechanisms is called the restriction-modification system (RM system). In this system, foreign DNA trying to enter the bacterial host is restricted by endonucleases that recognize specific base pairs within the DNA, while the DNA of the cell is protected from restriction due to methylase. RM systems have evolved to keep up with the ever-changing bacteria and phage. In general, these RM types differ in the nucleotide sequences that they recognize. However, there is an occasional slip where the endonuclease misses the DNA sequence of the phage and the phage DNA is able to enter the cell anyway, becoming methylated and protected against the endonuclease. This accident is what can spur the evolution of the RM system. Phage can acquire or use the enzyme from the host cell to protect their own DNA, or sometimes they will have proteins that dismantle the enzyme that is meant to restrict the phage DNA. Another option is for the phage to insert different base pairs into its DNA, thereby confusing the enzyme.

Another mechanism employed by bacteria is referred to as CRISPR. This stands for "clustered regularly interspersed palindromic repeats" which means that the immunity to phages by bacteria has been acquired via adding spacers of DNA that are identical to that of the DNA from the phage. Some phage have been found to be immune to this mechanism as well. In some way or another, the phage have managed to get rid of the sequence that would be replicated.

A third way that bacteria have managed to escape the effects of bacteriophage is by abortive infection. This is a last resort option- when the host cell has already been infected by the phage. This method is not ideal for the host cell, as it still leads to its death. The redeeming feature of this mechanism is the fact that it interferes with the phage processes and prevents it from then moving on to infect other cells.

Phage are also capable of interacting with species other than bacteria, e.g., such as phage-encoded exotoxin interaction with animals. Phage therapy is an example of applied phage community ecology.

Phage Ecosystem Ecology

An ecosystem consists of both the biotic and abiotic components of an environment. Abiotic entities are not alive and so an ecosystem essentially is a community combined with the non-living environment within which that ecosystem exists. Ecosystem ecology naturally differs from community ecology in terms of the impact of the community on these abiotic entities, and vice versa. In practice, the portion of the abiotic environment of most concern to ecosystem ecologists is inorganic nutrients and energy.

Phage impact the movement of nutrients and energy within ecosystems primarily by lysing bacteria. Phage can also impact abiotic factors via the encoding of exotoxins (a subset of which are capable of solubilizing the biological tissues of living animals). Phage ecosystem ecologists are primarily concerned with the phage impact on the global carbon cycle, especially within the context of a phenomenon known as the microbial loop.

REFERENCES

1. "Evolutionary Bioinformatics Online 2005". Libertas Academica.
2. "ICTV Official Taxonomy: Updates since the 8th Report". ICTV Official Taxonomy. ICTV Official Taxonomy. Retrieved 11 June 2014.
3. Bernardo P, Golden M, Akram M, et al. (October 2013). "Identification and characterisation of a highly divergent geminivirus: evolutionary and taxonomic

implications". Virus Res. 177 (1): 35–45. doi:10.1016/j.virusres.2013.07.006. PMID 23886668.

4. Abedon ST, Hyman P, Thomas C (December 2003). "Experimental examination of bacteriophage latent-period evolution as a response to bacterial availability". Appl. Environ. Microbiol. 69 (12): 7499–506. doi:10.1128/AEM.69.12.7499-7506.2003. PMC 310036Freely accessible. PMID 14660403.
5. Ackermann HW (1998). "Tailed bacteriophages: the order caudovirales". Adv Virus Res. Advances in Virus Research. 51: 135–201. doi:10.1016/S0065-3527(08)60785-X. ISBN 9780120398515. PMID 9891587.
6. Ackermann HW (2003). "Bacteriophage observations and evolution". Res Microbiol. 154 (4): 245–251. doi:10.1016/S0923-2508(03)00067-6. PMID 12798228.
7. Ackermann HW, Prangishvili D (2012). "Prokaryote viruses studied by electron microscopy". Arch Virol. 157 (10): 1843–9. doi:10.1007/s00705-012-1383-y. PMID 22752841.
8. Al Rwahnih M, Dave A, Anderson MM, Rowhani A, Uyemoto JK, Sudarshana M (October 2013). "Association of a DNA virus with grapevines affected by red blotch disease in California". Phytopathology Phytopathology. 103 (10): 1069–76. doi:10.1094/PHYTO-10-12-0253-R. PMID 23656312.
9. Andreani J, Aherfi S, Bou Khalil JY, Di Pinto F, Bitam I, Raoult D, Colson P, La Scola B (2016) Cedratvirus, a double-cork structured giant virus, is a distant relative of Pithoviruses. Viruses 8(11). pii: E300
10. Angly FE, Felts B, Breitbart M, Salamon P, Edwards RA, Carlson C, Chan AM, Haynes M, Kelley S, Liu H, Mahaffy JM, Mueller JE, Nulton J, Olson R, Parsons R, Rayhawk S, Suttle CA, Rohwer F (2006). "The marine viromes of four oceanic regions". PLoS Biol. 4 (11): e368. doi:10.1371/journal.pbio.0040368. PMC 1634881Freely accessible. PMID 17090214.
11. Baker ML, Jiang W, Rixon FJ, Chiu W (2005). "Common ancestry of herpesviruses and tailed DNA bacteriophages". J. Virol. 79 (23): 14967–70. doi:10.1128/JVI.79.23.14967-14970.2005. PMC 1287596Freely accessible. PMID 16282496.
12. Barksdale L, Arden SB (1974). "Persisting bacteriophage infections, lysogeny, and phage conversions". Annu. Rev. Microbiol. 28: 265–99. doi:10.1146/annurev.mi.28.100174.001405. PMID 4215366.
13. Bassami MR, Berryman D, Wilcox GE, Raidal SR (1998). "Psittacine beak and feather disease virus nucleotide sequence analysis and its relationship to porcine circovirus, plant circoviruses, and chicken anaemia virus". Virology. 249 (2): 453–9. doi:10.1006/viro.1998.9324. PMID 9791035.
14. Belyi VA, Levine AJ, Skalka AM (2010). "Sequences from ancestral single-stranded DNA viruses in vertebrate genomes: the parvoviridae and circoviridae are more than 40 to 50 million years old". J Virol. 84 (23): 12458–62. doi:10.1128/JVI.01789-10. PMC 2976387Freely accessible. PMID 20861255.
15. Benson SD, Bamford JK, Bamford DH, Burnett RM (1999). "Viral evolution revealed by bacteriophage PRD1 and human adenovirus coat protein structures".

Cell. 98 (6): 825–833. doi:10.1016/S0092-8674(00)81516-0. PMID 10499799.

16. Bézier A, Annaheim M, Herbinière J, Wetterwald C, Gyapay G, Bernard-Samain S, Wincker P, Roditi I, Heller M, Belghazi M, Pfister-Wilhem R, Periquet G, Dupuy C, Huguet E, Volkoff AN, Lanzrein B, Drezen JM (2009). "Polydnaviruses of braconid wasps derive from an ancestral nudivirus". Science. 323 (5916): 926–930. doi:10.1126/science.1166788. PMID 19213916.
17. Blinkova O, Victoria J, Li Y, Keele BF, Sanz C, Ndjango JB, Peeters M, Travis D, Lonsdorf EV, Wilson ML, Pusey AE, Hahn BH, Delwart EL (2010). "Novel circular DNA viruses in stool samples of wild-living chimpanzees". J Gen Virol. 91 (Pt 1): 74–86. doi:10.1099/vir.0.015446-0. PMC 2887567Freely accessible. PMID 19759238.
18. Breitbart M, Salamon P, Andresen B, et al. (October 2002). "Genomic analysis of uncultured marine viral communities". Proc. Natl. Acad. Sci. U.S.A. 99 (22): 14250–5. doi:10.1073/pnas.202488399. PMC 137870Freely accessible. PMID 12384570.
19. Buckling, Angus; Rainey, Paul B. (1 January 2002). "Antagonistic Coevolution between a Bacterium and a Bacteriophage". Proceedings: Biological Sciences. 269 (1494): 931–936. JSTOR 3067783.
20. Castrignano SB, Nagasse-Sugahara TK, Kisielius JJ, Ueda-Ito M, Brandão PE, Curti SP (December 2013). "Two novel circo-like viruses detected in human feces: complete genome sequencing and electron microscopy analysis". Virus Res. 178 (2): 364–73. doi:10.1016/j.virusres.2013.09.018. PMID 24055464.
21. Cheung AK, Ng TF, Lager KM, Alt DP, Delwart E, Pogranichniy RM (2015). "Identification of several clades of novel single-stranded circular DNA viruses with conserved stem-loop structures in pig feces". Arch. Virol. 160 (1): 353–8. doi:10.1007/s00705-014-2234-9. PMID 25248627.
22. Cheung AK, Ng TF, Lager KM, Alt DP, Delwart EL, Pogranichniy RM (2014). "Identification of a novel single-stranded circular DNA virus in pig feces". Genome Announc. 2 (2). doi:10.1128/genomeA.00347-14. PMC 4007987Freely accessible. PMID 24786952.
23. Cheung, A. K.; Ng, T. F.-f.; Lager, K. M.; Alt, D. P.; Delwart, E. L.; Pogranichniy, R. M. (2014). "Unique Circovirus-Like Genome Detected in Pig Feces". Genome Announcements. 2 (2): e00251–14. doi:10.1128/genomeA.00251-14. ISSN 2169-8287. PMC 3983299Freely accessible. PMID 24723710.
24. Colson P, de Lamballerie X, Fournous G, Raoult D (2012). "Reclassification of giant viruses composing a fourth domain of life in the new order Megavirales". Intervirology. 55 (5): 321–32. doi:10.1159/000336562. PMID 22508375.
25. Colson P, De Lamballerie X, Yutin N, et al. (December 2013). """Megavirales", a proposed new order for eukaryotic nucleocytoplasmic large DNA viruses". Archives of Virology. 158 (12): 2517–21. doi:10.1007/s00705-013-1768-6. PMC 4066373Freely accessible. PMID 23812617.
26. Cotmore SF, Agbandje-McKenna M, Chiorini JA, Mukha DV, Pintel DJ, Qiu J, Soderlund-Venermo M, Tattersall P, Tijssen P, Gatherer D, Davison AJ (2014).

"The family Parvoviridae". Arch. Virol. 159 (5): 1239–47. doi:10.1007/s00705-013-1914-1. PMC 4013247Freely accessible. PMID 24212889.

27. Curtis TP, Sloan WT, Scannell JW (August 2002). "Estimating prokaryotic diversity and its limits". Proc. Natl. Acad. Sci. U.S.A. 99 (16): 10494–9. doi:10.1073/pnas.142680199. PMC 124953Freely accessible. PMID 12097644.
28. Davison AJ (2002). "Evolution of the herpesviruses". Veterinary microbiology. 86 (1–2): 69–88. doi:10.1016/S0378-1135(01)00492-8. PMID 11888691.
29. Davison AJ (2010). "Herpesvirus systematics". Vet Microbiol. 143 (1–2): 52–69. doi:10.1016/j.vetmic.2010.02.014. PMC 2995426Freely accessible. PMID 20346601.
30. Dayaram A, Galatowitsch M, Harding JS, Argüello-Astorga GR, Varsani A (March 2014). "Novel circular DNA viruses identified in Procorduliagrayi and Xanthocnemiszealandica larvae using metagenomic approaches". Infect Genet Evol. 22: 134–41. doi:10.1016/j.meegid.2014.01.013. PMID 24462907.
31. Dayaram A, Goldstien S, Zawar-Reza P, Gomez C, Harding JS, Varsani A (2013). "whose replication associated protein (Rep) shares similarities with Rep-like sequences of bacterial origin". J Gen Virol. 94 (Pt 5): 1104–10. doi:10.1099/vir.0.050088-0. PMID 23364192.
32. Dayaram A, Opong A, Jäschke A, Hadfield J, Baschiera M, Dobson RC, Offei SK, Shepherd DN, Martin DP, Varsani A (2012). "Molecular characterisation of a novel cassava associated circular ssDNA virus". Virus Res. 166 (1–2): 130–5. doi:10.1016/j.virusres.2012.03.009. PMID 22465471.
33. Dayaram A, Potter KA, Pailes R, Marinov M, Rosenstein DD, Varsani A (2015). "Identification of diverse circular single-stranded DNA viruses in adult dragonflies and damselflies (Insecta: Odonata) of Arizona and Oklahoma, USA". Infect Genet Evol. 30: 278–287. doi:10.1016/j.meegid.2014.12.037. PMID 25577985.
34. Delwart E, Li L (2012). "Rapidly expanding genetic diversity and host range of the Circoviridae viral family and other Rep encoding small circular ssDNA genomes.". Virus Research. 164 (1–2): 114–121. doi:10.1016/j.virusres.2011.11.021. PMC 3289258Freely accessible. PMID 22155583.
35. Desnues C, Rodriguez-Brito B, Rayhawk S, Kelley S, Tran T, Haynes M, Liu H, Furlan M, Wegley L, Chau B, Ruan Y, Hall D, Angly FE, Edwards RA, Li L, Thurber RV, Reid RP, Siefert J, Souza V, Valentine DL, Swan BK, Breitbart M, Rohwer F (2008). "Biodiversity and biogeography of phages in modern stromatolites and thrombolites". Nature. 452 (7185): 340–3. doi:10.1038/nature06735. PMID 18311127.
36. Diemer GS, Stedman KM (2012). "A novel virus genome discovered in an extreme environment suggests recombination between unrelated groups of RNA and DNA viruses". Biology Direct. 7 (1): 13. doi:10.1186/1745-6150-7-13. PMC 3372434Freely accessible. PMID 22515485.
37. Federici BA, Bideshi DK, Tan Y, Spears T, Bigot Y (2009). "Ascoviruses: superb manipulators of apoptosis for viral replication and transmission". Curr Top Microbiol Immunol. Current Topics in Microbiology and Immunology.

328: 171–196. doi:10.1007/978-3-540-68618-7_5. ISBN 978-3-540-68617-0. PMID 19216438.

38. Gibbs MJ, Weiller GF (1999). "Evidence that a plant virus switched hosts to infect a vertebrate and then recombined with a vertebrate-infecting virus". Proc Natl Acad Sci USA. 96 (14): 8022–7. doi:10.1073/pnas.96.14.8022. PMC 22181Freely accessible. PMID 10393941.
39. Gronenborn B (2004). "Nanoviruses: genome organisation and protein function". Vet Microbiol. 98 (2): 103–9. doi:10.1016/j.vetmic.2003.10.015. PMID 14741122.
40. Grose C (2012). "Pangaea and the Out-of-Africa Model of Varicella-Zoster Virus Evolution and Phylogeography". Journal of Virology. 86 (18): 9558–65. doi:10.1128/JVI.00357-12. PMC 3446551Freely accessible. PMID 22761371.
41. Hanna ZR, Runckel C, Fuchs J, DeRisi JL, Mindell DP, Van Hemert C, Handel CM, Dumbacher JP (2015). "Isolation of a complete circular virus genome sequence from an Alaskan black-capped chickadee (Poecile atricapillus) gastrointestinal tract sample". Genome Announc. 3 (5): e01081–15. doi:10.1128/genomeA.01081-15. PMC 4582580Freely accessible. PMID 26404604.
42. Ilyina TV, Koonin EV (1992). "Conserved sequence motifs in the initiator proteins for rolling circle DNA replication encoded by diverse replicons from eubacteria, eucaryotes and archaebacteria". Nucleic Acids Res. 20 (13): 3279–85. doi:10.1093/nar/20.13.3279. PMC 312478Freely accessible. PMID 1630899.
43. ISSN 0092-8240 issue v62i0004 article 759
44. ISSN 0265-9247 issue v33i0001 article 43
45. Iyer LM, Balaji S, Koonin EV, Aravind L (2006). "Evolutionary genomics of nucleo-cytoplasmic large DNA viruses". Virus Res. 117 (1): 156–184. doi:10.1016/j.virusres.2006.01.009. PMID 16494962.
46. Jackson EW, Bistolas KS, Button JB, Hewson I (2016) Novel Circular Single-Stranded DNA Viruses among an Asteroid, Echinoid and Holothurian (Phylum: Echinodermata). PLoS One 17;11(11):e0166093
47. Jehle JA, Abd-Alla AM, Wang Y (2012). "Phylogeny and evolution of Hytrosaviridae". J Invertebr Pathol. 112 Suppl: S62–7. doi:10.1016/j.jip.2012.07.015. PMID 22841640.
48. Keller J, Leulliot N, Cambillau C, Campanacci V, Porciero S, Prangishvilli D, Forterre P, Cortez D, Quevillon-Cheruel S, van Tilbeurgh H (2007). "Crystal structure of AFV3-109, a highly conserved protein from crenarchaeal viruses". Virol J. 22 (4): 12. doi:10.1186/1743-422X-4-12. PMC 1796864Freely accessible. PMID 17241456.
49. Kim AR, Chung HC, Kim HK, Kim EO, Nguyen VG, Choi MG, Yang HJ, Kim JA, Park BK (February 2014). "Characterization of a complete genome of a circular single-stranded DNA virus from porcine stools in Korea". Virus Genes. 48 (1): 81–8. doi:10.1007/s11262-013-1003-2. PMID 24170425.
50. Knopf CW (1998). "Evolution of viral DNA-dependent DNA polymerases". Virus Genes. 16 (1): 47–58. doi:10.1023/A:1007997609122. PMID 9562890.

51. Koonin EV, Krupovic M, Yutin N (2015). "Evolution of double-stranded DNA viruses of eukaryotes: from bacteriophages to transposons to giant viruses". Ann. N. Y. Acad. Sci. 1341: 10–24. doi:10.1111/nyas.12728. PMC 4405056Freely accessible. PMID 25727355.

52. Krenz B, Thompson JR, Fuchs M, Perry KL (2012). "Complete genome sequence of a new circular DNA virus from grapevine". J Virol. 86 (14): 7715. doi:10.1128/JVI.00943-12. PMC 3416304Freely accessible. PMID 22733880.

53. Krupovic M (2012). "Recombination between RNA viruses and plasmids might have played a central role in the origin and evolution of small DNA viruses". BioEssays. 34 (10): 867–870. doi:10.1002/bies.201200083. PMID 22886750.

54. Krupovic M (2013). "Networks of evolutionary interactions underlying the polyphyletic origin of ssDNA viruses". Curr Opin Virol. 3 (5): 578–586. doi:10.1016/j.coviro.2013.06.010. PMID 23850154.

55. Krupovic M, Bamford DH (2008). "Virus evolution: how far does the double beta-barrel viral lineage extend?". Nature Reviews Microbiology. 6 (12): 941–8. doi:10.1038/nrmicro2033. PMID 19008892.

56. Krupovic M, Bamford DH, Koonin EV (2014). "Conservation of major and minor jelly-roll capsid proteins in Polinton (Maverick) transposons suggests that they are bona fide viruses". Biol Direct. 9: 6. doi:10.1186/1745-6150-9-6. PMC 4028283Freely accessible. PMID 24773695.

57. Krupovic M, Forterre P, Bamford DH (2010). "Comparative analysis of the mosaic genomes of tailed archaeal viruses and proviruses suggests common themes for virion architecture and assembly with tailed viruses of bacteria". J Mol Biol. 397 (1): 144–160. doi:10.1016/j.jmb.2010.01.037. PMID 20109464.

58. Krupovic M, Koonin EV (2014). "Evolution of eukaryotic single-stranded DNA viruses of the Bidnaviridae family from genes of four other groups of widely different viruses". Scientific Reports. 4: 5347. doi:10.1038/srep05347. PMC 4061559Freely accessible. PMID 24939392.

59. Krupovic M, Koonin EV (2015). "Polintons: a hotbed of eukaryotic virus, transposon and plasmid evolution". Nat Rev Microbiol. 13 (2): 105–115. doi:10.1038/nrmicro3389. PMID 25534808.

60. Krupovic M, Ravantti JJ, Bamford DH (2009). "Geminiviruses: a tale of a plasmid becoming a virus" (PDF). BMC Evol Biol. 9 (1): 112. doi:10.1186/1471-2148-9-112. PMC 2702318Freely accessible. PMID 19460138.

61. Labonté JM, Suttle CA (November 2013). "Previously unknown and highly divergent ssDNA viruses populate the oceans". ISME J. 7 (11): 2169–77. doi:10.1038/ismej.2013.110. PMC 3806263Freely accessible. PMID 23842650.

62. Lamberto I, Gunst K, Müller H, Zur Hausen H, de Villiers EM (2014). "Mycovirus-like DNA virus sequences from cattle serum and human brain and serum samples from multiple sclerosis patients". Genome Announc. 2 (4): e00848–14. doi:10.1128/genomeA.00848-14. PMC 4148726Freely accessible. PMID 25169858.

63. Legendre, M.; Bartoli, J.; Shmakova, L.; Jeudy, S.; Labadie, K.; Adrait, A.;

Lescot, M.; Poirot, O.; Bertaux, L.; Bruley, C.; Coute, Y.; Rivkina, E.; Abergel, C.; Claverie, J.-M. (2014). "Thirty-thousand-year-old distant relative of giant icosahedral DNA viruses with a pandoravirus morphology". Proc. Natl. Acad. Sci. U.S.A. To appear (11): 4274–9. doi:10.1073/pnas.1320670111. PMID 24591590.

64. Lenski, Richard E.; Levin, Bruce R. (1 January 1985). "Constraints on the Coevolution of Bacteria and Virulent Phage: A Model, Some Experiments, and Predictions for Natural Communities". The American Naturalist. 125 (4): 585–602. JSTOR 2461275.
65. Li W, Gu Y, Shen Q, Yang S, Wang X, Wan Y, Zhang W (2015). "A novel gemycircularvirus from experimental rats". Virus Genes. 51 (2): 302–5. doi:10.1007/s11262-015-1238-1. PMID 26303898.
66. Liu H, Fu Y, Xie J, Cheng J, Ghabrial SA, Li G, Peng Y, Yi X, Jiang D (2011). "Widespread endogenization of Densoviruses and Parvoviruses in animal and human genomes". J Virol. 85 (19): 9863–76. doi:10.1128/JVI.00828-11. PMC 3196449Freely accessible. PMID 21795360.
67. Male MF, Kami V, Kraberger S, Varsani A (2015). "Genome sequences of Poaceae-associated Gemycircularviruses from the Pacific Ocean island of Tonga". Genome Announc. 3 (5): e01144–15. doi:10.1128/genomeA.01144-15. PMC 4611678Freely accessible. PMID 26472826.
68. McGeoch DJ, Cook S (1994). "Molecular phylogeny of the alphaherpesvirinae subfamily and a proposed evolutionary timescale". J Mol Biol. 238 (1): 9–22. doi:10.1006/jmbi.1994.1264. PMID 8145260.
69. McGeoch DJ, Cook S, Dolan A, Jamieson FE, Telford EA (1995). "Molecular phylogeny and evolutionary timescale for the family of mammalian herpesviruses". J Mol Biol. 247 (3): 443–458. doi:10.1006/jmbi.1995.0152. PMID 7714900.
70. McGeoch DJ, Rixon FJ, Davison AJ (2006). "Topics in herpesvirus genomics and evolution". Virus Res. 117 (1): 90–104. doi:10.1016/j.virusres.2006.01.002. PMID 16490275.
71. Meehan BM, Creelan JL, McNulty MS, Todd D (1997). "Sequence of porcine circovirus DNA: affinities with plant circoviruses". J Gen Virol. 78 (Pt 1): 221–7. doi:10.1099/0022-1317-78-1-221. PMID 9010307.
72. Miller, R. V. & S. A. Ripp (2002). "Pseudolysogeny: A bacteriophage strategy for increasing longevity in situ". In Kado, Clarence I. & Syvanen, Michael. Horizontal gene transfer (2nd ed.). Boston: Academic Press. pp. 81–91. ISBN 0-12-680126-6.
73. Mochizuki T, Krupovic M, Pehau-Arnaudet G, Sako Y, Forterre P, Prangishvili D (2012). "Archaeal virus with exceptional virion architecture and the largest single-stranded DNA genome". Proc Natl Acad Sci U S A. 109 (33): 13386–91. doi:10.1073/pnas.1203668109. PMC 3421227Freely accessible. PMID 22826255.
74. Ng TF, Alavandi S, Varsani A, Burghart S, Breitbart M (2013). "Metagenomic identification of a nodavirus and a circular ssDNA virus in semi-purified viral nucleic acids from the hepatopancreas of healthy Farfantepenaeus duorarum shrimp". Dis Aquat Organ. 105 (3): 237–42. doi:10.3354/dao02628. PMID

23999707.

75. Ng TF, Chen LF, Zhou Y, Shapiro B, Stiller M, Heintzman PD, Varsani A, Kondov NO, Wong W, Deng X, Andrews TD, Moorman BJ, Meulendyk T, MacKay G, Gilbertson RL, Delwart E (2014). "Preservation of viral genomes in 700-y-old caribou feces from a subarctic ice patch". Proc. Natl. Acad. Sci. U.S.A. 111 (47): 16842–7. doi:10.1073/pnas.1410429111. PMC 4250163Freely accessible. PMID 25349412.

76. Ng TF, Manire C, Borrowman K, Langer T, Ehrhart L, Breitbart M (2009). "Discovery of a novel single-stranded DNA virus from a sea turtle fibropapilloma by using viral metagenomics". J Virol. 83 (6): 2500–9. doi:10.1128/JVI.01946-08. PMC 2648252Freely accessible. PMID 19116258.

77. Niagro FD, Forsthoefel AN, Lawther RP, Kamalanathan L, Ritchie BW, Latimer KS, Lukert PD (1998). "Beak and feather disease virus and porcine circovirus genomes: intermediates between the geminiviruses and plant circoviruses". Arch Virol. 143 (9): 1723–44. doi:10.1007/s007050050412. PMID 9787657.

78. Ogata H, Toyoda K, Tomaru Y, Nakayama N, Shirai Y, Claverie JM, Nagasaki K (2009). "Remarkable sequence similarity between the dinoflagellate-infecting marine girus and the terrestrial pathogen African swine fever virus". Virol J. 6 (1): 178. doi:10.1186/1743-422X-6-178. PMC 2777158Freely accessible. PMID 19860921.

79. Pennisi, E. (2013). "Ever-Bigger Viruses Shake Tree of Life". Science. 341 (6143): 226–7. doi:10.1126/science.341.6143.226. PMID 23868995.

80. Pham HT, Bergoin M, Tijssen P (2013). "Acheta domesticus volvovirus, a novel single-stranded circular DNA virus of the house cricket". Genome Announc. 1 (2): e0007913. doi:10.1128/genomeA.00079-13. PMC 3623006Freely accessible. PMID 23516206.

81. Pham HT, Iwao H, Bergoin M, Tijssen P (2013). "New Volvovirus Isolates from Acheta domesticus (Japan) and Gryllus assimilis (United States)". Genome Announc. 1 (3): e00328–13. doi:10.1128/genomeA.00328-13. PMC 3675518Freely accessible. PMID 23792751.

82. Pham HT, Yu Q, Boisvert M, Van HT, Bergoin M, Tijssen P (2014). "A circo-like virus isolated from Penaeus monodon shrimps". Genome Announc. 2 (1): e01172–13. doi:10.1128/genomeA.01172-13. PMC 3894284Freely accessible. PMID 24435870.

83. Phan TG, Kapusinszky B, Wang C, Rose RK, Lipton HL, Delwart EL (2011). "The fecal viral flora of wild rodents". PLoS Pathog. 7 (9): e1002218. doi:10.1371/journal.ppat.1002218. PMC 3164639Freely accessible. PMID 21909269.

84. Phan TG, Mori D, Deng X, Rajindrajith S, Ranawaka U, Fan Ng TF, Bucardo-Rivera F, Orlandi P, Ahmed K, Delwart E (2015). "Small circular single stranded DNA viral genomes in unexplained cases of human encephalitis, diarrhea, and in untreated sewage". Virology. 482: 98–104. doi:10.1016/j.virol.2015.03.011. PMC 4461510Freely accessible. PMID 25839169.

85. Phan TG, Vo NP, Bonkoungou IJ, Kapoor A, Barro N, O'Ryan M, Kapusinszky

B, Wang C, Delwart E (2012). "Acute diarrhea in West-African children: diverse enteric viruses and a novel parvovirus genus". J Virol. 86 (20): 11024–30. doi:10.1128/JVI.01427-12. PMC 3457132Freely accessible. PMID 22855485.

86. Pietilä MK, Atanasova NS, Manole V, Liljeroos L, Butcher SJ, Oksanen HM, Bamford DH (2012). "Virion Architecture Unifies Globally Distributed Pleolipoviruses Infecting Halophilic Archaea". Journal of Virology. 86 (9): 5067–79. doi:10.1128/JVI.06915-11. PMC 3347350Freely accessible. PMID 22357279.
87. Pietilä MK, Atanasova NS, Manole V, Liljeroos L, Butcher SJ, Oksanen HM, Bamford DH (2012). "Virion architecture unifies globally distributed pleolipoviruses infecting halophilic archaea". J Virol. 86 (9): 5067–79. doi:10.1128/JVI.06915-11. PMC 3347350Freely accessible. PMID 22357279.
88. Pietilä MK, Laurinavicius S, Sund J, Roine E, Bamford DH (2010). "The single-stranded DNA genome of novel archaeal virus Halorubrum pleomorphic virus 1 is enclosed in the envelope decorated with glycoprotein spikes". J Virol. 84 (2): 788–798. doi:10.1128/JVI.01347-09. PMC 2798366Freely accessible. PMID 19864380.
89. Prangishvili D, Garrett RA (2004). "Exceptionally diverse morphotypes and genomes of crenarchaeal hyperthermophilic viruses". Biochem Soc Trans. 32 (Pt 2): 204–8. doi:10.1042/BST0320204. PMID 15046572.
90. Rebrikov DV, Bulina ME, Bogdanova EA, Vagner LL, Lukyanov SA (2002). "Complete genome sequence of a novel extrachromosomal virus-like element identified in planarian Girardia tigrina". BMC Genomics. 13 (1): 15. doi:10.1186/1471-2164-3-15. PMC 3269984Freely accessible. PMID 22233149.
91. Reuter G, Boros A, Delwart E, Pankovics P (2014). "Novel circular single-stranded DNA virus from turkey faeces". Arch Virol. 159 (8): 2161–4. doi:10.1007/s00705-014-2025-3. PMID 24562429.
92. Rosario K, Dayaram A, Marinov M, Ware J, Kraberger S, Stainton D, Breitbart M, Varsani A (2012). "Diverse circular ssDNA viruses discovered in dragonflies (Odonata: Epiprocta)". J Gen Virol. 93 (12): 2668–81. doi:10.1099/vir.0.045948-0. PMID 22915694.
93. Rosario K, Duffy S, Breitbart M (2009). "Diverse circovirus-like genome architectures revealed by environmental metagenomics". J Gen Virol. 90 (Pt 10): 2418–24. doi:10.1099/vir.0.012955-0. PMID 19570956.
94. Roumagnac P, Granier M, Bernardo P, Deshoux M, Ferdinand R, Galzi S, Fernandez E, Julian C, Abt I, Filloux D, Mesléard F, Varsani A, Blanc S, Martin DP, Peterschmitt M (2015). "Alfalfa Leaf Curl Virus: an Aphid-Transmitted Geminivirus". J. Virol. 89 (18): 9683–8. doi:10.1128/JVI.00453-15. PMC 4542355Freely accessible. PMID 26109720.
95. Roux S, Enault F, Bronner G, Vaulot D, Forterre P, Krupovic M (2013). "Chimeric viruses blur the borders between the major groups of eukaryotic single-stranded DNA viruses". Nat Commun. 4: 2700. doi:10.1038/ncomms3700. PMID 24193254.

96. Roux S, Krupovic M, Poulet A, Debroas D, Enault F (2012). "Evolution and diversity of the Microviridae viral family through a collection of 81 new complete genomes assembled from virome reads". PLoS ONE. 7 (7): e40418. doi:10.1371/journal.pone.0040418. PMC 3394797Freely accessible. PMID 22808158.

97. Sapp J (September 2006). "Two faces of the prokaryote concept" (PDF). Int. Microbiol. 9 (3): 163–72. PMID 17061206. provides a history.

98. Sasaki M, Gonzalez G, Wada Y, Setiyono A, Handharyani E, Rahmadani I, Taha S, Adiani S, Latief M, Kholilullah ZA, Subangkit M, Kobayashi S, Nakamura I, Kimura T, Orba Y, Ito K, Sawa H (2016). "Divergent bufavirus harboured in megabats represents a new lineage of parvoviruses". Sci Rep. 6: 24257. doi:10.1038/srep24257. PMC 4845017Freely accessible. PMID 27113297.

99. Senčilo A, Jacobs-Sera D, Russell DA, Ko CC, Bowman CA, Atanasova NS, Österlund E, Oksanen HM, Bamford DH, Hatfull GF, Roine E, Hendrix RW (2013). "Snapshot of haloarchaeal tailed virus genomes". RNA Biol. 10 (5): 803–816. doi:10.4161/rna.24045. PMC 3737338Freely accessible. PMID 23470522.

100. Sencilo A, Paulin L, Kellner S, Helm M, Roine E (2012). "Related haloarchaeal pleomorphic viruses contain different genome types". Nucleic Acids Res. 40 (12): 5523–34. doi:10.1093/nar/gks215. PMC 3384331Freely accessible. PMID 22396526.

101. Shutt TE, Gray MW (2005). "Bacteriophage origins of mitochondrial replication and transcription proteins". Trends Genet. 22 (2): 90–95. doi:10.1016/j.tig.2005.11.007. PMID 16364493.

102. Sikorski A, Argüello-Astorga GR, Dayaram A, Dobson RC, Varsani A (2012). "Discovery of a novel circular single-stranded DNA virus from porcine faeces". Arch Virol. 158 (1): 283–9. doi:10.1007/s00705-012-1470-0. PMID 22972681.

103. Sikorski A, Dayaram A, Varsani A (2013). "Identification of a Novel Circular DNA Virus in New Zealand Fur Seal (Arctocephalus forsteri) Fecal Matter". Genome Announc. 1 (4): e00558–13. doi:10.1128/genomeA.00558-13. PMC 3738887Freely accessible. PMID 23929471.

104. Sikorski A, Kearvell J, Elkington S, Dayaram A, Argüello-Astorga GR, Varsani A (2013). "Novel ssDNA viruses discovered in yellow-crowned parakeet (Cyanoramphus auriceps) nesting material". Arch Virol. 158 (7): 1603–7. doi:10.1007/s00705-013-1642-6. PMID 23417396.

105. Sikorski A, Massaro M, Kraberger S, Young LM, Smalley D, Martin DP, Varsani A (2013). "Novel myco-like DNA viruses discovered in the faecal matter of various animals". Virus Res. 177 (2): 209–216. doi:10.1016/j.virusres.2013.08.008. PMID 23994297.

106. Simoliūnas E, Kaliniene L, Truncaitė L, Zajančkauskaitė A, Staniulis J, Kaupinis A, Ger M, Valius M, Meškys R, et al. (2013). "Klebsiella phage vB_KleM-RaK2—A giant singleton virus of the family Myoviridae". PLoS ONE. 8 (4): e60717. doi:10.1371/journal.pone.0060717. PMC 3622015Freely accessible. PMID 23593293.

107. Sinshemer RL (1959). "A single-stranded deoxyribonucleic acid from

bacteriophage φX174". Journal of Molecular Biology. 1: 43–IN6. doi:10.1016/S0022-2836(59)80006-1.

108. Sinshemer RL (1959). "Purification and properties of bacteriophage φX174". Journal of Molecular Biology. 1: 37–IN5. doi:10.1016/S0022-2836(59)80005-X.
109. Sogin ML, Morrison HG, Huber JA, et al. (August 2006). "Microbial diversity in the deep sea and the underexplored "rare biosphere"". Proc. Natl. Acad. Sci. U.S.A. 103 (32): 12115–20. doi:10.1073/pnas.0605127103. PMC 1524930Freely accessible. PMID 16880384.
110. Stern, Adi; Sorek, Rotem (2011). "The phage-host arms race: Shaping the evolution of microbes". BioEssays. 33 (1): 43–51. doi:10.1002/bies.201000071. PMC 3274958Freely accessible. PMID 20979102.
111. Sukhumsirichart W, Attasart P, Boonsaeng V, Panyim S (2006). "Complete nucleotide sequence and genomic organization of hepatopancreatic parvovirus (HPV) of Penaeus monodon". Virology. 346 (2): 266–277. doi:10.1016/j.virol.2005.06.052. PMID 16356523.
112. Summers WC (1991). "From culture as organism to organism as cell: historical origins of bacterial genetics". J Hist Biol. 24 (2): 171–90. doi:10.1007/bf00209428. PMID 11612551.
113. The term "prokaryotes" is useful to mean the sum of the bacteria and archaea but otherwise can be controversial, as discussed by Woese CR (June 2004). "A new biology for a new century". Microbiol. Mol. Biol. Rev. 68 (2): 173–86. doi:10.1128/MMBR.68.2.173-186.2004. PMC 419918Freely accessible. PMID 15187180. The Dismantling of Bacteriology and a Deconstruction of the Procaryote; see also pp. 103–4 of Sapp, Jan (2004). "Evolving biological organization". Microbial phylogeny and evolution: concepts and controversies. Oxford [Oxfordshire]: Oxford University Press. pp. 99–118. ISBN 0-19-516877-1.
114. Thézé J, Bézier A, Periquet G, Drezen JM, Herniou EA (2011). "Paleozoic origin of insect large dsDNA viruses". Proc Natl Acad Sci USA. 108 (38): 15931–5. doi:10.1073/pnas.1105580108. PMC 3179036Freely accessible. PMID 21911395.
115. This article on phage ecology was expanded from a stub during the writing of the first chapter of the edited monograph, Bacteriophage Ecology (forecasted publication date: March, 2008, Cambridge University Press), in order to be cited by that chapter especially as a repository of phage ecology review chapters and articles.
116. Tijssen P, Bergoin M (1995). "Densonucleosis viruses constitute an increasingly diversified subfamily among the parvoviruses". Seminars in Virology. 6 (5): 347–355. doi:10.1006/smvy.1995.0041.
117. Tomaru Y, Toyoda K, Suzuki H, Nagumo T, Kimura K, Takao Y (2013). "New single-stranded DNA virus with a unique genomic structure that infects marine diatom Chaetoceros setoensis". Sci Rep. 3: 3337. doi:10.1038/srep03337. PMC 3840382Freely accessible. PMID 24275766.

118. Uch R, Fournier PE, Robert C, Blanc-Tailleur C, Galicher V, Barre R, Jordier F, de Micco P, Raoult D, Biagini P (2015). "Divergent Gemycircularvirus in HIV-positive blood, France". Emerg Infect Dis. 21 (11): 2096–8. doi:10.3201/eid2111.150486. PMC 4622245Freely accessible. PMID 26488181.

119. van den Brand JM, van Leeuwen M, Schapendonk CM, Simon JH, Haagmans BL, Osterhaus AD, Smits SL (2012). "Metagenomic Analysis of the Viral Flora of Pine Marten and European Badger Feces". Journal of Virology. 86 (4): 2360–5. doi:10.1128/JVI.06373-11. PMC 3302375Freely accessible. PMID 22171250.

120. Villarreal LP, DeFilippis VR (2000). "A hypothesis for DNA viruses as the origin of eukaryotic replication proteins". J Virol. 74 (15): 7079–84. doi:10.1128/JVI.74.15.7079-7084.2000. PMC 112226Freely accessible. PMID 10888648.

121. Wang Y, Bininda-Emonds OR, van Oers MM, Vlak JM, Jehle JA (2011). "The genome of Oryctes rhinoceros nudivirus provides novel insight into the evolution of nuclear arthropod-specific large circular double-stranded DNA viruses". Virus Genes. 42 (3): 444–456. doi:10.1007/s11262-011-0589-5. PMID 21380757.

122. Wang Y, Jehle JA (2009). "Nudiviruses and other large, double-stranded circular DNA viruses of invertebrates: new insights on an old topic". J Invertebr Pathol. 101 (3): 187–193. doi:10.1016/j.jip.2009.03.013. PMID 19460388.

123. Weinbauer MG (May 2004). "Ecology of prokaryotic viruses". FEMS Microbiol. Rev. 28 (2): 127–81. doi:10.1016/j.femsre.2003.08.001. PMID 15109783.

124. Whitman WB, Coleman DC, Wiebe WJ (June 1998). "Prokaryotes: the unseen majority". Proc. Natl. Acad. Sci. U.S.A. 95 (12): 6578–83. doi:10.1073/pnas.95.12.6578. PMC 33863Freely accessible. PMID 9618454.

125. Wilson WH, Van Etten JL, Allen MJ (2009). "The Phycodnaviridae: the story of how tiny giants rule the world". Curr Top Microbiol Immunol. Current Topics in Microbiology and Immunology. 328: 1–42. doi:10.1007/978-3-540-68618-7_1. ISBN 978-3-540-68617-0. PMC 2908299Freely accessible. PMID 19216434.

126. Wommack KE, Colwell RR (March 2000). "Virioplankton: viruses in aquatic ecosystems". Microbiol. Mol. Biol. Rev. 64 (1): 69–114. doi:10.1128/MMBR.64.1.69-114.2000. PMC 98987Freely accessible. PMID 10704475.

127. Xie Y, Wu P, Liu P, Gong H, Zhou X (2010). "Characterization of alphasatellites associated with monopartite begomovirus/betasatellite complexes in Yunnan, China". Virol J. 7 (1): 178. doi:10.1186/1743-422X-7-178. PMC 2922188Freely accessible. PMID 20678232.

128. Yoon HS, Price DC, Stepanauskas R, Rajah VD, Sieracki ME, Wilson WH, Yang EC, Duffy S, Bhattacharya D, et al. (2011). "Single-cell genomics reveals organismal interactions in uncultivated marine protists". Science. 332 (6030): 714–7. doi:10.1126/science.1203163. PMID 21551060.

129. You L, Suthers PF, Yin J (April 2002). "Effects of Escherichia coli physiology on growth of phage T7 in vivo and in silico". J. Bacteriol. 184 (7): 1888–94. doi:10.1128/JB.184.7.1888-1894.2002. PMC 134924Freely accessible. PMID 11889095.

130. Yu X, Li B, Fu Y, Jiang D, Ghabrial SA, Li G, Peng Y, Xie J, Cheng J, Huang J, Yi X (2010). "A geminivirus-related DNA mycovirus that confers hypovirulence to a plant pathogenic fungus". Proc Natl Acad Sci USA. 107 (18): 8387–92. doi:10.1073/pnas.0913535107. PMC 2889581Freely accessible. PMID 20404139.
131. Yutin N, Koonin EV (2012). "Hidden evolutionary complexity of Nucleo-Cytoplasmic Large DNA viruses of eukaryotes". Virol J. 9 (1): 161. doi:10.1186/1743-422X-9-161. PMC 3493329Freely accessible. PMID 22891861.
132. Yutin N, Koonin EV (2013). "Pandoraviruses are highly derived phycodnaviruses". Biol. Direct. 8: 25. doi:10.1186/1745-6150-8-25. PMC 3924356Freely accessible. PMID 24148757.
133. Yutin N, Wolf YI, Koonin EV (2014). "Origin of giant viruses from smaller DNA viruses not from a fourth domain of cellular life". Virology. 466–467: 38–52. doi:10.1016/j.virol.2014.06.032. PMC 4325995Freely accessible. PMID 25042053.
134. Yutin N, Wolf YI, Raoult D, Koonin EV (2009). "Eukaryotic large nucleo-cytoplasmic DNA viruses: clusters of orthologous genes and reconstruction of viral genome evolution". Virol. J. 6 (1): 223. doi:10.1186/1743-422X-6-223. PMC 2806869Freely accessible. PMID 20017929.
135. Yutin, Natalya; Raoult, Didier; Koonin, Eugene V (2013). "Virophages, polintons, and transpovirons: a complex evolutionary network of diverse selfish genetic elements with different reproduction strategies". Virology Journal. 10 (1): 158. doi:10.1186/1743-422X-10-158. ISSN 1743-422X. PMC 3671162Freely accessible. PMID 23701946.
136. Zhou C, Zhang S, Gong Q, Hao A (2015). "A novel gemycircularvirus in an unexplained case of child encephalitis". Virol. J. 12: 197. doi:10.1186/s12985-015-0431-0. PMC 4657213Freely accessible. PMID 26596706.
137. Zillig W, Prangishvilli D, Schleper C, Elferink M, Holz I, Albers S, Janekovic D, Götz D (1996). "Viruses, plasmids and other genetic elements of thermophilic and hyperthermophilic Archaea". FEMS Microbiol Rev. 18 (2–3): 225–236. doi:10.1111/j.1574-6976.1996.tb00239.x. PMID 8639330.

CHAPTER 7

Pathogenic Bacteria

Chapter Contents

- Introduction
- Diseases
- Mechanisms
- Identification
- Treatment
- List of Genera of Pathogenic Bacteria and Microscopy Features
- Acinetobacter Baumannii
- Pseudomonas Aeruginosa
- Moraxella Catarrhalis
- Biochemistry

Historically, bacteria have been the cause of some of the most deadly diseases and widespread epidemics of human civilization. Smallpox and malaria, diseases caused by other microbes, have killed more humans than bacterial diseases, but diseases such as tuberculosis, typhus, plague, diphtheria, typhoid, cholera, dysentery and pneumonia have taken a large toll of humanity. At the beginning of the Twentieth Century, pneumonia, tuberculosis and diarrhea were the three leading causes of death.

INTRODUCTION

Pathogenic bacteria are bacteria that can cause infection. This deals with human pathogenic bacteria.

Although most bacteria are harmless or often beneficial, several are pathogenic. One of the bacterial diseases with the highest disease burden is tuberculosis, caused by the bacterium *Mycobacterium tuberculosis*, which kills about 2 million people a year, mostly in sub-Saharan Africa. Pathogenic bacteria contribute to other globally important diseases, such as pneumonia, which can be caused by bacteria such as *Streptococcus* and *Pseudomonas*, and foodborne illnesses, which can be caused by bacteria such as *Shigella*, *Campylobacter*, and *Salmonella*. Pathogenic bacteria also cause infections such as tetanus, typhoid fever, diphtheria, syphilis, and leprosy. Pathogenic bacteria are also the cause of high infant mortality rates in developing countries.

Koch's postulates are the standard to establish a causative relationship between a microbe and a disease.

DISEASES

Each species has specific effect and causes symptoms in people who are infected. Some, if not most people who are infected with a pathogenic bacteria do not have symptoms. Immunocompromised individuals are more susceptible to pathogenic bacteria.

Pathogenic Susceptibility

Some pathogenic bacteria cause disease under certain conditions, such entry through the skin via a cut, through sexual activity or an compromised immune function. *Streptococcus* and *Staphylococcus* are part of the normal skin microbiota and typically reside on healthy skin or in the nasopharangeal region. Yet these species can potentially initiate skin infections. They are also able to cause sepsis, pneumonia, meningitis. These infections can become quite serious creating a systemic inflammatory response resulting in massive vasodilation, shock, and death. Other bacteria are opportunistic pathogens and cause disease mainly in people suffering from immunosuppression or cystic fibrosis Examples of these opportunistic pathogens include *Pseudomonas aeruginosa*, *Burkholderia cenocepacia*, and *Mycobacterium avium*.

Intracellular

Obligate intracellular parasites (e.g. Chlamydophila, Ehrlichia, Rickettsia) have the ability to only grow and replicate inside other cells. Even these intracellular infections may be asymptomatic, requiring an incubation period. An example of this *Rickettsia* which causes typhus. Another causes Rocky Mountain spotted fever.

Chlamydia is a phylum of intracellular parasites. These pathogens can cause pneumonia or urinary tract infection and may be involved in coronary heart disease.

Other groups of intracellular bacterial pathogens include *Salmonella*, *Neisseria*, *Brucella*, *Mycobacterium*, *Nocardia*, *Listeria*, *Francisella*, *Legionella*, and *Yersinia pestis*. These can exist intracellularly, but can exist outside of host cells.

Infections in Specific Tissue

Bacterial pathogens often cause infection in specific areas of the body. Others are generalists.

- Bacterial vaginosis is caused by bacteria that change the vaginal microbiota caused by an overgrowth of bacteria that crowd out the Lactobacilli species that maintain healthy vaginal microbial populations.
- Other non-bacterial vaginal infections include: yeast infection (candidiasis), *Trichomonas vaginalis* (trichomoniasis).
- Bacterial meningitis is a bacterial inflammation of the meninges, that is, the

protective membranes covering the brain and spinal cord.

- Bacterial pneumonia is a bacterial infection of the lungs.
- Urinary tract infection is predominantly caused by bacteria. Symptoms include the strong and frequent sensation or urge to urinate, pain during urination, and urine that is cloudy. The main causal agent is *Escherichia coli*. Urine is typically sterile but contains a variety of salts, and waste products. Bacteria can ascend into the bladder or kidney and causing cystitis and nephritis.
- Bacterial gastroenteritis is caused by enteric, pathogenic bacteria. These pathogenic species are usually distinct from the usually harmless bacteria of the normal gut flora. But a different strain of the same species may be pathogenic. The distinction is sometimes difficult as in the case of *Escherichia*.
- Bacterial skin infections include:
    - Impetigo is a highly contagious bacterial skin infection commonly seen in children. It is caused by *Staphylococcus aureus*, and *Streptococcus pyogenes*.
    - Erysipelas is an acute streptococcus bacterial infection of the deeper skin layers that spreads via with lymphatic system.
    - Cellulitis is a diffuse inflammation of connective tissue with severe inflammation of dermal and subcutaneous layers of the skin. Cellulitis can be caused by normal skin flora or by contagious contact, and usually occurs through open skin, cuts, blisters, cracks in the skin, insect bites, animal bites, burns, surgical wounds, intravenous drug injection, or sites of intravenous catheter insertion. In most cases it is the skin on the face or lower legs that is affected, though cellulitis can occur in other tissues.

MECHANISMS

Nutrients

Iron is required for humans, as well as the growth of most bacteria. To obtain free iron, some pathogens secrete proteins called siderophores, which take the iron away from iron-transport proteins by binding to the iron even more tightly. Once the iron-siderophore complex is formed, it is taken up by siderophore receptors on the bacterial surface and then that iron is brought into the bacterium.

Direct Damage

Once pathogens attach to host cells, they can cause direct damage as the pathogens use the host cell for nutrients and produce waste products. As pathogens multiply and divide inside host cells, the cells usually rupture and the intercellular bacteria are released. Some bacteria such as *E. coli*, *Shigella*, *Salmonella*, and *Neisseria gonorrhoeae*, can induce host epithelial cells to engulf them in a process resembling phagocytosis. The pathogens can then disrupt host cells as they pass through them and be extruded from host cells by a reverse phagocytosis process, enabling them to enter other host cells. Some bacteria can also penetrate host cells by excreting enzymes and by their own motility; such penetration can itself damage the host cell.

Toxin Production

Toxins are poisonous substances that are produced by certain microorganisms and are often the primary factor contributing to the pathogenic properties of the microorganisms. Endotoxins are the lipid portions of lipopolysaccharides that are part of the outer membrane of the cell wall of gram negative bacteria. Endotoxins are released when the bacteria lyses, which is why after antibiotic treatment symptoms can at first worsen as the bacteria are killed and they release their endotoxins. Exotoxins are proteins produced inside pathogenic bacteria as part of their growth and metabolism, most common in gram positive bacteria. The exotoxins are released when the bacteria die and the cell wall breaks apart. Exotoxins are highly specific in the effects on body tissues and work by destroying particular parts of the host cell or by inhibiting certain metabolic functions. Exotoxins are among the most lethal known substances, only 1 mg of the botulinum exotoxin is enough to kill one million guinea pigs. Diseases caused this way are often caused by minute amounts of exotoxins, not by the bacteria themselves.

IDENTIFICATION

Typically identification is done by growing the organism in a wide range of cultures which can take up to 48 hours. The growth is then visually or genomically identified. The cultured organism is then subjected to antibiotics to observe reaction to help further identify species and strain.

TREATMENT

Bacterial infections may be treated with antibiotics, which are classified as bacteriocidal if they kill bacteria or bacteriostatic if they just prevent bacterial growth. There are many types of antibiotics and each class inhibits a process that is different in the pathogen from that found in the host. For example, the antibiotics chloramphenicol and tetracyclin inhibit the bacterial ribosome but not the structurally different eukaryotic ribosome, so they exhibit selective toxicity. Antibiotics are used both in treating human disease and in intensive farming to promote animal growth. Both uses may be contributing to the rapid development of antibiotic resistance in bacterial populations. Phage therapy can also be used to treat certain bacterial infections. Infections can be prevented by antiseptic measures such as sterilizing the skin prior to piercing it with the needle of a syringe and by proper care of indwelling catheters. Surgical and dental instruments are also sterilized to prevent infection by bacteria. Disinfectants such as bleach are used to kill bacteria or other pathogens on surfaces to prevent contamination and further reduce the risk of infection. Bacteria in food are killed by cooking to temperatures above 73 °C (163 °F).

LIST OF GENERA OF PATHOGENIC BACTERIA AND MICROSCOPY FEATURES

Many genera contain pathogenic bacteria species. They often possess characteristics that help to classify and organize them into groups. The following is a partial listing.

Genus	Species	Gram staining	Shape	**Oxygen requirement**	**Intra/ Extracellular**
Bacillus	Bacillus anthracis Bacillus cereus	Positive	Rods	Facultative anaerobic	Extracellular
Bartonella	Bartonella henselae Bartonella quintana	Negative	Rods	Aerobic	Facultative intracellular
Bordetella	Bordetella pertussis	Negative	Small coccobacilli	Aerobic	Extracellular
Borrelia	Borrelia burgdorferi Borrelia garinii Borrelia afzelii Borrelia recurrentis	Negative, stains poorly	spirochete	Anaerobic	Extracellular
Brucella	Brucella abortus Brucella canis Brucella melitensis Brucella suis	Negative	coccobacilli	Aerobic	Intracellular
Campylobacter	Campylobacter jejuni	Negative	Spirochete Bacillus	microaerophilic	extracellular
Chlamydia and *Chlamydophila*	Chlamydia pneumoniae Chlamydia trachomatis Chlamydophila psittaci	(not Gram-stained)	Small, round, ovoid	Facultative or strictly aerobic	Obligate intracellular
Clostridium	Clostridium botulinum Clostridium difficile Clostridium perfringens Clostridium tetani	Positive	Large, blunt-ended rods	Obligate anaerobic	extracellular
Corynebacterium	Corynebacterium diphtheriae	Positive (unevenly)	bacilli	Mostly facultative anaerobic	extracellular
Enterococcus	Enterococcus faecalis Enterococcus faecium	Positive	Cocci	Facultative Anaerobic	extracellular

Escherichia	Escherichia coli	Negative	Bacillus	Facultative anaerobic	extracellular or intracellular
Francisella	Francisella tularensis	Negative	coccobacillus	strictly aerobic	Facultative intracellular
Haemophilus	Haemophilus influenzae	Negative	coccobacilli to long and slender filaments		extracellular
Helicobacter	Helicobacter pylori	Negative	Spirochete	Microaerophile	extracellular
Legionella	Legionella pneumophila	Negative, stains poorly	cocobacilli	aerobic	facultative intracellular
Leptospira	Leptospira interrogans Leptospira santarosai Leptospira weilii Leptospira noguchii	Negative, stains poorly	Spirochete	Strictly aerobic	extracellular
Listeria	Listeria monocytogenes	Positive, darkly	Slender, short rods	Facultative Anaerobic	intracellular
Mycobacterium	Mycobacterium leprae Mycobacterium tuberculosis Mycobacterium ulcerans	(none)	Long, slender rods	aerobic	extracellular
Mycoplasma	Mycoplasma pneumoniae	(none)	'fried egg' appearance, no cell wall	Mostly facultative anaerobic; *M. pneumoniae* strictly aerobic	extracellular
Neisseria	Neisseria gonorrhoeae Neisseria meningitidis	Negative	Kidney bean-shaped	aerobic	*Gonococcus*: facultative intracellular *N. meningitidis*: extracellular
Pseudomonas	Pseudomonas aeruginosa	Negative	rods	Obligate aerobic	extracellular
Rickettsia	Rickettsia rickettsii	Negative, stains poorly	Small, rod-like coccobacillary	Aerobic	Obligate intracellular

Salmonella	Salmonella typhi Salmonella typhimurium	Negative	Bacillus shape	Facultative anaerobica	Facultative intracellular
Shigella	Shigella sonnei	Negative	rods	Facultative anaerobic	extracellular
Staphylococcus	Staphylococcus aureus Staphylococcus epidermidis Staphylococcus saprophyticus	Positive, darkly	Round cocci	Facultative anaerobic	extracellular, facultative intracellular
Streptococcus	Streptococcus agalactiae Streptococcus pneumoniae Streptococcus pyogenes	Positive	ovoid to spherical	Facultative anaerobic	extracellular
Treponema	Treponema pallidum	Negative, stains poorly	Spirochete	Aerobic	extracellular
Ureaplasma	Ureaplasma urealyticum	Stains poorly	indistinct, 'fried egg' appearance, no cell wall	anaerobic	extracellular
Vibrio	Vibrio cholerae	Negative	Spiral with single polar flagellum	Facultative anaerobic	extracellular
Yersinia	Yersinia pestis Yersinia enterocolitica Yersinia pseudotuberculosis	Negative, bipolarly	Small rods	Facultative Anaerobe	Intracellular

List of species of pathogenic bacteria and clinical characteristics

This is description of the more common genera and species presented with their clinical characteristics and treatments.

Species of human pathogenic bacteria				
Species	Transmission	Diseases	Treatment	Prevention
Actinomyces israelii	Oral flora	Actinomycosis: painful abscesses in the mouth, lungs, or gastrointestinal tract.	Prolonged penicillin G and drainage	

Bacillus anthracis		Contact with cattle, sheep, goats and horses Spores enter through inhalation or through abrasions	Anthrax: pulmonary, gastrointestinal and/or cutaneous symptoms.	In early infection: Penicillin Doxycycline Ciprofloxacin Raxibacumab	Anthrax vaccine Autoclaving of equipment
Bacteroides fragilis		Gut flora	Abscesses in gastrointestinal tract, pelvic cavity and lungs	metronidazole	Wound care Aspiration prevention
Bordetella pertussis		Contact with respiratory droplets expelled by infected human hosts.	Whooping cough Secondary bacterial pneumonia	Macrolides such as erythromycin, before paroxysmal stage	Pertussis vaccine, such as in DPT vaccine
Borrelia	*B. burgdorferi* *B. garinii* *B. afzelii*	Ixodes ticks reservoir in deer and mice	Lyme disease (B. burgdorferi) Relapsing fever	Early stages of Lyme disease: doxycycline amoxicillin ceftriaxone in neurological involvement Chronic Lyme disease: penicillin G Relapsing fever: doxycycline	Wearing clothing that limits skin exposure to ticks. Insect repellent. Avoid areas where ticks are found.
Brucella	*B. abortus* *B. canis* *B. melitensis* *B. suis*	Direct contact with infected animal Oral, by ingestion of unpasteurized milk or milk products	Brucellosis	doxycycline streptomycin or gentamicin	
Campylobacter jejuni		Fecal-oral from animals (mammals and fowl) Uncooked meat (especially poultry) Contaminated water	Enteritis, bloody diarrhea Guillain–Barré syndrome	Treat symptoms Fluoroquinolone such as ciprofloxacin in severe cases	Good hygiene Avoiding contaminated water Pasteurizing milk and milk products Cooking meat (especially poultry)

Chlamydia	*C. pneumoniae*	Respiratory droplets	Atypical pneumonia	Doxycycline Erythromycin	None
	C. trachomatis	vaginal sex oral sex anal sex Vertical from mother to newborn(ICN) Direct or contaminated surfaces and flies (trachoma)	Trachoma Neonatal conjunctivitis Neonatal pneumonia Nongonococcal urethritis (NGU) Urethritis Pelvic inflammatory disease Epididymitis Prostatitis Lymphogranuloma venereum (LGV)	Erythromycin (adults) Doxycycline (infants and pregnant women)	Erythromycin or silver nitrate in newborn's eyes Safe sex Abstinence
Chlamydophila psittaci		Inhalation of dust with secretions or feces from birds (e.g. parrots)	Psittacosis	Tetracycline Doxycycline Erythromycin	-
Clostridium	*C. botulinum*	Spores from soil, persevere in canned food, smoked fish and honey	Botulism: Mainly muscle weakness and paralysis	Antitoxin Penicillin Hyperbaric oxygen Mechanical ventilation	Proper food preservation techniques
	C. difficile	Gut flora, overgrowing when other flora is depleted	Pseudomembranous colitis	Discontinuing responsible antibiotic Vancomycin or metronidazole if severe	Fecal bacteriotherapy
	C. perfringens	Spores in soil Vaginal flora and gut flora	Anaerobic cellulitis Gas gangrene Acute food poisoning	Gas gangrene: Debridement or amputation Hyperbaric medicine High doses of doxycycline or penicillin G and clindamycin Food poisoning: Supportive care is sufficient	Appropriate food handling
	C. tetani	Spores in soil, skin penetration through wounds	Tetanus	Tetanus immune globulinSedatives Muscle relaxants Mechanical ventilation Penicillin or metronidazole	Tetanus vaccine (such as in the DPT vaccine)
Corynebacterium diptheriae		respiratory droplets part of human flora	Diphtheria	Horse serum antitoxin Erythromycin Penicillin	DPT vaccine
Ehrlichia	*E. canis* *E. chaffeensis*	Dog tick	Ehrlichiosis	doxycycline rifampin	

Enterococcus	*E. faecalis* *E. faecium*	Part of gut flora, opportunistic or entering through GI tract or urinary system wounds	bacterial endocarditis biliary tract infections urinary tract infections	Ampicillin (combined with aminoglycoside in endocarditis) Vancomycin	No vaccine Hand washing and other nosocomial prevention
Escherichia	*E. coli* (generally)	Gut flora, and in urinary tract Spreading extraintestinally or proliferating in the GI tract	Diarrhea Urinary tract infections (UTI) Meningitis in infants Hospital-acquired pneumonia Hospital-acquired sepsis	**UTI:** (resistance-tests are required first) Co-trimoxazole Fluoroquinolone, e.g. ciprofloxacin Meningitis: Cephalosporin (e.g. cefotaxime) and gentamicin combination Diarrhea: Antibiotics above shorten duration Electrolyte and fluid replacement	(no vaccine or preventive drug) Cooking ground beef and pasteurizing milk against O157:H7 Hand washing and disinfection
	Enterotoxigenic *E. coli* (ETEC)	Fecal-oral through food and water Direct physical contact	Traveller's diarrhea		
	Enteropathogenic *E. coli*	Vertical, in utero or at birth	Diarrhea in infants		
	Enteroinvasive E.coli (EIEC)	Fecal-oral	bloody diarrhea and fever		
	Enterohemorrhagic (EHEC), including *E. coli* O157:H7	Reservoir in cattle	bloody diarrhea Hemolytic-uremic syndrome		
Francisella tularensis		vector-borne by arthropods Infected wild or domestic animals, birds or house pets	Tularemia: Fever, ulceration at entry site and/or lymphadenopathy. Can cause severe pneumonia.	Streptomycin Gentamicin	Avoiding insect vectors Precautions when handling wild animals or animal products
Haemophilus influenzae		Droplet contact Human flora of e.g. upper respiratory tract	Bacterial meningitis Upper respiratory tract infections Pneumonia,bronchitis Septic arthritis in infants	**Meningitis:** (resistance-tests are required first) Third generation cephalosporin, e.g. cefotaxime or ceftriaxone Ampicillin and sulbactam combination	Hib vaccine to infants Rifampin prophylactically
Helicobacter pylori		Colonizing stomach Unclear person-to-person transmission	Peptic ulcer Chronic gastritis Risk factor for gastric carcinoma and gastric B-cell lymphoma	Tetracycline, metronidazole and bismuth salt combination	(No vaccine or preventive drug)
Klebsiella pneumoniae		Mouth, skin, and gut flora. Pneumonia upon aspiration	Klebsiella pneumonia, with significant lung necrosis and hemoptysis Hospital-acquired Urinary tract infection and sepsis	3rd generation cephalosporin ciprofloxacin	hand hygiene.

Legionella pneumophila		Droplet contact, from e.g. cooling towers, humidifiers, air conditioners and water distribution systems	Legionnaire's Disease Pontiac fever	Macrolides, such as erythromycin Fluoroquinolones Rifampin	(no vaccine or preventive drug) Heating water
Leptospira species		Food and water contaminated by urine from infected wild or domestic animals. *Leptospira* survives for weeks in fresh water and moist soil.	Leptospirosis	Penicillin G Tetracycline, e.g. doxycycline	Vaccine not widely used Doxycycline Prevention of exposure Rodent control
Listeria monocytogenes		Raw milk or cheese, ground meats, poultry Vertically to newborn or fetus	Listeriosis: Meningitis Sepsis	Ampicillin Co-trimoxazole	(no vaccine) Proper food preparation and handling
Mycobacterium	M. leprae	Prolonged human-human contact, e.g. through exudates from skin lesions to abrasion of other person	Leprosy (Hansen's disease)	Tuberculoid form: Dapsone and rifampin Lepromatous form: Clofazimine	BCG vaccine shows some effects
	M. tuberculosis	Droplet contact	Tuberculosis	(difficult, see Tuberculosis treatment for more details) Standard "short" course: First 2 months, combination: Isoniazid Rifampicin Pyrazinamide Ethambutol Further 4 months, combination: Isoniazid Rifampicin	BCG vaccine Isoniazid
Mycoplasma pneumoniae		Human flora Respiratory droplets	Mycoplasma pneumonia	Doxycycline and erythromycin	

Neisseria	N. gonorrhoeae	Sexually transmitted vertical in birth	Gonorrhea Urethritis (men) Pelvic inflammatory disease (women) Ophthalmia neonatorum Septic arthritis	Uncomplicated gonorrhea: Ceftriaxone Tetracycline, e.g. doxycycline if also chlamydia is suspected Spectinomycin for resistance or patient allergy to cephalosporin Ophthalmia neonatorum: Erythromycin + ceftriaxone	(No vaccine) Safe sex Erythromycin into eyes of newborn at risk
	N. meningitidis	Droplet transmission	Meningococcal disease including meningitis Sepsis, including Waterhouse-Friderichsen syndrome	Penicillin G Ceftriaxone	NmVac4-A/C/Y/W-135 vaccine Rifampin
Pseudomonas aeruginosa		Opportunistic; Infects damaged tissues or people with immunodeficiency.	Pseudomonas infection: Pneumonia Urinary tract infection Corneal infection Endocarditis Osteomyelitis Burn wound infection Sepsis Malignant external otitis	Anti-pseudomonal penicillins such as ticarcillin Aminoglycoside	(no vaccine) Topical silver sulfadiazine for burn wounds
Nocardia asteroides		In soil	Nocardiosis	TMP/SMX	
Rickettsia rickettsii		Wood or dog tick	Rocky mountain spotted fever	Doxycycline Chloramphenicol	(no preventive drug or approved vaccine) Vector control, such as clothing Prompt removal of attached ticks

Salmonella	S typhi	Fecal-oral route, through food or water	Typhoid fever type salmonellosis (fever, abdominal pain, hepatosplenomegaly, rose spots) Chronic carrier state	Ceftriaxone Fluoroquinolones, e.g. ciprofloxacin	Ty21a and ViCPS vaccines Hygiene and food preparation
	Other *Salmonella* species e.g. S. typhimurium	Fecal-oral Food contaminated by fowl (e.g. uncooked eggs) or turtles	Salmonellosis with gastroenteritis Paratyphoid fever Osteomyelitis in people with sickle cells Sepsis	Fluid and electrolyte replacement for diarrhea Antibiotics (in neonates and immuno-compromised): Ciprofloxacin Ceftriaxone TMP/SMX Azithromycin	(No vaccine or preventive drug) Proper sewage disposal Food preparation Good personal hygiene
Shigella	*S. sonnei* *S. dysenteriae*	Fecal-oral	Shigellosis (bacillary dysentery)	Fluid and electrolyte replacement Fluoroquinolonesuch as ciprofloxacin if severe	Protection of water and food supplies Vaccines are in trial stage
Staphylococcus	aureus	Human flora on mucosae in e.g. anterior nares, skin and vagina, entering through wound	Coagulase-positive staphylococcal infections: Skin infections, including impetigo Acute infective endocarditis Septis Necrotizing pneumonia Meningitis Osteomyelitis Toxinoses Scalded skin syndrome Toxic shock syndrome Staphylococcal food poisoning	Incision and drainage of localized lesions Nafcillin, oxacillin, methicillin Vancomycin for Methicillin-resistant (MRSA)	(no vaccine or preventive drug) Barrier precautions, washing hands and fomite disinfection in hospitals
	epidermidis	Human flora in skin, anterior nares and mucous membranes	Infections of implanted prostheses (e.g. heart valves and joints) and catheters	Vancomycin	None
	saprophyticus	Part of normal vaginal flora	Cystitis in women	TMP/SMX or norfloxacin	None

Streptococcus	*agalactiae*	Human flora in vagina, urethral mucous membranes, rectum Vertically during childbirth Sexually	Neonatal meningitis Neonatal sepsis Neonatal pneumonia Endometritis in postpartum women Opportunistic infections with septicemia and pneumonia	Penicillin G Aminoglycoside in case of lethal infection	None
	pneumoniae	Respiratory droplets Human flora in nasopharynx(spreading in immunocompromised)	Acute bacterial pneumonia & meningitis in adults Otitis media and sinusitis in children Sepsis	Penicillin G	23-serotype vaccine for adults (PPV) Heptavalent conjugated vaccine for children (PCV)
	pyogenes	Respiratory droplets Direct physical contact with impetigo lesions	Streptococcal pharyngitis Sepsis Scarlet fever Rheumatic fever Impetigo and erysipelas Puerperal fever Necrotizing fasciitis Poststreptococcal glomerulonephritis	Penicillin G or V Macrolide, e.g. clarithromycin or erythromycin in penicillin allergy Drainage and debridement for necrotizing fasciitis	No vaccine Rapid antibiotic treatment helps prevent rheumatic fever
	viridans	Oral flora, penetration through abrasions	Subacute bacterial endocarditis Dental cavities Abscesses of brain and liver	Penicillin G	
Treponema pallidum		Sexual	Syphilis Congenital syphilis	Penicillin G Doxycycline if penicillin allergy	No preventive drug or vaccine Safe sex Antibiotics to pregnant women if risk of transmitting to child
Vibrio cholerae		Fecal-oral route Contaminated water and raw seafood	Cholera: Severe "rice water" diarrhea	Fluid and electrolyte replacement Doxycycline	Proper sanitation Adequate food preparation
Yersinia pestis		Fleas from animals Ingestion of animal tissues Respiratory droplets	Plague: Bubonic plague Pneumonic plague	Streptomycin primarily Tetracyclin Supportive therapy for shock	Plague vaccine Minimize exposure to rodents and fleas

ACINETOBACTER BAUMANNII

Acinetobacter baumannii is a typically short, almost round, rod-shaped (coccobacillus) Gram-negative bacterium. It can be an opportunistic pathogen in humans, affecting people with compromised immune systems, and is becoming increasingly important as a hospital-derived (nosocomial) infection. While other species of the genus *Acinetobacter* are often found in soil samples (leading to the common misconception that *A. baumannii* is a soil organism, too), it is almost exclusively isolated from hospital environments. Although occasionally it has been found in environmental soil and water samples, its natural habitat is still not known. Bacteria of this genus lack flagella, whip-like structures many bacteria use for locomotion, but exhibit twitching or swarming motility. This may be due to the activity of type IV pili, pole-like structures that can be extended and retracted. Motility in *A. baumannii* may also be due to the excretion of exopolysaccharide, creating a film of high-molecular-weight sugar chains behind the bacterium to move forward. Clinical microbiologists typically differentiate members of the *Acinetobacter* genus from other Moraxellaceae by performing an oxidase test, as *Acinetobacter* spp. are the only members of the Moraxellaceae to lack cytochrome c oxidases. *A. baumannii* is part of the ACB complex (*A. baumannii*, *A. calcoaceticus*, and *Acinetobacter* genomic species 13TU). Members of the ACB complex are difficult to determine the specific species, and comprise the most clinically relevant members of the genus. *A. baumannii* has also been identified as an ESKAPE pathogen (*Enterococcus faecium*, *Staphylococcus aureus*, *Klebsiella pneumoniae*, *Acinetobacter baumannii*, *Pseudomonas aeruginosa*, and *Enterobacter* species), a group of pathogens with a high rate of antibiotic resistance that are responsible for the majority of nosocomial infections. Colloquially, *A. baumannii* is referred to as 'Iraqibacter› due to its seemingly sudden emergence in military treatment facilities during the Iraq War. It has continued to be an issue for veterans and soldiers who served in Iraq and Afghanistan. Multidrug-resistant *A. baumannii* has spread to civilian hospitals in part due to the transport of infected soldiers through multiple medical facilities.

Virulence Factors and Determinants

Many microbes, including *A. baumannii*, have several properties that allow them to be more successful as pathogens. These properties may be virulence factors such as toxins or toxin delivery systems which directly affect the host cell. They may also be virulence determinants, which are qualities contributing to a microbe's fitness and allow it to survive the host environment, but that do not affect the host directly. These characteristics are just some of the known factors which make *A. baumannii* effective as a pathogen:

AbaR resistance islands

Pathogenicity islands, relatively common genetic structures in bacterial pathogens, are composed of two or more adjacent genes that increase a pathogen's virulence. They may contain genes that encode toxins, coagulate blood, or as in this case, allow the bacteria to resist antibiotics. AbaR-type resistance islands are typical of drug-resistant *A. baumannii*, and different variations may be present in a given strain. Each consists of a transposon backbone of about 16.3 Kb that facilitates horizontal gene transfer. Transposons allow portions of genetic material to be excised from one spot in the genome and integrate into another. This makes horizontal gene transfer of this and similar pathogenicity islands more likely because, when genetic material is taken up by a new bacterium, the transposons allow the pathogenicity island to integrate into the new microorganism›s genome. In this case, it would grant the new microorganism the potential to resist certain antibiotics. AbaRs contain several genes for antibiotic resistance, all flanked by insertion sequences. These genes provide resistance to aminoglycosides, aminocyclitols, tetracycline, and chloramphenicol.

Beta-lactamase

A. baumannii has been shown to produce at least one beta-lactamase, which is an enzyme responsible for cleaving the four-atom lactam ring typical of beta-lactam antibiotics. Beta-lactam antibiotics are structurally related to penicillin, which inhibits synthesis of the bacterial cell wall. The cleaving of the lactam ring renders these antibiotics harmless to the bacteria. The beta-lactamase OXA-23 was found to be flanked by insertion sequences, suggesting it was acquired by horizontal gene transfer.

Biofilm formation

A. baumannii has been noted for its apparent ability to survive on artificial surfaces for an extended period of time, therefore allowing it to persist in the hospital environment. This is thought to be due to its ability to form biofilms. For many biofilm-forming bacteria, the process is mediated by flagella. However, for *A. baumannii*, this process seems to be mediated by pili. Further, disruption of the putative pili chaperone and usher genes *csuC* and *csuE* were shown to inhibit biofilm formation. The formation of biofilms has been shown to alter the metabolism of microorganisms within the biofilm, consequently reducing their sensitivity to antibiotics. This may be because less nutrients are available deeper within the biofilm. A slower metabolism can prevent the bacteria from taking up an antibiotic or performing a vital function fast enough for particular antibiotics to have an effect. They also provide a physical barrier against larger molecules and may prevent desiccation of the bacteria.

Capsule

Many virulent bacteria possess the ability to generate a protective capsule around each individual cell. This capsule, made of long chains of sugars, provides an extra physical barrier between antibiotics, antibodies, and complement. The association of increased virulence with presence of a capsule was classically demonstrated in Griffith›s experiment. A gene cluster responsible for secretion of the polysaccharide capsule has been identified and shown to inhibit the antibiotic effect of complement when grown on ascites fluid. A decrease in killing associated with loss of capsule production was then demonstrated using a rat virulence model.

Efflux pumps

Efflux pumps are protein machines that use energy to pump antibiotics and other small molecules that get into the bacterial cytoplasm and the periplasmic space out of the cell. By constantly pumping antibiotics out of the cell, bacteria can increase the concentration of a given antibiotic required to kill them or inhibit their growth when the target of the antibiotic is inside the bacterium. *A. baumannii* is known to have two major efflux pumps which decrease its susceptibility to antimicrobials. The first, AdeB, has been shown to be responsible for aminoglycoside resistance. The second, AdeDE, is responsible for efflux of a wide range of substrates, including tetracycline, chloramphenicol, and various carbapenems.

Small RNA

Bacterial small RNAs are noncoding RNAs that regulate various cellular processes. Three sRNAs, AbsR11, AbsR25, and AbsR28, have been experimentally validated in the MTCC 1425 (ATCC15308) strain, which is a (multidrug-resistant) strain showing resistance to 12 antibiotics. AbsR25 sRNA could play a role in the efflux pump regulation and drug resistance.

OMPA

Adhesion can be a critical determinant of virulence for bacteria. The ability to attach to host cells allows bacteria to interact with them in various ways, whether by type III secretion system or simply by holding on against the prevailing movement of fluids. Outer membrane protein A has been shown to be involved in the adherence of *A. baumannii* to epithelial cells. This allows the bacteria to invade the cells through the zipper mechanism. The protein was also shown to localize to the mitochondria of epithelial cells and cause necrosis by stimulating the production of reactive oxygen species.

Course of Treatment for Infection

Because most infections are now resistant to multiple drugs, determining what susceptibilities the particular strain has is necessary to for treatment to be successful. Traditionally, infections were treated with imipenem or meropenem, but a steady rise in carbapenem-resistant *A. baumannii* has been noted. Consequently, treatment methods often fall back on polymyxins, particularly colistin. Colistin is considered a drug of last resort because it often causes kidney damage, among other side effects. Prevention methods in hospitals focus on increased hand-washing and more diligent sterilization procedures.

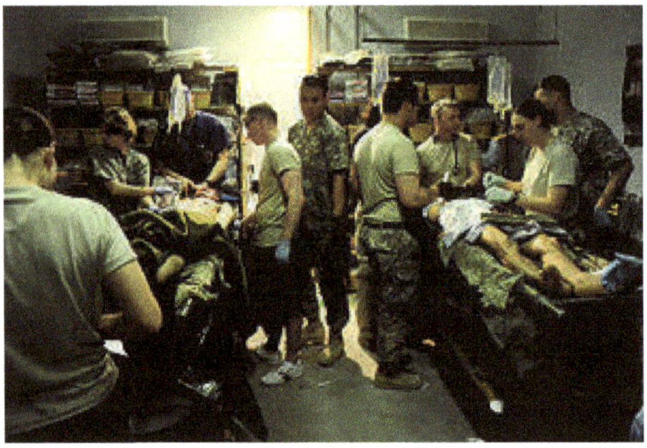

Traumatic injuries, like those from improvised explosive devices, leave large open areas contaminated with debris that are vulnerable to becoming infected with *A. baumannii*.

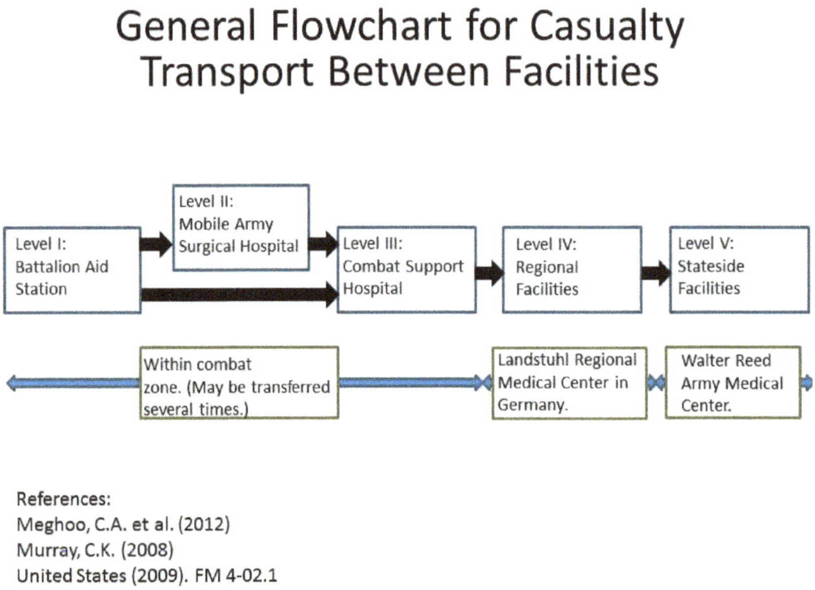

The logistics of transporting wounded soldiers result in patients visiting several facilities where they may acquire *A. baumannii* infections.

Occurrence in Veterans Injured in Iraq and Afghanistan

Soldiers in Iraq and Afghanistan are at risk for traumatic injury due to gunfire and improvised explosive devices. Previously, infection was thought to occur due to contamination with *A. baumannii* at the time of injury. Subsequent studies have shown, although *A. baumannii* may be infrequently isolated from the natural environment, the infection is more likely nosocomially acquired, likely due to the ability of *A. baumannii* to persist on artificial surfaces for extended periods, and the several facilities to which injured soldiers are exposed during the casualty-evacuation process. Injured soldiers are first taken to level-I facilities, where they are stabilized. Depending on the severity of the injury, the soldiers may then be transferred to a level-II facility, which consists of a forward surgical team, for additional stabilization. Depending on the logistics of the locality, the injured soldiers may transfer between these facilities several times before finally being taken to a major hospital within the combat zone (level III). Generally after 1–3 days, when the patients are stabilized, they are transferred by air to a regional facility (level IV) for additional treatment. For soldiers serving in Iraq or Afghanistan, this is typically Landstuhl Regional Medical Center in Germany. Finally, the injured soldiers are transferred to hospitals in their home country for rehabilitation and additional treatment. This repeated exposure to many different medical environments seems to be the reason *A. baumannii* infections have become increasingly common. Multidrug-resistant *A. baumannii* is a major factor in complicating the treatment and rehabilitation of injured soldiers, and has led to additional deaths.

Incidence of *A. baumannii* in hospitals

The importation of *A. baumannii* and subsequent presence in hospitals has been well documented. *A. baumannii* is usually introduced into a hospital by a colonized patient. Due to its ability to survive on artificial surfaces and resist desiccation, it can remain and possibly infect new patients for some time. *A baumannii* growth is suspected to be favored in hospital settings due to the constant use of antibiotics by patients in the hospital. Acinetobacter can be spread by person-to-person contact or contact with contaminated surfaces.In a study of European intensive care units in 2009, *A. baumannii* was found to be responsible for 19.1% of ventilator-associated pneumonia cases.

Documented case studies

Country	**Reference**
Australia	
Brazil	
China	
Germany	
India	
South Korea	
United Kingdom	
United States	

Studies show that A. baumannii are derivers from the skins of patients, causing a reoccurrence of A. baumannii in hospital setting.

PSEUDOMONAS AERUGINOSA

Pseudomonas aeruginosa is a common Gram-negative, rod-shaped bacterium that can cause disease in plants and animals, including humans. A species of considerable medical importance, *P. aeruginosa* is a prototypical "multidrug resistant (MDR) pathogen recognised for its ubiquity, its intrinsically advanced antibiotic resistance mechanisms, and its association with serious illnesses – especially nosocomial infections such as ventilator-associated pneumonia and various sepsis syndromes.

The organism is considered opportunistic insofar as serious infection is often superimposed upon acute or chronic morbidity – most notably cystic fibrosis and traumatic burns – or found in immunocompromised individuals, but the organism does produce a range of clinically important infections in the immunocompetent and/or in situations where no pre-existing vulnerability is required e.g. hot tub folliculitis. In all infections produced by *P. aeruginosa,* treatment is dually complicated by the organism's resistance profile, which may lead to treatment failure and/or expose patients to untoward adverse effects from advanced antibiotic drug regimens. This dilemma is a central clinical problem in the field of antimicrobial resistance.

It is citrate, catalase, and oxidase positive. It is found in soil, water, skin flora, and most man-made environments throughout the world. It thrives not only in normal atmospheres, but also in hypoxic atmospheres, thus has colonized many natural and artificial environments. It uses a wide range of organic material for food; in animals, its versatility enables the organism to infect damaged tissues or those with reduced immunity. The symptoms of such infections are generalized inflammation and sepsis. If such colonizations occur in critical body organs, such as the lungs, the urinary tract, and kidneys, the results can be fatal. Because it thrives on moist surfaces, this bacterium is also found on and in medical equipment, including catheters, causing cross-infections in hospitals and clinics. It is implicated in hot-tub rash. It is also able to decompose hydrocarbons and has been used to break down tarballs and oil from oil spills. *P. aeruginosa* is not extremely virulent in comparison with other major pathogenic bacterial species – for example *Staphylococcus aureus* and *Streptococcus pyogenes* – though *P. aeruginosa* is capable of extensive colonization, and can aggregate into enduring biofilms. *P. aeruginosa* does not fare especially well under suboptimal atmospheric conditions.

P. aeruginosa is among the Gram-negative bacilli commonly isolated from the exoskeletons and/or droppings of the cosmopolitan peridomestic cockroaches – including *Periplaneta americana* and *Blatella germanica* – which are often pervasive in households, as well as hospital settings. The importance of *P. americana* (and other vermin) as a potential reservoir or vector of *P. aeruginosa* continues to be studied.

Nomenclature

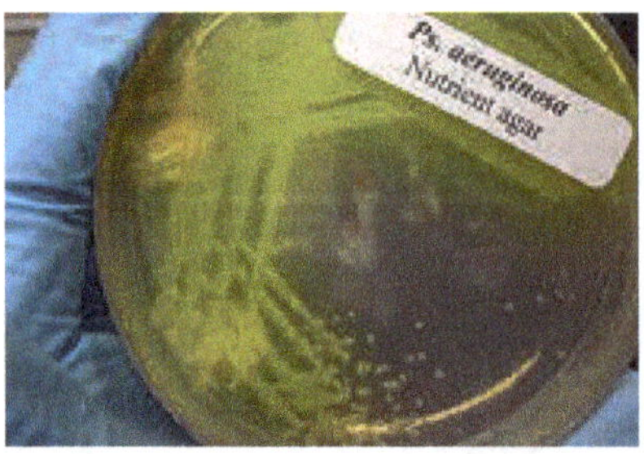

The word *Pseudomonas* means "false unit", from the Greek *pseudo* (Greek: ψευδο, false) and (Latin: *monas*, from Greek: μονος, a single unit). The stem word *mon* was used early in the history of microbiology to refer to germs, e.g., kingdom Monera.

The species name *aeruginosa* is a Latin word meaning verdigris ("copper rust"), referring to the blue-green color of laboratory cultures of the species. This blue-green pigment is a combination of two metabolites of *P. aeruginosa*, pyocyanin (blue) and pyoverdine (green), which impart the blue-green characteristic color of cultures. Another assertion is that the word may be derived from the Greek prefix *ae-* meaning "old or aged", and the suffix *ruginosa* means wrinkled or bumpy.

The names pyocyanin and pyoverdine are from the Greek, with *pyo-*, meaning "pus", *cyanin*, meaning "blue", and *verdine*, meaning "green". Pyoverdine in the absence of pyocyanin is a fluorescent-yellow color.

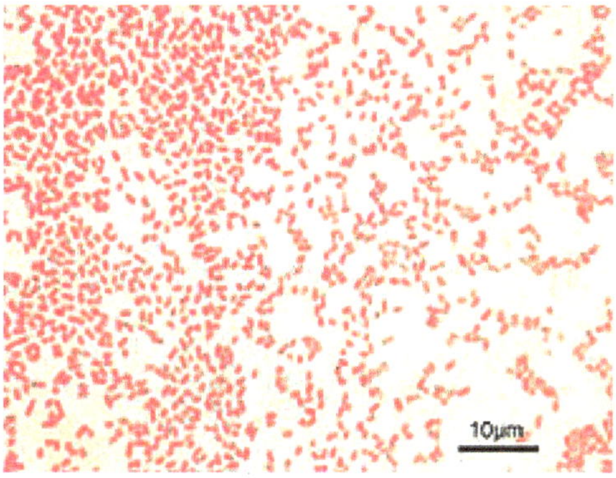

Gram-stained *P. aeruginosa* bacteria (pink-red rods)

Biology

Host Range and Symptoms of P. aeruginosa

P. aeruginosa is a pathogen that could be described as an archetype for opportunistic behavior. Its host range is extremely broad, and its ability to infect mammals like humans, invertebrates like nematodes, and a variety of plant species is a way in which it is unique from other plant pathogens. It is opportunistic because it attacks hosts with compromised defense systems, this could be due to previous disease or other environmental or biological factors. Certain strains of P. aeruginosa are able to infect the roots of plant species like Arabidopsis and sweet basil to cause the disease root rot. Symptoms of this disease include decaying root tissue with necrotic black patches on root tips. Often times the roots are brown or discolored and can be slimy, secondary symptoms include wilting and yellowing of plant leaves. There are other strains are able to cause soft rot in lettuce, symptoms of this include watery or soft feeling to plant tissues. Water lesions symptomatic of soft rot are caused by the release of pectate and other degrading enymes that bind plant cells and cause structures to fall apart.[citation needed]

Genome

The genome of *P. aeruginosa* is relatively large (5.5–6.8 Mb) and encodes between 5,500 and 6,000 open reading frames, depending on the strain; 5,021 genes are present across the first five genomes analyzed, with at least 70% sequence identity. This set of genes is the *P. aeruginosa* core genome.

strain:	VRFPA04	C3719	PAO1	PA14	PACS2
genome size (bp)	6,818,030	6,222,097	6,264,404	6,537,648	6,492,423
ORFs	5,939	5,578	5,571	5,905	5,676

Metabolism

P. aeruginosa is a facultative anaerobe, as it is well adapted to proliferate in conditions of partial or total oxygen depletion. This organism can achieve anaerobic growth with nitrate or nitrite as a terminal electron acceptor. When oxygen, nitrate, and nitrite are absent, it is able to ferment arginine and pyruvate by substrate-level phosphorylation. Adaptation to microaerobic or anaerobic environments is essential for certain lifestyles of *P. aeruginosa*, for example, during lung infection in cystic fibrosis patients, where thick layers of lung mucus and alginate surrounding mucoid bacterial cells can limit the diffusion of oxygen. *P. aeruginosa* growth within the human body can be asymptomatic until the bacteria form a biofilm, which overwhelms the immune system. These biofilms are found in the lungs of cystic fibrosis patients, and a leading cause of death among them.

Pathogenesis

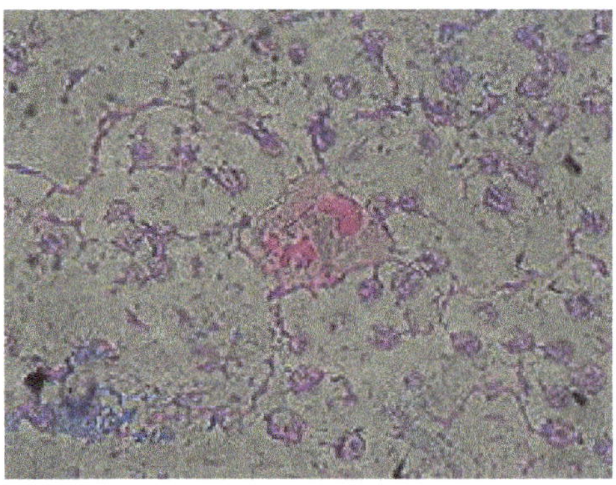

Phagocytosis of *P. aeruginosa* by neutrophil in patient with bloodstream infection (Gram stain)

An opportunistic, nosocomial pathogen of immunocompromised individuals, *P. aeruginosa* typically infects the airway, urinary tract, burns, and wounds, and also causes other blood infections.

Infections	Details and common associations	High-risk groups
Pneumonia	Diffuse bronchopneumonia	Cystic fibrosis patients
Septic shock	Associated with a purple-black skin lesion ecthyma gangrenosum	Neutropenic patients
Urinary tract infection	Urinary tract catheterization	
Gastrointestinal infection	Necrotising enterocolitis	Premature infants and neutropenic cancer patients
Skin and soft tissue infections	Hemorrhage and necrosis	Burns victims and patients with wound infections

It is the most common cause of infections of burn injuries and of the outer ear (otitis externa), and is the most frequent colonizer of medical devices (e.g., catheters). *Pseudomonas* can be spread by equipment that gets contaminated and is not properly cleaned or on the hands of healthcare workers. *Pseudomonas* can, in rare circumstances, cause community-acquired pneumonias, as well as ventilator-associated pneumonias, being one of the most common agents isolated in several studies. Pyocyanin is a virulence factor of the bacteria and has been known to cause death in *C. elegans* by oxidative stress. However, salicylic acid can inhibit pyocyanin production. One in ten hospital-acquired infections is from *Pseudomonas*. Cystic fibrosis patients are also predisposed to *P. aeruginosa* infection of the lungs. *P. aeruginosa* may also be a common cause of "hot-tub rash" (dermatitis), caused by lack of proper, periodic attention to water quality. Since these bacteria like moist environments, such as hot tubs and swimming pools, they can cause skin rash or swimmer›s ear. *Pseudomonas* is also a common cause of postoperative infection in radial keratotomy surgery patients. The organism is also associated with the skin lesion ecthyma gangrenosum. *P. aeruginosa* is frequently associated with osteomyelitis involving puncture wounds of the foot, believed to result from direct inoculation with *P. aeruginosa* via the foam padding found in tennis shoes, with diabetic patients at a higher risk.

Toxins

P. aeruginosa uses the virulence factor exotoxin A to inactivate eukaryotic elongation factor 2 via ADP-ribosylation in the host cell, much as the diphtheria toxin does. Without elongation factor 2, eukaryotic cells cannot synthesize proteins and necrotise. The release of intracellular contents induces an immunologic response in immunocompetent patients. In addition *P. aeruginosa* uses an exoenzyme, ExoU, which degrades the plasma membrane of eukaryotic cells, leading to lysis. Increasingly, it is becoming recognized that the iron-acquiring siderophore, pyoverdine, also functions as a toxin by removing iron from mitochondria, inflicting damage on this organelle.

Phenazines

Phenazines are redox-active pigments produced by *P. aeruginosa*. These pigments are involved in quorum sensing, virulence, and iron acquisition. *P. aeruginosa* produces several pigments all produced via a biosynthetic pathway. Pyocyanin, 1-Hydroxyphenazine,

Phenazine-1-Carboxamide, 5-methylphenazine-1-carboxylic acid betaine, and Aeruginosin A. Two operons are involved in phenazine biosynthesis: *phzA1B1C1D1E1F1G1* and *phzA2B2C2D2E2F2G2*. These operons convert a chorismic acid to the phenazines mentioned above. Three key genes, *phzH*, *phzM*, and *phzS* convert phenazine-1-carboxylic acid to the phenazines mentioned above. Though phenazine biosynthesis is well studied, questions remain as to the final structure of the brown phenazine pyomelanin.

When pyocyanin biosynthesis is inhibited, a decrease in *P. aeruginosa* pathogenicity is observed *in vitro*. This suggests that pyocyanin is most responsible for the initial colonization of *P. aeruginosa in vivo*.

Triggers

With low phosphate levels, *P. aeruginosa* has been found to activate from benign symbiont to express lethal toxins inside the intestinal tract and severely damage or kill the host, which can be mitigated by providing excess phosphate instead of antibiotics.

Plants and Invertebrates

In higher plants, *P. aeruginosa* induces soft rot, for example in *Arabidopsis thaliana* (Thale cress) and *Lactuca sativa* (lettuce). It is also pathogenic to invertebrate animals, including the nematode *Caenorhabditis elegans*, the fruit fly *Drosophila* and the moth *Galleria mellonella*. The associations of virulence factors are the same for plant and animal infections.

Quorum Sensing

Regulation of gene expression can occur through cell-cell communication or quorum sensing (QS) via the production of small molecules called autoinducers. The extracellular accumulation of these molecules signals to bacteria to alter gene expression and coordinate behavior. *P. aeruginosa* employs three interconnected QS systems — lasRl, rhlRl, and PQS — that each produce unique signaling molecules. Detection of these molecules indicates *P. aeruginosa* is growing as biofilm within the lungs of cystic fibrosis patients. QS is known to control expression of a number of virulence factors, including the pigment pyocyanin. Another form of gene regulation that allows the bacteria to rapidly adapt to surrounding changes is through environmental signaling. Recent studies have discovered anaerobiosis can significantly impact the major regulatory circuit of QS. This important link between QS and anaerobiosis has a significant impact on production of virulence factors of this organism. Garlic experimentally blocks quorum sensing in *P. aeruginosa*.

Biofilms and Treatment Resistance

Biofilms of *P. aeruginosa* can cause chronic opportunistic infections, which are a serious problem for medical care in industrialized societies, especially for immunocompromised patients and the elderly. They often cannot be treated effectively with traditional antibiotic therapy. Biofilms seem to protect these bacteria from adverse environmental factors. *P. aeruginosa* can cause nosocomial infections and is considered a model organism for the study of antibiotic-resistant bacteria. Researchers consider it important to learn more about the molecular mechanisms that cause the switch from planktonic growth to a biofilm phenotype and about the role of QS in treatment-resistant bacteria such as *P. aeruginosa*. This should contribute to better clinical management of chronically infected patients, and should lead to the development of new drugs.

Many genes and factors affect biofilm formation in *P. aeruginosa*. One of the main gene operons responsible for the initiation and maintaining the biofilm is the PSL operon. This 15-gene operon is responsible for the cell-cell and cell-surface interactions required for cell communication. It is also responsible for the sequestering of the extracellular polymeric substance matrix. This matrix is composed of nucleic acids, amino acids, carbohydrates, and various ions. This matrix is one of the main resistance mechanisms in the biofilms of *P. aeruginosa*.

Cdi-GMP is a major contributor to biofilm adherent properties. This signalling molecule in high quantities makes superadherent biofilms. When suppressed, the biofilms are less adherent and easier to treat. Polysaccharide synthesis locus (PSL) and cdi-GMP form a negative feedback loop. PSL stimulates cdi-GMP production, while high cd-GMP turns on the operon and increases activity of the operon.

Recent studies have shown that the dispersed cells from *P. aeruginosa* biofilms have lower c-di-GMP levels and different physiologies from those of planktonic and biofilm cells. Such dispersed cells are found to be highly virulent against macrophages and *C. elegans*, but highly sensitive towards iron stress, as compared with planktonic cells.

Recently, scientists have been examining the possible genetic basis for *P. aeruginosa* resistance to antibiotics such as tobramycin. One locus identified as being an important genetic determinant of the resistance in this species is *ndvB*, which encodes periplasmic glucans that may interact with antibiotics and cause them to become sequestered into the periplasm. These results suggest a genetic basis exists behind bacterial antibiotic resistance, rather than the biofilm simply acting as a diffusion barrier to the antibiotic.

Diagnosis

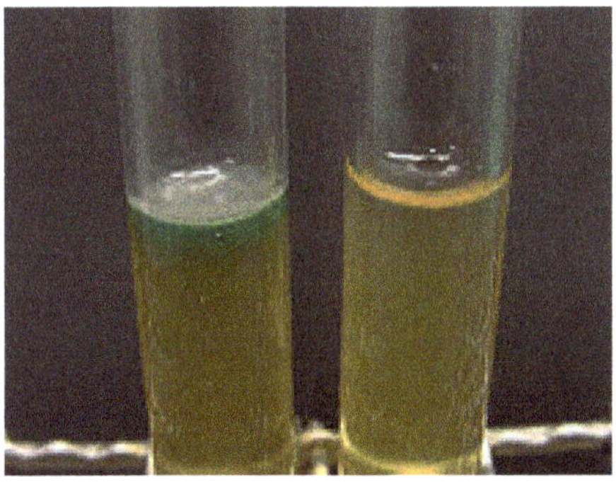

Production of pyocyanin, water-soluble green pigment of *P. aeruginosa* (left tube)

Depending on the nature of infection, an appropriate specimen is collected and sent to a bacteriology laboratory for identification. As with most bacteriological specimens, a Gram stain is performed, which may show gram-negative rods and/or white blood cells. *P. aeruginosa* produces colonies with a characteristic "grape-like" or "fresh-tortilla" odor on bacteriological media. In mixed cultures, it can be isolated as clear colonies on MacConkey agar (as it does not ferment lactose) which will test positive for oxidase. Confirmatory tests include production of the blue-green pigment pyocyanin on cetrimide agar and growth at 42 °C. A TSI slant is often used to distinguish nonfermenting *Pseudomonas* species from enteric pathogens in faecal specimens.

When *P. aeruginosa* is isolated from a normally sterile site (blood, bone, deep collections), it is generally considered dangerous, and almost always requires treatment. [*citation needed*] However, *P. aeruginosa* is frequently isolated from nonsterile sites (mouth swabs, sputum, etc.), and, under these circumstances, it may represent colonization and not infection. The isolation of *P. aeruginosa* from nonsterile specimens should, therefore, be interpreted cautiously, and the advice of a microbiologist or infectious diseases physician/pharmacist should be sought prior to starting treatment. Often, no treatment is needed.

Treatment

Many *P. aeruginosa* isolates are resistant to a large range of antibiotics and may demonstrate additional resistance after unsuccessful treatment. It should usually be possible to guide treatment according to laboratory sensitivities, rather than choosing an antibiotic empirically. If antibiotics are started empirically, then every effort should be made to obtain cultures (before administering first dose of antibiotic), and the choice of antibiotic used should be reviewed when the culture results are available.

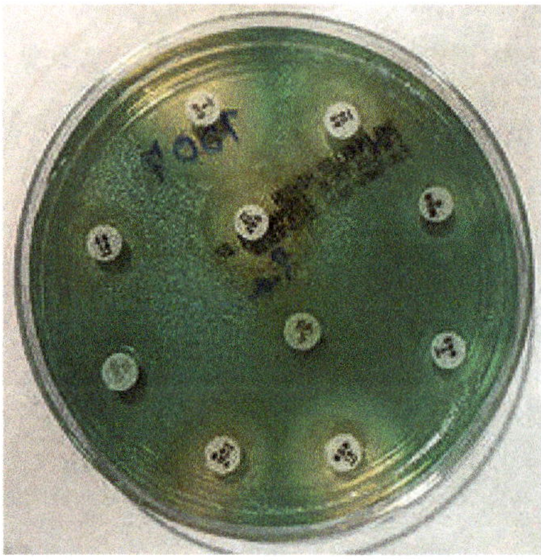

The antibiogram of *P. aeruginosa* on Mueller-Hinton agar

Due to widespread resistance to many common first-line antibiotics, carbapenems, polymyxins, and more recently tigecycline were considered to be the drugs of choice; however, resistance to these drugs has also been reported. Despite this, they are still being used in areas where resistance has not yet been reported. Use of β-lactamase inhibitors such as sulbactam has been advised in combination with antibiotics to enhance antimicrobial action even in the presence of a certain level of resistance. Combination therapy after rigorous antimicrobial susceptibility testing has been found to be the best course of action in the treatment of multidrug-resistant *P. aeruginosa*. Some next-generation antibiotics that are reported as being active against *P. aeruginosa* include doripenem, ceftobiprole, and ceftaroline. However, these require more clinical trials for standardization. Therefore, research for the discovery of new antibiotics and drugs against P. *aeruginosa* is very much needed. Antibiotics that may have activity against *P. aeruginosa* include:

- aminoglycosides (gentamicin, amikacin, tobramycin, but *not* kanamycin)
- quinolones (ciprofloxacin, levofloxacin, but not moxifloxacin)
- cephalosporins (ceftazidime, cefepime, cefoperazone, cefpirome, ceftobiprole, but not cefuroxime, cefotaxime, or ceftriaxone)
- antipseudomonal penicillins: carboxypenicillins (carbenicillin and ticarcillin), and ureidopenicillins (mezlocillin, azlocillin, and piperacillin). *P. aeruginosa* is intrinsically resistant to all other penicillins.
- carbapenems (meropenem, imipenem, doripenem, but not ertapenem)
- polymyxins (polymyxin B and colistin)
- monobactams (aztreonam)

As fluoroquinolone is one of the few antibiotics widely effective against *P. aeruginosa*, in some hospitals, its use is severely restricted to avoid the development of resistant strains. On the rare occasions where infection is superficial and limited (for example, ear infections or nail infections), topical gentamicin or colistin may be used.

Antibiotic Resistance

One of the most worrisome characteristics of *P. aeruginosa* is its low antibiotic susceptibility, which is attributable to a concerted action of multidrug efflux pumps with chromosomally encoded antibiotic resistance genes (e.g., *mexAB*, *mexXY*, etc.) and the low permeability of the bacterial cellular envelopes. In addition to this intrinsic resistance, *P. aeruginosa* easily develops acquired resistance either by mutation in chromosomally encoded genes or by the horizontal gene transfer of antibiotic resistance determinants. Development of multidrug resistance by *P. aeruginosa* isolates requires several different genetic events, including acquisition of different mutations and/or horizontal transfer of antibiotic resistance genes. Hypermutation favours the selection of mutation-driven antibiotic resistance in *P. aeruginosa* strains producing chronic infections, whereas the clustering of several different antibiotic resistance genes in integrons favors the concerted acquisition of antibiotic resistance determinants. Some recent studies have shown phenotypic resistance associated to biofilm formation or to the emergence of small-colony variants may be important in the response of *P. aeruginosa* populations to antibiotics treatment.

Mechanisms underlying antibiotic resistance have been found to include production of antibiotic-degrading or antibiotic-inactivating enzymes, outer membrane proteins to evict the antibiotics and mutations to change antibiotic targets. Presence of antibiotic-degrading enzymes such as extended-spectrum β-lactamases like PER-1, PER-2, VEB-1, AmpC cephalosporinases, carbapenemases like serine oxacillinases, metallo-b-lactamases, OXA-type carbapenemases, aminoglycoside-modifying enzymes, among others have been reported. *P. aeruginosa* can also modify the targets of antibiotic action, for example methylation of 16S rRNA to prevent aminoglycoside binding and modification of DNA, or topoisomerase to protect it from the action of quinolones. *P. aeruginosa* has also been reported to possess multidrug efflux pumps like AdeABC and AdeDE efflux systems that confer resistance against number of antibiotic classes. An important factor found to be associated with antibiotic resistance is the decrease in the virulence capabilities of the resistant strain. Such findings have been reported in the case of rifampicin-resistant and colistin-resistant strains, in which decrease in infective ability, quorum sensing and motility have been documented. Mutations in DNA gyrase are commonly associated with antibiotic resistance in *P. aeruginosa has*. These mutations, when combined with others, confer high resistance without hindering survival. Additionally, genes involved in cyclic-di-GMP signaling may contribute to resistance. When grown *in vitro* conditions designed to mimic a cystic fibrosis patient's lungs, these genes mutate repeatedly.

Prevention

Probiotic prophylaxis may prevent colonization and delay onset of *Pseudomonas* infection in an ICU setting. Immunoprophylaxis against *Pseudomonas* is being investigated. The risk of contracting 'P. aeruginosa *can be reduced by avoiding pools, hot tubs, and other bodies of standing water; regularly disinfecting and/or replacing equipment that regularly encounters moisture (such as contact lens equipment and solutions); and washing one›s hands often (which is protective against many other pathogens as well). However, even the best hygiene practices cannot totally protect an individual against* P. aeruginosa, *given how common ‹P. aeruginosa* is in the environment.

Experimental therapies

Phage therapy against *P. aeruginosa* has been investigated as a possible effective treatment, which can be combined with antibiotics, has no contraindications and minimal adverse effects. Phages are produced as sterile liquid, suitable for intake, applications etc. Phage therapy against ear infections caused by *P. aeruginosa* was reported in the journal *Clinical Otolaryngology* in August 2009.

Research

Experimental evolution

In 2013, Joao Xavier published on an experiment in which *P. aeruginosa*, when subjected to repeated rounds of conditions in which it needed to swarm to acquire food, developed the ability to "hyperswarm" at speeds 25% faster than baseline organisms, by developing multiple flagella, whereas the baseline organism has a single flagellum. This result was notable in the field of experimental evolution in that it was highly repeatable.

Identification

Test	Results
Gram Stain	-
Oxidase	+
Indole Production	-
Methyl Red	-
Voges-Proskaeur	-
Citrate	+
Hydrogen Sulfide Production	-
Urea Hydrolysis	+
Phenylalanine Deaminase	-
Lysine Decarboxylase	-
Motility	+
Gelatin Hydrolysis	+
Acid from lactose	-
acid from glucose	-
acid from maltose	-
acid from mannitol	+
acid from sucrose	-
nitrate reduction	+
DNAse	-
Lipase	+
Pigment	+ (bluish green pigmentation)
Catalase	+

P. aeruginosa is a Gram-negative, aerobic (and at times facultatively anaerobic), bacillus with unipolar motility. It has been identified as an opportunistic pathogen of both humans and plants. *P. aeruginosa* is the type species of the genus *Pseudomonas*.

In certain conditions, *P. aeruginosa* can secrete a variety of pigments, including pyocyanin (blue-green), pyoverdine (yellow-green and fluorescent), and pyorubin (red-brown). These can be used to identify the organism.

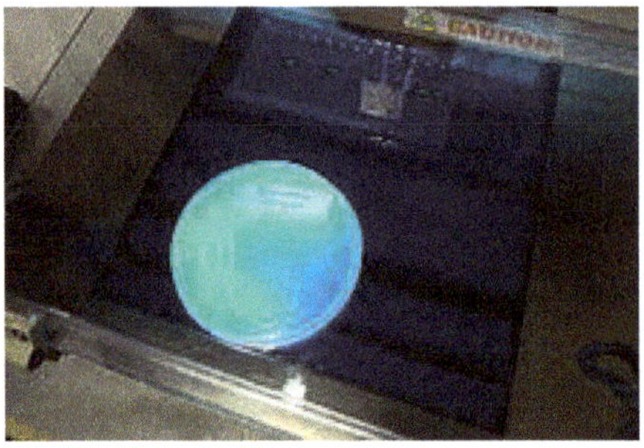

Pseudomonas aeruginosa fluorescence under UV illumination

P. aeruginosa is often preliminarily identified by its pearlescent appearance and grape-like or tortilla-like odor *in vitro*. Definitive clinical identification of *P. aeruginosa* often includes identifying the production of both pyocyanin and fluorescein, as well as its ability to grow at 42 °C. *P. aeruginosa* is capable of growth in diesel and jet fuels, where it is known as a hydrocarbon-using microorganism, causing microbial corrosion. It creates dark, gellish mats sometimes improperly called algae because of their appearance. [*citation needed*]

Pseudomonas *aeruginosa* as a Plant Pathogen

Host Range and Symptoms of P. aeruginosa

P. *aeruginosa* is a pathogen that could be described as an archetype for opportunistic behavior. Its host range is extremely broad, and its ability to infect mammals like humans, invertebrates like nematodes, and a variety of plant species is a way in which it is unique from other plant pathogens. It is opportunistic because it attacks hosts with compromised defense systems, this could be due to previous disease or other environmental or biological factors.

Certain strains of P. *aeruginosa* are able to infect the roots of plant species like Arabidopsis and sweet basil to cause the disease root rot. Symptoms of this disease include decaying root tissue with necrotic black patches on root tips. Often times the roots are brown or discolored and can be slimy, secondary symptoms include wilting and yellowing of plant leaves. There are other strains are able to cause soft rot in lettuce, symptoms of this include watery or soft feeling to plant tissues. Water lesions symptomatic of soft rot are caused by the release of pectate and other degrading enymes that bind plant cells and cause structures to fall apart.

Pathogenicity of P. aeruginosa

P. *aeruginosa* is a gram negative bacterium, its host range is extremely broad in that it is able to cause disease in mammals, non-mammalian animals like nematodes, and plants as well. P. aeruginosa is known to cause root rot in plant species, characterized by a softening and degrading of root tissues as well as black necrotic regions on root tips. How the pathogen is actually able to enter and infect the host has been studied extensively. To analyze the mechanisms the bacteria uses to infect hosts, we can examine its interactions with a plant species, namely Sweet basil (Ocimum basilicum). The pathogen is able to enter host plants via wounds or natural openings, sweet basil has evolved a way to detect infection of the pathogen, and upon entry the plant roots secrete excessive amounts of rosmarinic acid, a compound that has been shown to have antibacterial properties able to combat cells of P. *aeruginosa*. To counter this plant defense response, the pathogen has developed the ability to form a biofilm layer. These biofilms are an organized structure of attached cell colonies encased by an extracellular polymeric matrix, and are able to protect the bacterium from the effects of rosmarinic acid. The biofilms layers act as a means of resistance to the harsh environmental conditions created by the host plant. The pathogen can then go on to continue other processes, like the output of degradation enzymes that allow the bacteria to collect nutreince from plant cells. This sort of arms race between pathogen and host, where new genes arise that are able to confer some sort of resistance or tool to the organism's advantage is known as the gene for gene concept, these sort of interactions are common across many different sorts of pathogen and host relationships.

Importance of P. aeruginosa

Certain strains of P. *aeruginosa* are able to cause soft rot in host plants, and therefore are a member of the bacterial soft rot pathogens, perhaps the most notable of these bacterial soft rot pathogens being Erwinia caratova. Soft rots commonly affect crops such as potato, carrot, tomato, and cucurbis, as well as cruciferous crops such as cabbage. More recently, there have been new reports of P. aeruginosa causing soft rot in onions. On a global scale, soft rots cause more crop losses than any other bacterial disease. In some cases, yield losses can be up to 100% due to substandard storage facility conditions. The problem of yield losses can be exacerbated when we take a look at how it affects different markets.

A lack of available produce can lead to increases of produce prices, which can then go on to have other economic effects. All of these host crops carry enormous economic importance, onions, for example, where it has been estimated that 6.7 million acres are grown globally are known to be a household staple world wide. This crop is especially important for the developing economies of countries like, Egypt, Iran, and India, India being the world leader in onion production. This of course is just an example of the importance of one crop affected by P. *aeruginosa*, when we consider its ability to infect a range of hosts the need to control the pathogen becomes more clear. Understanding of these sorts of diseases is crucial in fighting them, and especially in the case of P. *aeruginosa*, where the pathogen has developed defenses that confer resistance to antibiotics, it is important to fully understand these bacterial mechanisms so we can develop new ways in treating them. With a growing global population, yield losses become more and more problematic

MORAXELLA CATARRHALIS

Moraxella catarrhalis is a fastidious, nonmotile, Gram-negative, aerobic, oxidase-positive diplococcus that can cause infections of the respiratory system, middle ear, eye, central nervous system, and joints of humans. It causes the infection of the host cell by sticking to the host cell using trimeric autotransporter adhesins.

Epidemiology

M. catarrhalis is a human pathogen with an affinity for the human upper respiratory tract. Other primates, such as macaques, might become infected by this bacterium.

M. catarrhalis was previously placed in a separate genus named *Branhamella*. The rationale for this was that other members of the genus *Moraxella* are rod-shaped and rarely caused infections in humans. However, results from DNA hybridization studies and 16S rRNA sequence comparisons were used to justify inclusion of the species *M. catarrhalis* in the genus *Moraxella*. As a consequence, the name *Moraxella catarrhalis* is currently preferred for these bacteria. Nevertheless, some in the medical field continue to call these bacteria *Branhamella catarrhalis*.

Moraxella is named after Victor Morax, a Swiss ophthalmologist who first described this genus of bacteria. *Catarrhalis* is derived from catarrh, from the Greek meaning "to flow down" (*cata-* implies down; *-rrh* implies flow), describing the profuse discharge from eyes and nose typically associated with severe inflammation in colds.

Genetics

The whole genome sequence of *M. catarrhalis* CCUG 353 type strain was deposited and published in DNA Data Bank of Japan, European Nucleotide Archive, and GenBank in 2016 under the accession number LWAH00000000.

Clinical significance

These bacteria are known to cause otitis media, bronchitis, sinusitis, and laryngitis. Elderly patients and long-term heavy smokers with chronic pulmonary disease should be aware that *M. catarrhalis* is associated with bronchopneumonia, as well as exacerbations of existing chronic obstructive pulmonary disease.

The peak rate of colonisation by *M. catarrhalis* appears to occur around 2 years of age, with a striking difference in colonization rates between children and adults (very high to very low).

M. catarrhalis has recently been gaining attention as an emerging human pathogen. It has been identified as an important cause in bronchopulmonary infection, causing infection through pulmonary aspiration in the upper pulmonary tract. Additionally, it causes bacterial pneumonia, especially in adults with a compromised immune system. It has also been known to cause infective exacerbations in adults with chronic lung disease, and it is an important cause in acute sinusitis, maxillary sinusitis, bacteremia, meningitis, conjunctivitis, acute purulent irritation of chronic bronchitis, urethritis, septicemia (although this is rare), septic arthritis (which is also a rare occurrence),and acute laryngitis in adults and acute otitis media in children. *M. catarrhalis* is an opportunistic pulmonary invader, and causes harm especially in patients who have compromised immune systems or any underlying chronic disease.

Link with Bacteremia

M. catarrhalis has also been linked with septic arthritis in conjunction with bacteremia. Although cases of bacteremia cased by *M. catarrhalis* have been reported before, this was the first instance in which bacteremia caused by *M. catarrhalis* was also associated with septic arthritis. A microbiological evaluation of the patient (a 41-year-old male) revealed that *M. catarrhalis* was the cause of the disease rather than *Neisseria* as was previously believed. This was also the second case of *M. catarrhalis* causing septic arthritis (although in the first case, no mention of bacteremia was made).

Along with its relation to septic arthritis, bacteremia is also caused by *M. catarrhalis* infection, which can range in severity from a slight fever to lethal sepsis and an associated respiratory tract infection is usually also identified. Bacteremia infections caused by *M. catarrhalis* have a 21% mortality rate among patients. However, this may have been due to a lack of knowledge about the bacterium because of its recent recognition as a pathogen.

Infection of high-grade bacteremia was linked with the development of endocarditis. However, the patients without endocarditis has been related to the background of each patient, especially the existence of other illnesses and any possible immune impairments they may have. Also, although bacteremia caused by *M. catarrhalis* has been infrequently reported, this may be due to a misdiagnosis or oversight because *M. catarrhalis* was only recently (1990s) identified as an important pathogen. Many chronic diseases in patients with *M. catarrhalis* bacteremia can be linked to the patients with immune defects or respiratory debility. Likewise, respiratory debility in patients with bacteremic pneumonia caused by *M. catarrhalis* infection can be linked with increased rates of pharyngeal colonization, enhancement of bacterial adherence to abnormal epithelium, and increased susceptibility of pulmonary parenchyma to infection.

Antibiotic Resistance

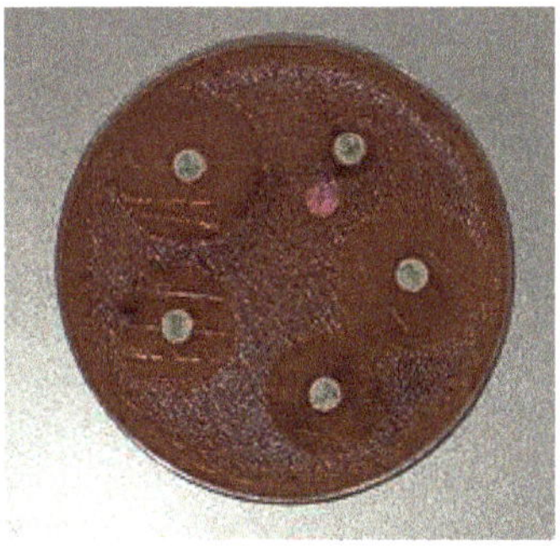

Antibiotic sensitivity test: This strain shows resistance to ampicillin because it produces the enzyme β-lactamase. This is confirmed by the disc labelled β turning red.

M. catarrhalis can be treated with antibiotics, but it is commonly resistant to penicillin, ampicillin, and amoxicillin.

Current research priorities involve trying to find a suitable vaccine for this genotypically diverse organism, as well as determining factors involved with virulence, e.g. complement resistance. Lipooligosaccharide is considered one possible virulence factor. Since the recent recognition of *M. catarrhalis* as an important pathogenic microbe, development of a possible antibiotic has been ongoing. A fraction of *M. catarrhalis* strains seemed to be resistant to ampicillin, which makes ampicillin and amoxicillin inappropriate choices of antibiotic against it. Although all strains of *M. catarrhalis* were susceptible to cotrimoxazole, erythromycin, sulfadimidine, and tetracycline, they were also resistant to trimethoprim. One of the reasons for the resistance of *M. catarrhalis* to ampicillin and trimethoprim is because of the beta-lactamase production, which allows resistance to ampicillin. Also, the resistance of *M. catarrhalis* to other antibiotics may be attributed to beta-lactamase, as well, because the use of these antibiotics has triggered an increase in development of beta-lactamase, which resists antibiotics.

However, a 1994 study has identified a large protein on the surface of *M. catarrhalis* that may serve as a target for protective antibodies. This UspA (the designated antigen) protein is the first surface-exposed protein on *M. catarrhalis* that can be a target for biologically active antibodies, and therefore lead to a vaccination. This protein was also present in all of the strains tested. The large size of the exposed protein macromolecule makes it similar to *Neisseria gonorrhoeae* outer membrane protein macromolecular complex, which implies that UspA may be a single polypeptide chain.

Active immunization, in a study, of *M. catarrhalis* in the respiratory tract allowed the control of the growth of *M. catarrhalis* and led to the development of serum antigens. Also, an enhanced ability exists in the test subjects (mice) to clear *M. catarrhalis* from their lungs. Likewise, passive immunization of *M. catarrhalis* from the mice respiratory tracts also enhanced the mice's ability to clear the microbes from their lungs, which means that serum antibodies likely play a large role in the immunization and protection of the respiratory tract. Along with outer membrane proteins that are consistent among different strains of *M. catarrhalis*, a sort of subclass-specific IgG antibody response to certain outer membrane proteins may also exist. Therefore, the outer membrane antigens of *M. catarrhalis* also provide a possible vaccine source. Also, a bactericidal serum antibody has also been developed in response to the diseases caused by *M. catarrhalis*.

Treatment

Treatment options include antibiotic therapy or a so-called "watchful waiting" approach. The great majority of clinical isolates of this organism produce beta-lactamases, so are resistant to penicillin. Resistance to trimethoprim, trimethoprim-sulfamethoxazole (TMP-SMX), clindamycin, and tetracycline have been reported. It is susceptible to fluoroquinolones, most second- and third-generation cephalosporins, erythromycin, and amoxicillin-clavulanate.

Vaccine Development

Currently, no vaccine is known in the US against *M. catarrhalis* infection. It is a significant cause of respiratory tract infections against which a vaccine is sought. Several outer membrane proteins are currently under investigation as potential vaccine antigens, including the porin M35.

BIOCHEMISTRY

During the first reported case of *M. catarrhalis* causing bacteremia that was associated with septic arthritis, the microbe was cultured, which revealed much about the morphology of its colonies, as well as *M. catarrhalis* itself. *M. catarrhalis* is a large, kidney-shaped, Gram-negative diplococcus. It can be cultured on blood and chocolate agar plates after an aerobic incubation at 37°C for 24 hours. Cultures revealed gray-white hemispheric colonies about 1 mm in diameter. These colonies were fragile and easy to crumble, and appeared to have a waxy surface.

The hockey puck test was applied to these *M. catarrhalis* colonies, in which a wooden stick is used to try to push the colonies across the plate. The *M. catarrhalis* colonies scored positively on this test, which means they could be slid across the plate. The colonies did not demonstrate hemolysis, and were not able to ferment glucose, sucrose, maltose, or lactose. They were able to produce DNase. Cultures of the *M. catarrhalis* tested positive for oxidase and nitrate reduction, which is characteristic of *M. catarrhalis*. Many laboratories also perform a butyrate esterase test and a beta-lactamase test. Both tests should be positive and can help to rapidly identify it from a culture.

The recognition of *M. catarrhalis* as a pathogen has led to studies for possible antibodies against it, which have led to a wider understanding of theits composition. The outer membrane protein (OMP) profiles of different strains of *M. catarrhalis* are extremely similar to each other. Analyses of these OMP profiles with monoclonal antibodies (MAbs) revealed that a few proteins with similar molecular masses in the different strains have cross-reactive epitopes. Also, a surface-exposed protein on *M. catarrhalis* has an unusually high molecular mass. An 80-kDa OMP on *M. catarrhalis* is immunogenic and common to all nonencapsulated strands of *M. catarrhalis*, which suggests it may be used as an antigen for immunization.

REFERENCES

1. Acinetobacter in Healthcare Settings. CDC. Retrieved April 8, 2013.
2. Army Medical Logistics (PDF). FM 4-02.1. United States. Retrieved April 8, 2013.
3. Abbo, A; Navon-Venezia, S; Hammer-Muntz, O; Krichali, T; et al. (January 2005). Multidrug-resistant Acinetobacter baumannii. Emerging Infectious Diseases. 11 (1): 22–9. doi:10.3201/eid1101.040001. PMID 15705318.
4. Adams, D; Yee, L; Rimmer, JA; Williams, R; Martin, H; Ovington, C (Feb 10–23, 2011). Investigation and management of an A. Baumannii outbreak in ICU.. British Journal of Nursing. 20 (3): 140, 142, 144–7. doi:10.12968/bjon.2011.20.3.140. PMID 21378633.
5. Aivazova, V; Kainer, F; Friese, K; Mylonas, I (January 2010). Acinetobacter baumannii infection during pregnancy and puerperium.. Archives of Gynecology and Obstetrics. 281 (1): 171–4. doi:10.1007/s00404-009-1107-z. PMID 19462176.
6. Antunes, LCS; Visca, P; Towner, KJ (2014). Acinetobacter baumannii: evolution of a global pathogen. Pathogens and Disease. 71 (3): 292–301. doi:10.1111/2049-

632X.12125. PMID 24376225.

7. Chau, SL; Chu, YW; Houang, ET (October 2004). Novel resistance-nodulation-cell division efflux system AdeDE in Acinetobacter genomic DNA group 3.. Antimicrobial Agents and Chemotherapy. 48 (10): 4054–5. doi:10.1128/aac.48.10.4054-4055.2004. PMID 15388479.
8. Choi, CH; Lee, JS; Lee, YC; Park, TI; Lee, JC (Dec 10, 2008). Acinetobacter baumannii invades epithelial cells and outer membrane protein A mediates interactions with epithelial cells.. BMC Microbiology. 8: 216. doi:10.1186/1471-2180-8-216. PMID 19068136.
9. Dijkshoorn, L; Nemec, A; Seifert, H (December 2007). An increasing threat in hospitals: multidrug-resistant Acinetobacter baumannii.. Nature Reviews Microbiology. 5 (12): 939–51. doi:10.1038/nrmicro1789. PMID 18007677.
10. Drummond, Katie. Pentagon to Troop-Killing Superbugs: Resistance Is Futile. Wired.com. Condé Nast. Retrieved 8 April 2013.
11. Duan, X; Yang, L; Xia, P (March 2010). Septic arthritis of the knee caused by antibiotic-resistant Acinetobacter baumannii in a gout patient: a rare case report.. Archives of Orthopaedic and Trauma Surgery. 130 (3): 381–4. doi:10.1007/s00402-009-0958-x. PMID 19707778.
12. Espinal, P; Martí, S; Vila, J (January 2012). Effect of biofilm formation on the survival of Acinetobacter baumannii on dry surfaces.. The Journal of Hospital Infection. 80 (1): 56–60. doi:10.1016/j.jhin.2011.08.013. PMID 21975219.
13. Farrugia, DN; Elbourne, LD; Hassan, KA; Eijkelkamp, BA; Tetu, SG; Brown, MH; Shah, BS; Peleg, AY; Mabbutt, BC; Paulsen, IT (2013). The Complete Genome and Phenome of a Community-Acquired Acinetobacter baumannii. PLoS ONE. 8 (3): e58628. Bibcode:2013PLoSO...858628F. doi:10.1371/journal.pone.0058628. PMC 3602452. PMID 23527001.
14. Fitzpatrick, MA; Esterly, JS; Postelnick, MJ; Sutton, SH (Jul–Aug 2012). Successful treatment of extensively drug-resistant Acinetobacter baumannii peritoneal dialysis peritonitis with intraperitoneal polymyxin B and ampicillin-sulbactam. Annals of Pharmacotherapy. 46 (7–8): e17. doi:10.1345/aph.1r086. PMID 22811349.
15. Garrity, edited by G. (2000). Bergey›s Manual of Systematic Bacteriology Vol. 2, Pts. A & B: The Proteobacteria. (2nd ed., rev. ed.). New York: Springer. p. 454. ISBN 0-387-95040-0.
16. Gerner-Smidt, P (October 1992). Ribotyping of the Acinetobacter calcoaceticus-Acinetobacter baumannii complex.. Journal of Clinical Microbiology. 30 (10): 2680–5. PMID 1383266.
17. Gionco, B; Pelayo, JS; Venancio, EJ; Cayô, R; Gales, AC; Carrara-Marroni, FE (October 2012). Detection of OXA-231, a new variant of blaOXA-143, in Acinetobacter baumannii from Brazil: a case report.. The Journal of Antimicrobial Chemotherapy. 67 (10): 2531–2. doi:10.1093/jac/dks223. PMID 22736746.
18. Gusten, WM; Hansen, EA; Cunha, BA (Jan–Feb 2002). Acinetobacter baumannii pseudomeningitis.. Heart & Lung. 31 (1): 76–8. doi:10.1067/mhl.2002.120258.

PMID 11805753.

19. Higgins, PG; Pérez-Llarena, FJ; Zander, E; Fernández, A; Bou, G; Seifert, H (Feb 25, 2013). OXA-235, a novel Class D Beta-Lactamase Involved in Resistance to Carbapenems in Acinetobacter baumannii.. Antimicrobial Agents and Chemotherapy. 57 (5): 2121–6. doi:10.1128/AAC.02413-12. PMID 23439638.
20. Hong, KB; Oh, HS; Song, JS; Lim, JH; Kang, DK; Son, IS; Park, JD; Kim, EC; Lee, HJ; Choi, EH (July 2012). Investigation and control of an outbreak of imipenem-resistant Acinetobacter baumannii Infection in a Pediatric Intensive Care Unit.. The Pediatric Infectious Disease Journal. 31 (7): 685–90. doi:10.1097/inf.0b013e318256f3e6. PMID 22466324.
21. http://www.cdc.gov/HAI/organisms/acinetobacter.html
22. Jeong, HL; Yeom, JS; Park, JS; Seo, JH; Park, ES; Lim, JY; Park, CH; Woo, HO; Youn, HS (Jul–Aug 2011). Acinetobacter baumannii isolation in cerebrospinal fluid in a febrile neonate. The Turkish journal of Pediatrics. 53 (4): 445–7. PMID 21980849.
23. John, TM; Jacob, CN; Ittycheria, CC; George, AM; Jacob, AG; Subramaniyam, S; Puthiyaveettil, J; Jayaprakash, R (March 2012). Macrophage activation syndrome following Acinetobacter baumannii sepsis.. International Journal of Infectious Diseases. 16 (3): e223–4. doi:10.1016/j.ijid.2011.12.002. PMID 22285540.
24. Jones, A; Morgan, D; Walsh, A; Turton, J; Livermore, D; Pitt, T; Green, A; Gill, M; Mortiboy, D (June 2006). Importation of multidrug-resistant Acinetobacter spp infections with casualties from Iraq. The Lancet infectious diseases. 6 (6): 317–8. doi:10.1016/S1473-3099(06)70471-6. PMID 16728314.
25. Kleinman, HK; McGarvey, ML; Hassell, JR; Star, VL; Cannon, FB; Laurie, GW; Martin, GR (Jan 28, 1986). Basement membrane complexes with biological activity.. Biochemistry. 25 (2): 312–8. doi:10.1021/bi00350a005. PMID 2937447.
26. Koulenti, D; Lisboa, T; Brun-Buisson, C; Krueger, W; Macor, A; Sole-Violan, J; Diaz, E; Topeli, A; DeWaele, J; Carneiro, A; Martin-Loeches, I; Armaganidis, A; Rello, J (August 2009). EU-VAP/CAP Study, Group. Spectrum of practice in the diagnosis of nosocomial pneumonia in patients requiring mechanical ventilation in European intensive care units.. Critical Care Medicine. 37 (8): 2360–8. doi:10.1097/ccm.0b013e3181a037ac. PMID 19531951.
27. Lee, JS; Choi, CH; Kim, JW; Lee, JC (June 2010). Acinetobacter baumannii outer membrane protein A induces dendritic cell death through mitochondrial targeting.. Journal of Microbiology. 48 (3): 387–92. doi:10.1007/s12275-010-0155-1. PMID 20571958.
28. Lee, SY; Lee, JW; Jeong, DC; Chung, SY; Chung, DS; Kang, JH (August 2008). Multidrug-resistant Acinetobacter meningitis in a 3-year-old boy treated with i.v. colistin.. Pediatrics International. 50 (4): 584–5. doi:10.1111/j.1442-200x.2008.02677.x. PMID 18937759.
29. Lee, YK; Kim, JK; Oh, SE; Lee, J; Noh, JW (December 2009). Successful antibiotic lock therapy in patients with refractory peritonitis.. Clinical Nephrology. 72 (6): 488–91. doi:10.5414/cnp72488. PMID 19954727.

30. Luke, NR; Sauberan, SL; Russo, TA; Beanan, JM; Olson, R; Loehfelm, TW; Cox, AD; St Michael, F; Vinogradov, EV; Campagnari, AA (May 2010). Identification and characterization of a glycosyltransferase involved in Acinetobacter baumannii lipopolysaccharide core biosynthesis.. Infection and Immunity. 78 (5): 2017–23. doi:10.1128/iai.00016-10. PMID 20194587.

31. Magnet, S; Courvalin, P; Lambert, T (December 2001). Resistance-nodulation-cell division-type efflux pump involved in aminoglycoside resistance in Acinetobacter baumannii strain BM4454.. Antimicrobial Agents and Chemotherapy. 45 (12): 3375–80. doi:10.1128/aac.45.12.3375-3380.2001. PMID 11709311.

32. Martins, N; Martins, IS; de Freitas, WV; de Matos, JA; Magalhães, AC; Girão, VB; Dias, RC; de Souza, TC; Pellegrino, FL; Costa, LD; Boasquevisque, CH; Nouér, SA; Riley, LW; Santoro-Lopes, G; Moreira, BM (June 2012). Severe infection in a lung transplant recipient caused by donor-transmitted carbapenem-resistant Acinetobacter baumannii.. Transplant Infectious Disease. 14 (3): 316–20. doi:10.1111/j.1399-3062.2011.00701.x. PMID 22168176.

33. McQueary, CN; Kirkup, BC; Si, Y; Barlow, M; Actis, LA; Craft, DW; Zurawski, DV (June 2012). Extracellular stress and lipopolysaccharide modulate Acinetobacter baumannii surface-associated motility.. Journal of Microbiology. 50 (3): 434–43. doi:10.1007/s12275-012-1555-1. PMID 22752907.

34. Meghoo, CA; Dennis, JW; Tuman, C; Fang, R (May 2012). Diagnosis and management of evacuated casualties with cervical vascular injuries resulting from combat-related explosive blasts.. Journal of Vascular Surgery. 55 (5): 1329–36; discussion 1336–7. doi:10.1016/j.jvs.2011.11.125. PMID 22325667.

35. Murray, CK (March 2008). Epidemiology of infections associated with combat-related injuries in Iraq and Afghanistan.. The Journal of Trauma. 64 (3 Suppl): S232–8. doi:10.1097/ta.0b013e318163c3f5. PMID 18316967.

36. Ng, J; Gosbell, IB; Kelly, JA; Boyle, MJ; Ferguson, JK (November 2006). Cure of multiresistant Acinetobacter baumannii central nervous system infections with intraventricular or intrathecal colistin: case series and literature review.. The Journal of Antimicrobial Chemotherapy. 58 (5): 1078–81. doi:10.1093/jac/dkl347. PMID 16916866.

37. O›Shea, MK (May 2012). Acinetobacter in modern warfare.. International Journal of Antimicrobial Agents. 39 (5): 363–75. doi:10.1016/j.ijantimicag.2012.01.018. PMID 22459899.

38. Patel, JA; Pacheco, SM; Postelnick, M; Sutton, S (Aug 15, 2011). Prolonged triple therapy for persistent multidrug-resistant Acinetobacter baumannii ventriculitis.. American Journal of Health-System Pharmacy. 68 (16): 1527–31. doi:10.2146/ajhp100234. PMID 21817084.

39. Pencavel, TD; Singh-Ranger, G; Crinnion, JN (May 2006). Conservative treatment of an early aortic graft infection due to Acinetobacter baumanii.. Annals of Vascular Surgery. 20 (3): 415–7. doi:10.1007/s10016-006-9030-2. PMID 16602028.

40. Piparsania, S; Rajput, N; Bhatambare, G (Sep–Oct 2012). Intraventricular

polymyxin B for the treatment of neonatal meningo-ventriculitis caused by multi-resistant Acinetobacter baumannii--case report and review of literature.. The Turkish Journal of Pediatrics. 54 (5): 548–54. PMID 23427525.

41. Post, V; White, PA; Hall, RM (June 2010). Evolution of AbaR-type genomic resistance islands in multiply antibiotic-resistant Acinetobacter baumannii.. The Journal of Antimicrobial Chemotherapy. 65 (6): 1162–70. doi:10.1093/jac/dkq095. PMID 20375036.

42. Rice, LB (Apr 15, 2008). Federal funding for the study of antimicrobial resistance in nosocomial pathogens: no ESKAPE.. The Journal of Infectious Diseases. 197 (8): 1079–81. doi:10.1086/533452. PMID 18419525.

43. Schulte, B; Goerke, C; Weyrich, P; Gröbner, S; Bahrs, C; Wolz, C; Autenrieth, IB; Borgmann, S (December 2005). Clonal spread of meropenem-resistant Acinetobacter baumannii strains in hospitals in the Mediterranean region and transmission to South-west Germany.. The Journal of Hospital Infection. 61 (4): 356–7. doi:10.1016/j.jhin.2005.05.009. PMID 16213625.

44. Seputiene, V.; Povilonis, J.; Suziedeliene, E. (30 January 2012). Novel Variants of AbaR Resistance Islands with a Common Backbone in Acinetobacter baumannii Isolates of European Clone II. Antimicrobial Agents and Chemotherapy. 56 (4): 1969–1973. doi:10.1128/AAC.05678-11. PMC 3318354. PMID 22290980.

45. Sharma, A; Shariff, M; Thukral, SS; Shah, A (October 2005). Chronic community-acquired Acinetobacter pneumonia that responded slowly to rifampicin in the anti-tuberculous regime.. The Journal of Infection. 51 (3): e149–52. doi:10.1016/j.jinf.2004.12.003. PMID 16230195.

46. Sharma, Rajnikant; Arya, Sankalp; Patil, Supriya Deepak; Sharma, Atin; Jain, Pradeep Kumar; Navani, Naveen Kumar; Pathania, Ranjana (2014-01-01). Identification of novel regulatory small RNAs in Acinetobacter baumannii. PloS One. 9 (4): e93833. doi:10.1371/journal.pone.0093833. ISSN 1932-6203. PMC 3976366. PMID 24705412.

47. Spapen, H; Jacobs, R; Van Gorp, V; Troubleyn, J; et al. (May 25, 2011). Renal and neurological side effects of colistin in critically ill patients. Annals of Intensive Care. 1 (1): 14. doi:10.1186/2110-5820-1-14. PMID 21906345.

48. Su, CH; Wang, JT; Hsiung, CA; Chien, LJ; et al. (2012). Increase of carbapenem-resistant Acinetobacter baumannii infection in acute care hospitals in Taiwan: Association with hospital antimicrobial usage. PLOS ONE. 7 (5): e37788. Bibcode:2012PLoSO...737788S. doi:10.1371/journal.pone.0037788. PMC 3357347. PMID 22629456.

49. Sullivan, DR; Shields, J; Netzer, G (June 2010). Fatal case of multi-drug resistant Acinetobacter baumannii necrotizing fasciitis.. The American Surgeon. 76 (6): 651–3. PMID 20583528.

50. Superti, SV; Martins Dde, S; Caierão, J; Soares Fda, S; Prochnow, T; Zavascki, AP (Mar–Apr 2009). Indications of carbapenem resistance evolution through heteroresistance as an intermediate stage in Acinetobacter baumannii after carbapenem administration.. Revista do Instituto de Medicina Tropical de Sao

Paulo. 51 (2): 111–3. doi:10.1590/s0036-46652009000200010. PMID 19390741.

51. Tjoa E, Moehario LH, Rukmana A, Rohsiswatmo R (2013). Acinetobacter baumannii: Role in Blood Stream Infection in Neonatal Unit, Dr. Cipto Mangunkusumo Hospital, Jakarta, Indonesia. International Journal of Microbiology. 2013: 180763. doi:10.1155/2013/180763.

52. to:a b Wagner, JA; Nenoff, P; Handrick, W; Renner, R; Simon, J; Treudler, R (February 2011). [Necrotizing fasciitis caused by Acinetobacter baumannii : A case report].. Der Hautarzt; Zeitschrift für Dermatologie, Venerologie, und verwandte Gebiete. 62 (2): 128–30. doi:10.1007/s00105-010-1962-3. PMID 20835812.

53. Tomaras, AP; Dorsey, CW; Edelmann, RE; Actis, LA (December 2003). Attachment to and biofilm formation on abiotic surfaces by Acinetobacter baumannii: involvement of a novel chaperone-usher pili assembly system.. Microbiology. 149 (Pt 12): 3473–84. doi:10.1099/mic.0.26541-0. PMID 14663080.

54. Werneck, JS; Picão, RC; Carvalhaes, CG; Cardoso, JP; Gales, AC (February 2011). OXA-72-producing Acinetobacter baumannii in Brazil: a case report.. The Journal of Antimicrobial Chemotherapy. 66 (2): 452–4. doi:10.1093/jac/dkq462. PMID 21131320.

55. Worthington, RJ; Richards, JJ; Melander, C (Oct 7, 2012). Small molecule control of bacterial biofilms.. Organic & Biomolecular Chemistry. 10 (37): 7457–74. doi:10.1039/c2ob25835h. PMID 22733439.

56. Wu, YC; Hsieh, TC; Sun, SS; Wang, CH; Yen, KY; Lin, YY; Kao, CH (November 2009). Unexpected cloud-like lesion on gallium-67 scintigraphy: detection of subcutaneous abscess underneath the skin with normal appearance in a comatose patient in an intensive care setting.. The American Journal of the Medical Sciences. 338 (5): 388. doi:10.1097/maj.0b013e3181a6dd36. PMID 19770790.

57. Xiao, SC; Zhu, SH; Xia, ZF; Ma, B; Cheng, DS (November 2009). Successful treatment of a critical burn patient with obstinate hyperglycemia and septic shock from pan-drug-resistant strains.. Medical Science Monitor. 15 (11): CS163–5. PMID 19865060.

58. Yeom, J; Shin, JH; Yang, JY; Kim, J; Hwang, GS (2013). (1)H NMR-Based Metabolite Profiling of Planktonic and Biofilm Cells in Acinetobacter baumannii 1656-2.. PLoS ONE. 8 (3): e57730. Bibcode:2013PLoSO...857730Y. doi:10.1371/journal.pone.0057730. PMC 3590295. PMID 23483923.

59. Zhao, WS; Liu, GY; Mi, ZH; Zhang, F (March 2011). Coexistence of blaOXA-23 with armA and novel gyrA mutation in a pandrug-resistant Acinetobacter baumannii isolate from the blood of a patient with haematological disease in China.. The Journal of Hospital Infection. 77 (3): 278–9. doi:10.1016/j.jhin.2010.11.006. PMID 21281989.

CHAPTER 8

Human Microbiota

Chapter Contents

Human microbiome, the full array of microorganisms (the microbiota) that live on and in humans and, more specifically, the collection of microbial genomes that contribute to the broader genetic portrait, or metagenome, of a human. The genomes that constitute the human microbiome represent a remarkably diverse array of microorganisms that includes bacteria, archaea (primitive single-celled organisms), fungi, and even some protozoans and nonliving viruses.

INTRODUCTION

The **human microbiota** is the aggregate of microorganisms, a microbiome that resides on or within a number of tissues and biofluids, including the skin, mammary glands, placenta, seminal fluid, uterus, ovarian follicles, lung, saliva, oral mucosa, conjunctiva, and gastrointestinal tracts. They include bacteria, fungi, and archaea. Micro-animals which live on the human body are excluded. The human microbiome refers to their genomes.

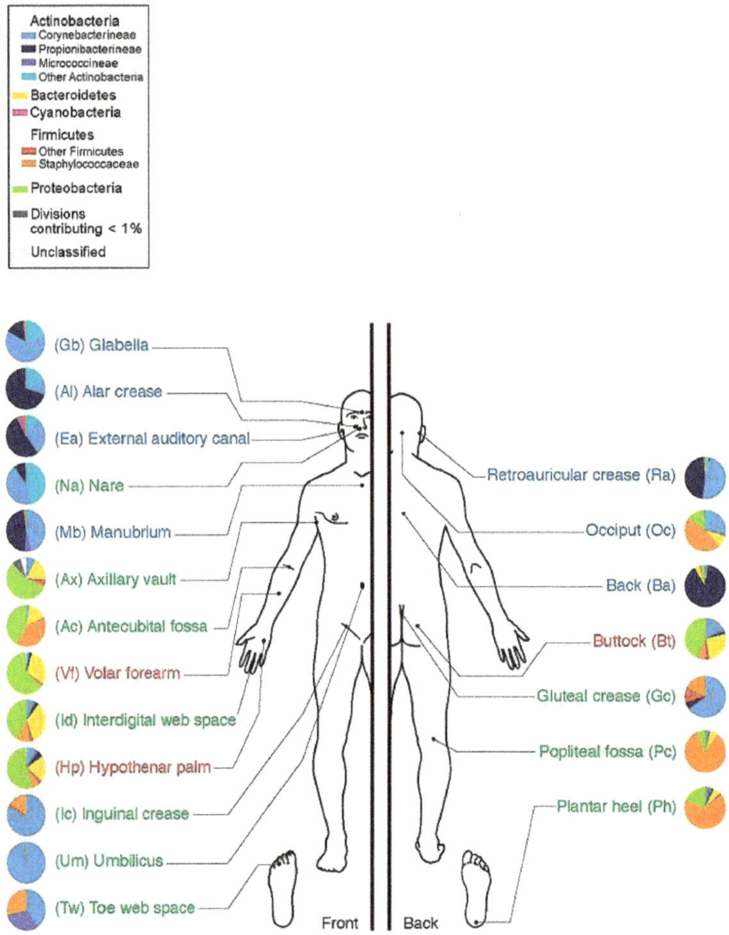

Graphic depicting the human skin microbiota, with relative prevalences of various classes of bacteria.

Humans are colonized by many microorganisms; the traditional estimate was that humans live with ten times more non-human cells than human cells; more recent estimates have lowered that to 3:1 and even to approximately the same number; all the numbers are estimates. Some microbiota that colonize humans have not merely a commensal (a non-harmful coexistence), but rather a mutualistic relationship with their human hosts.[700] Conversely, some non-pathogenic microbiota can harm human hosts via the metabolites that they produce, like trimethylamine. Certain microbiota perform tasks that are known to be useful for the human host; for most, the role is not well understood. Those that are expected to be present, and that under normal circumstances do not cause disease, are deemed *normal flora* or *normal microbiota*.

The Human Microbiome Project took on the project of sequencing the genome of the human microbiota, focusing particularly on the microbiota that normally inhabit the skin, mouth, nose, digestive tract, and vagina. It reached a milestone in 2012 when it published initial results.

TERMINOLOGY

Though widely known as *flora or microflora*, this is a misnomer in technical terms, since the word root *flora* pertains to plants, and *biota* refers to the total collection of organisms in a particular ecosystem. Recently, the more appropriate term *microbiota* is applied, though its use has not eclipsed the entrenched use and recognition of *flora* with regard to bacteria and other microorganisms. Both terms are being used in different literature.

RELATIVE NUMBERS

As of 2014, it was often reported in popular media and in the scientific literature that there are about 10 times as many microbial cells in the human body than there are human cells; this figure was based on estimates that the human microbiome includes around 100 trillion bacterial cells and an adult human typically has around 10 trillion human cells. In 2014 the American Academy of Microbiology published an FAQ that emphasized that the number of microbial cells and the number of human cells are both estimates, and noted that recent research had arrived at a new estimate of the number of human cells at around 37 trillion cells, meaning that the ratio of microbial to human cells is probably about 3:1. In 2016 another group published a new estimate of ratio as being roughly 1:1 (1.3:1, with an uncertainty of 25% and a variation of 53% over the population of standard 70 kg males).

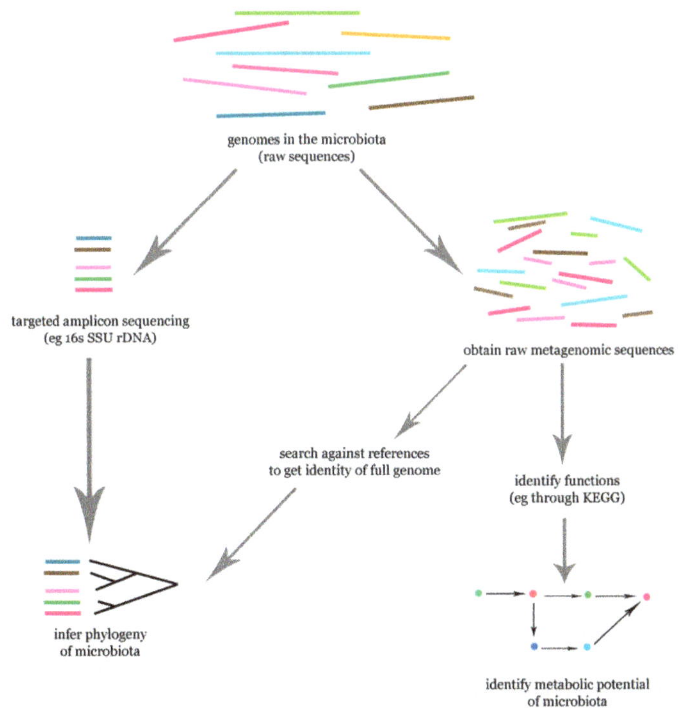

Flowchart illustrating how the human microbiome is studied on the DNA level.

The problem of elucidating the human microbiome is essentially identifying the members of a microbial community which includes bacteria, eukaryotes, and viruses. This is done primarily using DNA-based studies, though RNA, protein and metabolite based studies are also performed. DNA-based microbiome studies typically can be categorized as either targeted amplicon studies or more recently shotgun metagenomic studies. The former focuses on specific known marker genes and is primarily informative taxonomically, while the latter is an entire metagenomic approach which can also be used to study the functional potential of the community. One of the challenges that is present in human microbiome studies but not in other metagenomic studies is to avoid including the host DNA in the study.

Aside from simply elucidating the composition of the human microbiome, one of the major questions involving the human microbiome is whether there is a core, that is, whether there is a subset of the community that is shared among most humans. If there is a core, then it would be possible to associate certain community compositions with disease states, which is one of the goals of the Human Microbiome Project. It is known that the human microbiome is highly variable both within a single subject and between different individuals. For example, the gut microbiota of humans is markedly dissimilar between individuals, a phenomenon which is also observed in mice.

On 13 June 2012, a major milestone of the Human Microbiome Project (HMP) was announced by the NIH director Francis Collins. The announcement was accompanied with a series of coordinated articles published in Nature and several journals in the Public Library of Science (PLoS) on the same day. By mapping the normal microbial make-up of healthy humans using genome sequencing techniques, the researchers of the HMP have created a reference database and the boundaries of normal microbial variation in humans. From 242 healthy U.S. volunteers, more than 5,000 samples were collected from tissues from 15 (men) to 18 (women) body sites such as mouth, nose, skin, lower intestine (stool), and vagina. All the DNA, human and microbial, were analyzed with DNA sequencing machines. The microbial genome data were extracted by identifying the bacterial specific ribosomal RNA, 16S rRNA. The researchers calculated that more than 10,000 microbial species occupy the human ecosystem and they have identified 81 – 99% of the genera.

TYPES

Bacteria

Populations of microbes (such as bacteria and yeasts) inhabit the skin and mucosal surfaces in various parts of the body. Their role forms part of normal, healthy human physiology, however if microbe numbers grow beyond their typical ranges (often due to a compromised immune system) or if microbes populate (such as through poor hygiene or injury) areas of the body normally not colonized or sterile (such as the blood, or the lower respiratory tract, or the abdominal cavity), disease can result (causing, respectively, bacteremia/sepsis, pneumonia, and peritonitis).

The Human Microbiome Project found that individuals host thousands of bacterial types, different body sites having their own distinctive communities. Skin and vaginal sites showed smaller diversity than the mouth and gut, these showing the greatest richness. The bacterial makeup for a given site on a body varies from person to person, not only in type, but also in abundance. Bacteria of the same species found throughout the mouth are of multiple subtypes, preferring to inhabit distinctly different locations in the mouth. Even the enterotypes in the human gut, previously thought to be well-understood, are from a broad spectrum of communities with blurred taxon boundaries. It is estimated that 500 to 1,000 species of bacteria live in the human gut but belong to just a few phyla: Firmicutes and Bacteroidetes dominate but there are also Proteobacteria, Verrumicrobia, Actinobacteria, Fusobacteria and Cyanobacteria.

A number of types of bacteria, such as *Actinomyces viscosus* and *A. naeslundii*, live in the mouth, where they are part of a sticky substance called plaque. If this is not removed by brushing, it hardens into calculus (also called tartar). The same bacteria also secrete acids that dissolve tooth enamel, causing tooth decay.

The vaginal microflora consist mostly of various lactobacillus species. It was long thought that the most common of these species was *Lactobacillus acidophilus*, but it has later been shown that *L. iners* is in fact most common, followed by *L. crispatus*. Other lactobacilli found in the vagina are *L. jensenii, L. delbruekii* and *L. gasseri*. Disturbance of the vaginal flora can lead to infections such as bacterial vaginosis or candidiasis ("yeast infection").

Archaea

Archaea are present in the human gut, but, in contrast to the enormous variety of bacteria in this organ, the numbers of archaeal species are much more limited. The dominant group are the methanogens, particularly *Methanobrevibacter smithii* and *Methanosphaera stadtmanae*. However, colonization by methanogens is variable, and only about 50% of humans have easily detectable populations of these organisms.

As of 2007, no clear examples of archaeal pathogens were known, although a relationship has been proposed between the presence of some methanogens and human periodontal disease.

Fungi

Fungi, in particular yeasts, are present in the human gut. The best-studied of these are *Candida* species due to their ability to become pathogenic in immunocompromised and even in healthy hosts. Yeasts are also present on the skin, such as *Malassezia* species, where they consume oils secreted from the sebaceous glands.

Viruses

Viruses, especially bacterial viruses (bacteriophages), colonize various body sites. These colonized sites include the skin, gut, lungs, and oral cavity. Virus communities have been associated with some diseases, and do not simply reflect the bacterial communities.

ANATOMICAL AREAS

Skin

A study of twenty skin sites on each of ten healthy humans found 205 identified genera in nineteen bacterial phyla, with most sequences assigned to four phyla: Actinobacteria (51.8%),

Firmicutes (24.4%), Proteobacteria (16.5%), and Bacteroidetes (6.3%). A large number of fungal genera are present on healthy human skin, with some variability by region of the body; however, during pathological conditions, certain genera tend to dominate in the affected region. For example, *Malassezia* is dominant in atopic dermatitis and *Acremonium* is dominant on dandruff-afflicted scalps.

The skin acts as a barrier to deter the invasion of pathogenic microbes. The human skin contains microbes that reside either in or on the skin and can be residential or transient. Resident microorganism types vary in relation to skin type on the human body. A majority of microbes reside on superficial cells on the skin or prefer to associate with glands. These glands such as oil or sweat glands provide the microbes with water, amino acids, and fatty acids. In addition, resident bacteria that associated with oil glands are often Gram-positive and can be pathogenic.

Conjunctiva

A small number of bacteria and fungi are normally present in the conjunctiva. Classes of bacteria include Gram-positive cocci (e.g., *Staphylococcus* and Streptococcus) and Gram-negative rods and cocci (e.g., *Haemophilus* and *Neisseria*) are present. Fungal genera include *Candida*, *Aspergillus*, and *Penicillium*. The lachrymal glands continuously secrete, keeping the conjunctiva moist, while intermittent blinking lubricates the conjunctiva and washes away foreign material. Tears contain bactericides such as lysozyme, so that microorganisms have difficulty in surviving the lysozyme and settling on the epithelial surfaces.

Gut

This diagram shows the biosynthesis of bioactive compounds (indole and certain derivatives) from tryptophan by bacteria in the gut. Indole is produced from tryptophan by bacteria that express tryptophanase.*Clostridium sporogenes* metabolizes indole into 3-indolepropionic acid (IPA), a highly potent neuroprotectiveantioxidant that scavenges hydroxyl radicals. In the intestine, IPA binds to pregnane X receptors (PXR) in intestinal cells, thereby facilitating mucosal homeostasis and barrier function. Following absorption from the intestine and distribution to the brain, IPA confers a neuroprotective effect against cerebral ischemia and Alzheimer's disease. *Lactobacillus* species metabolize tryptophan into indole-3-aldehyde (I3A) which acts on the aryl hydrocarbon receptor (AhR) in intestinal immune cells, in turn increasing interleukin-22 (IL-22) production. Indole itself acts as a glucagon-like peptide-1 (GLP-1) secretagogue in intestinal L cells and as a ligand for AhR. Indole can also be metabolized by the liver into indoxyl sulfate, a compound that is toxic in high concentrations and associated with vascular disease and renal dysfunction. AST-120 (activated charcoal), an intestinal sorbent that is taken by mouth, adsorbs indole, in turn decreasing the concentration of indoxyl sulfate in blood plasma.

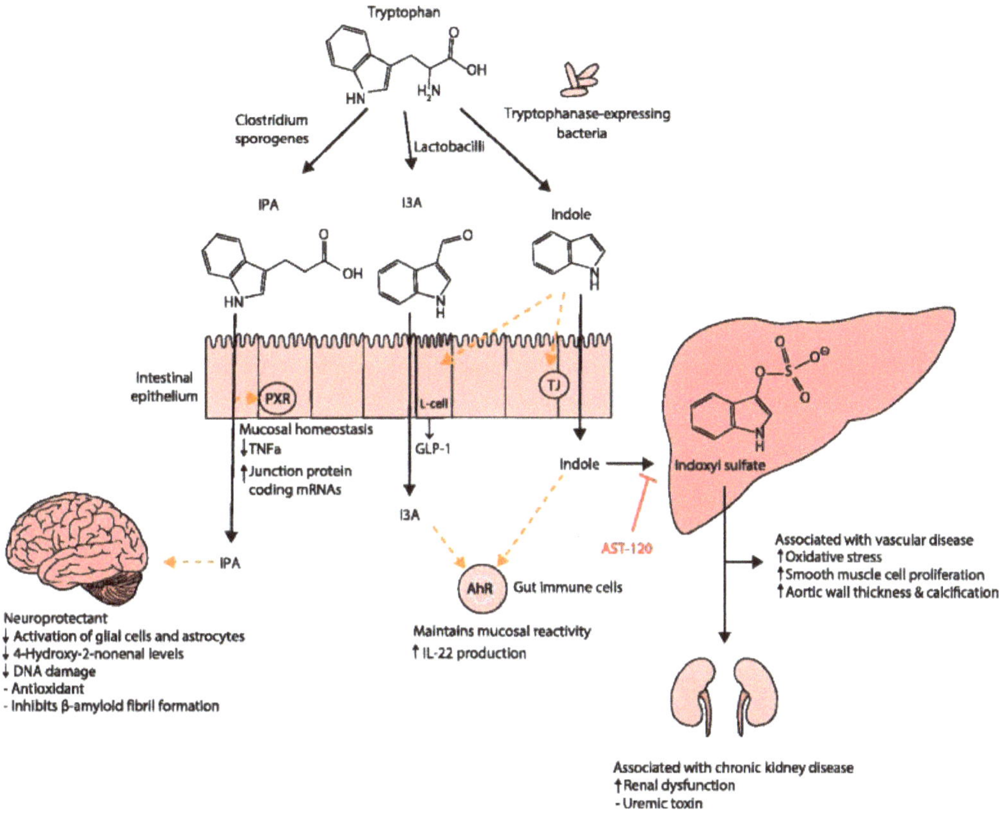

***Tryptophan metabolism by human gastrointestinal microbiota** (v · t · e)*

The gut flora has the largest numbers of bacteria and the greatest number of species compared to other areas of the body. In humans the gut flora is established at one to two years after birth, and by that time the intestinal epithelium and the intestinal mucosal barrier that it secretes have co-developed in a way that is tolerant to, and even supportive of, the gut flora and that also provides a barrier to pathogenic organisms. The relationship between some gut flora and humans is not merely commensal (a non-harmful coexistence), but rather a mutualistic relationship. Some human gut microorganisms benefit the host by fermentating dietary fiber into short-chain fatty acids (SCFAs), such as acetic acid and butyric acid, which are then absorbed by the host. Intestinal bacteria also play a role in synthesizing vitamin B and vitamin K as well as metabolizing bile acids, sterols, and xenobiotics. The systemic importance of the SCFAs and other compounds they produce are like hormones and the gut flora itself appears to function like an endocrine organ, and dysregulation of the gut flora has been correlated with a host of inflammatory and autoimmune conditions.

The composition of human gut flora changes over time, when the diet changes, and as overall health changes. A systematic review of 15 human randomized controlled trials from July 2016 found that certain commercially available strains of probiotic bacteria from the *Bifidobacterium* and *Lactobacillus* genera (*B. longum*, *B. breve*, *B. infantis*, *L. helveticus*, *L. rhamnosus*, *L. plantarum*, and *L. casei*), when taken by mouth in daily doses of 10^9–10^{10} colony forming units (CFU) for 1–2 months, possess treatment efficacy (i.e., improved behavioral outcomes) in certain central nervous system disorders – including anxiety, depression, autism spectrum disorder, and obsessive–compulsive disorder – and improved certain aspects of memory.

Vagina

Vaginal microbiota refers to those species and genera that colonize the lower reproductive tract of women. These organisms play an important role in protecting against infections and maintaining vaginal health. The most abundant vaginal microorganisms found in premenopausal women are from the genus *Lactobacillus*, which suppress pathogens by producing hydrogen peroxide and lactic acid. Bacterial species composition and ratios vary depending on the stage of the menstrual cycle. Ethnicity also influences vaginal flora. The occurrence of hydrogen peroxide-producing lactobacilli is lower in African American women and vaginal pH is higher. Other influential factors such as sexual intercourse and antibiotics have been linked to the loss of lactobacilli. Moreover, studies have found that sexual intercourse with a condom does appear to change lactobacilli levels, and does increase the level of *Escherichia coli* within the vaginal flora. Changes in the normal, healthy vaginal microbiota is an indication of infections, such as candidiasis or bacterial vaginosis. *Candida albicans* inhibits the growth of *Lactobacillus* species, while *Lactobacillus* species which produce hydrogen peroxide inhibit the growth and virulence of *Candida albicans* in both the vagina and the gut.

Fungal genera that have been detected in the vagina include *Candida*, *Pichia*, *Eurotium*, *Alternaria*, *Rhodotorula*, and *Cladosporium*, among others.

Placenta

Until recently the placenta was considered to be a sterile organ but commensal, nonpathogenic bacterial species and genera have been identified that reside in the placental tissue.

Uterus

Until recently, the upper reproductive tract of women was considered to be a sterile environment. A variety of microorganisms inhabit the uterus of healthy, asymptomatic women of reproductive age. The microbiome of the uterus differs significantly from that of the vagina and gastrointestinal tract.

Oral cavity

The environment present in the human mouth allows the growth of characteristic microorganisms found there. It provides a source of water and nutrients, as well as a moderate temperature. Resident microbes of the mouth adhere to the teeth and gums to resist mechanical flushing from the mouth to stomach where acid-sensitive microbes are destroyed by hydrochloric acid.

Anaerobic bacteria in the oral cavity include: *Actinomyces*, *Arachnia*, *Bacteroides*, *Bifidobacterium*, *Eubacterium*, *Fusobacterium*, *Lactobacillus*, *Leptotrichia*, *Peptococcus*, *Peptostreptococcus*, *Propionibacterium*, *Selenomonas*, *Treponema*, and *Veillonella*. Genera of fungi that are frequently found in the mouth include *Candida*, *Cladosporium*, *Aspergillus*, *Fusarium*, *Glomus*, *Alternaria*, *Penicillium*, and *Cryptococcus*, among others. Bacteria accumulate on both the hard and soft oral tissues in biofilms. Bacterial adhesion is particularly important for oral bacteria. Oral bacteria have evolved mechanisms to sense their environment and evade or modify the host. Bacteria occupy the ecological niche provided by both the tooth surface and gingival epithelium. However, a highly efficient innate host defense system constantly monitors the bacterial colonization and prevents bacterial invasion of local tissues. A dynamic equilibrium exists between dental plaque bacteria and the innate host defense system. Of particular interest is the role of oral microorganisms in the two major dental diseases: dental caries and periodontal disease. Additionally, research has correlated poor oral heath and the resulting ability of the oral microbiota to invade the body to affect cardiac health as well as cognitive function.

Lung

Much like the oral cavity, the upper and lower respiratory system possess mechanical deterrents to remove microbes. Goblet cells produce mucous which traps microbes and moves them out of the respiratory system via continuously moving ciliated epithelial cells. In addition, a bactericidal effect is generated by nasal mucus which contains the enzyme lysozyme.

Nonetheless, the upper and lower respiratory tract appears to have their own set of microbiota. Pulmonary bacterial microbiota belong to 9 major bacterial genera: *Prevotella*, *Sphingomonas*, *Pseudomonas*, *Acinetobacter*, *Fusobacterium*, *Megasphaera*, *Veillonella*, *Staphylococcus*, and *Streptococcus*. Some of the bacteria considered "normal biota" in the respiratory tract can cause serious disease especially in immunocompromised individuals; these include *Streptococcus pyogenes*, *Haemophilus influenzae*, *Streptococcus pneumoniae*, *Neisseria meningitidis*, and *Staphylococcus aureus*.

Fungal genera that compose the pulmonary mycobiome include *Candida*, *Malassezia*, *Neosartorya*, *Saccharomyces*, and *Aspergillus*, among others.

Unusual distributions of bacterial and fungal genera in the respiratory tract is observed in people with cystic fibrosis. Their bacterial flora often contains antibiotic-resistant and slow-growing bacteria, and the frequency of these pathogens changes in relation to age.

DISEASE

Communities of microflora have been shown to change their behavior in diseased individuals.

Cancer

Although cancer is generally a disease of host genetics and environmental factors, microorganisms are implicated in ~20% of human malignancies. Mucosal microbes can become part of the tumor microenvironment (TME) of aerodigestive tract malignancies. Intratumoral microbes can affect cancer growth and spread. Gut microbiota also detoxify dietary components, reducing inflammation and balancing host cell growth and proliferation. Coley›s toxins were one of the earliest forms of cancer bacteriotherapy. Synthetic biology employs designer microbes and microbiota transplants against tumors. Microbes and the microbiota affect carcinogenesis in three broad ways: (i) altering the balance of tumor cell proliferation and death, (ii) regulating immune system function and (iii) influencing metabolism of host-produced factors, foods and pharmaceuticals.

Modes of Action

Ten microbes are designated by the International Agency for Research on Cancer (IARC) as human carcinogens. Most of these microbes colonize large percentages of the human population, although only genetically susceptible individuals develop cancer. Tumors arising at boundary surfaces, such as the skin, oropharynx and respiratory, digestive and urogenital tracts, harbor a microbiota, which complicates cancer-microbe causality. Substantial microbe presence at a tumor site does not establish association or causal links. Instead, microbes may find the tumor's oxygen tension or nutrient profile supportive. Decreased populations of specific microbes may also increase risks.

Human oncoviruses can drive carcinogenesis by integrating oncogenes into host genomes. Human papillomaviruses (HPV) express oncoproteins such as E6 and E7. Viral integration selectively amplifies host genes in pathways with established cancer roles.

Microbes affect genomic stability, resistance to cell death and proliferative signaling. Many bacteria can damage DNA, to kill competitors/survive. These defense factors can lead to mutational events that contribute to carcinogenesis. Examples include colibactin encoded by the *pks* locus (expressed by B2 group *Escherichia coli* as well as by other Enterobacteriaceae), *Bacteroides fragilis* toxin (Bft) produced by enterotoxigenic *B. fragilis* and cytolethal distending toxin (CDT) produced by several ε- and γ-proteobacteria. Colibactin is of interest in colorectal carcinogenesis, given the detection of pks^{+} *E. coli* in human colorectal cancers and the ability of colibactin-expressing *E. coli* to potentiate intestinal tumorigenesis in mice. Data also support a role for enterotoxigenic *B. fragilis* in both human and animal models of colon tumors. Both colibactin and CDT can cause double-stranded DNA damage in mammalian cells. In contrast, Bft acts indirectly by eliciting high levels of reactive oxygen species (ROS), which in turn damage host DNA. Chronically high ROS levels can outpace DNA repair mechanisms, leading to DNA damage and mutations.

β-catenin

Several microbes possess proteins that engage host pathways involved in carcinogenesis. The Wnt/β-catenin signaling pathway, which regulates cells' polarity, growth and differentiation, is one example and is altered in many malignancies. Multiple cancer-associated bacteria can influence β-catenin signaling. Oncogenic type 1 strains of *Helicobacter pylori* express CagA, which is injected directly into the cytoplasm of host cells and modulates β-catenin to drive gastric cancer. This modulation leads to up-regulation of cellular proliferation, survival and migration genes, as well as angiogenesis—all processes central to carcinogenesis. Oral microbiota *Fusobacterium nucleatum* is associated with human colorectal adenomas and adenocarcinomas and amplified intestinal tumorigenesis in mice. *F. nucleatum* expresses FadA, a bacterial cell surface adhesion component that binds host E-cadherin, activating β-catenin. Enterotoxigenic *B. fragilis*, which is enriched in some human colorectal cancers, can stimulate E-cadherin cleavage via Btf, leading to β-catenin activation. *Salmonella* Typhi strains that maintain chronic infections secrete AvrA, which can activate epithelial β-catenin signaling and are associated with hepatobiliary cancers. Several of these bacteria are normal microbiota constituents. The presence of these cancer-potentiating microbes and their access to E-cadherin in evolving tumors demonstrate that a loss of appropriate boundaries and barrier maintenance between host and microbe is a critical step in the development of some tumors.

Inflammation

Mucosal surface barriers are subject to environmental insult and must rapidly repair to maintain homeostasis. Compromised host or microbiota resiliency also reduce resistance to malignancy. Cancer and inflammatory disorders can then arise. Once barriers are breached, microbes can elicit proinflammatory or immunosuppressive programs.

Inflammation, whether high-grade as in inflammatory disorders or low-grade as in malignancies and obesity, drive a tumor-permissive milieu. Pro-inflammatory factors such as reactive oxygen and nitrogen species, cytokines and chemokines can also drive tumor growth and spread. Tumors can up-regulate and activate pattern recognition receptors (e.g. toll-like receptors), driving feedforward loops of activation of cancer-associated inflammation regulator NF-κB. Cancer-associated microbes appear to activate NF-κB signaling within the TME. The activation of NF-κB by *F. nucleatum* may be the result of pattern recognition receptor engagement or FadA engagement of E-cadherin. Other pattern recognition receptors, such as nucleotide-binding oligomerization domain–like receptor (NLR) family members *NOD-2*, *NLRP3*, *NLRP6* and *NLRP12*, may play a role in mediating colorectal cancer.

Immune system TME engagement is not restricted to the innate immune system. Once the innate immune system is activated, adaptive immune responses ensue, often with tumor progression. The interleukin-23 (IL-23)–IL-17 axis, tumor necrosis factor–α (TNF-α)–TNF receptor signaling, IL-6–IL-6 family member signaling, and STAT3 activation all represent innate and adaptive pathways contributing to tumor progression and growth.

The microbiota adapts to host changes such as inflammation. Adaptation shift microbiota to a vulnerable tissue site. Genotoxin azoxymethane and colon barrier–disrupting agent dextransodium sulfate independently result in colon tumors in susceptible mouse strains; combining them accelerates tumorigenesis.

Perturbations to a host immune system coupled with inflammatory stimulus may enrich bacterial clades that attach to host surfaces, invade host tissue, or trigger host inflammatory mediators. Fecal microbiota from *NOD2*- or *NLRP6*-deficient mice acquire features that enhance the susceptibility of wild-type mice to caCRC. In mice, gut microbiota modulate colon tumorigenesis, independent of genetic deficiencies. Germ-free mice developed more tumors when colonized from donors with caCRC, once followed by treatments that induced caCRC.

LUNG MICROBIOME

The **lung microbiota** (or pulmonary microbial community) is a complex variety of microbes found in the lower respiratory tract particularly on the mucus layer and the epithelial surfaces (the **lung microbiome** refer to their genomes). These lung microbes include bacteria, fungi, viruses and bacteriophages. The bacterial part of microbiome has been addressed more deeply. It consists of 9 core genera: *Prevotella*, *Sphingomonas*, *Pseudomonas*, *Acinetobacter*, *Fusobacterium*, *Megasphaera*, *Veillonella*, *Staphylococcus*, and *Streptococcus*. They are aerobes as well as anaerobes and aerotolerant bacteria. The microbial communities are highly variable in particular individuals and compose of about 140 distinct families. The bronchial tree for instance contains a mean of 2000 bacterial genomes per cm^2 surface. The harmful or potentially harmful bacteria are also detected routinely in respiratory specimens. The most significant are *Moraxella catarrhalis*, *Haemophilus influenzae*, and *Streptococcus pneumoniae*. They are known to cause respiratory disorders under particular conditions namely if the human immune system is impaired. The mechanism by which they persist in the lower airways in healthy individuals is unknown.

Fungal genera that are commonly found in the pulmonary microbiome include *Candida*, *Malassezia*, *Neosartorya*, *Saccharomyces*, and *Aspergillus*, among others.

Role of the Epithelial Barrier

The airway epithelium together with alveolar macrophages and dendritic cells play a major role in the initial recognition of bacterial products getting into the lower airways with the air. Since some of these products are potent proinflammatory stimuli it is extremely important for the immune system to distinguish between pathogens and non-pathogenic commensals. This prevents the development of constant inflammation and forms tolerance against harmless microbiota.

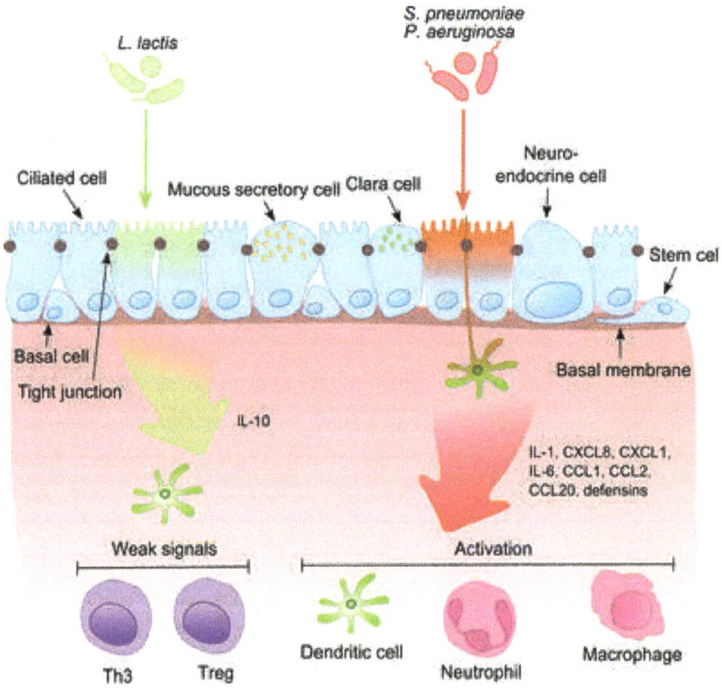

Mechanisms underlying inflammation. The airway epithelium has a complex structure consisting of at least seven diverse cell types interacting with each other by means of tight junctions. Epithelial cells can transmit immunostimulatory signals to underlying tissues taking part in the mechanisms of innate and adaptive immune response. The key transmitters of these signals are dendritic cells. Once pathogenic bacteria (e.g., *S. pneumoniae*, *P. aeruginosa*) have activated particular pattern recognition receptors on/in epithelial cells, the proinflammatory signaling pathways are activated. This results mainly in IL-1, IL-6 and IL-8 production. These cytokines induce chemotaxis to the site of infection in its target cells (e.g., neutrophils, dendritic cells and macrophages). On the other hand, representatives of standard microbiota induce only weak signals preventing inflammation. The mechanism of distinguishing between harmless and harmful bacteria on the molecular as well as on physiological levels is not completely understood.

This process becomes much more intriguing when taking into account that commensals often share their surface molecules with pathogens. Epithelial cells are equipped with very sensitive recognition tools - toll like receptors (TLRs), nucleotide-binding oligomerization domain (NOD)-like receptors (NLRs) and retinoic acid-inducible gene (RIG)-I-like receptors (RLRs) which recognize a broad variety of microbial structural components. After recognition of pathogenic bacteria proinflammatory pathways are activated and cellular components of the adaptive and innate immunity are recruited to the infection site. One key regulator in this process is the NF-κB which translocates from the cytoplasm into the nucleus and activates pro-inflammatory genes in epithelial cells and macrophages. The DNA-binding protein complex recognizes a discrete nucleotide sequence (5'-GGG ACT TTC T-3') in the upstream region of a variety of response genes. The activation of NF-κB by a number of stimuli: bacterial cell walls or inflammatory cytokines results in its translocation to the nucleus.

In contrast, harmless bacteria do not cause the translocation of NF-κB into the nucleus thus preventing the inflammation although they can express the same microbe-associated molecular patterns (MAMPs). One possible mechanism explaining this effect was suggested by Neish showing that non-pathogenic *S. typhimurium* PhoPc and *S. pullorum* are able to prohibit the ubiquitination of NF-κB inhibitor molecule nuclear factor of NF-κB light polypeptide gene enhancer in B-cells inhibitor alpha (IκB-κ). Another explanation of commensal tolerance of the epithelium refers to the post-translational modification of a protein by the covalent attachment of one or more ubiquitin (Ub) monomers. The inhibition of ubiquitination leads to reduction of inflammation, because only polyubiquitinated (IκB-κ is targeted for degradation by the 26 S proteasome, allowing NF-κB translocation to the nucleus and activation the transcription of effector genes (for example IL-8). Probiotic bacteria such as *Lactobacilli* are able to modulate the activity of the Ub-proteasome system via inducing reactive oxygen species (ROS) production in epithelial cells. In mammalian cells, ROS have been shown to serve as critical second messengers in multiple signal transduction pathways in response to proinflammatory cytokines. Bacterially induced ROS causes oxidative inactivation of the catalytic cysteine residue of Ub 12 resulting in incomplete but transient loss of cullin-1 neddylation and consequent effects on NF-κB and β-catenin signaling. Another commensal species, *B. thetaiotaomicron*, attenuates pro-inflammatory cytokine expression by promoting nuclear export of NF-κB subunit RelA, through a peroxisome proliferator activated receptor γ (PPAR-γ)-dependent pathway. PPAR-γ target transcriptionally active Rel A and induce early nuclear clearance limiting the duration of NF-κB action.

The balance between pathogens and commensals is extremely important in the maintenance of homeostasis in the respiratory tract.

Physiology

The airways are continually exposed to a multitude of microorganisms, some of which are able to persist and even colonize respiratory tract. This is possible due to the presence of nutrients, oxygen, and optimal growth temperature. There are several host-derived nutrient sources for microbial residents: secretions from airway epithelial cells (especially goblet cells), secretions from submucosal glands and transudate from plasma. Moreover, the pool of available nutrients is increased by the activities of some members of the microbiota. Macromolecular components of respiratory secretions (proteins, glycoproteins, lipids, nucleic acids) are converted to nutrients (e.g. carbohydrates, amino acids). Thus, the metabolic activity of present bacteria allow for the colonization of new species. The commensal bacteria are nonpathogenic and defend our airways against the pathogens. There are several possible mechanisms. Commensals are the native competitors of pathogenic bacteria, because they tend to occupy the same ecological niche inside the human body. Secondly, they are able to produce antibacterial substances called bacteriocins which inhibit the growth of pathogens.

Genera *Bacillus*, *Lactobacillus*, *Lactococcus*, *Staphylococcus*, *Streptococcus*, and *Streptomyces* are the main producers of bacteriocins in respiratory tract. Moreover, commensals are known to induce Th1 response and anti-inflammatory interleukin (IL)-10, antimicrobial peptides, FOXP3, secretory immunoglobulin A (sIgA) production.

Clinical Significance

Changes in microbial community composition seem to play a role in progression of such pulmonary disorders as chronic obstructive pulmonary disease (COPD), asthma, and cystic fibrosis. For example, presence of such genera as *Mycoplasma*, *Pseudomonas*, and *Staphylococcus* is correlated with stable COPD state. On the other hand, *Prevotella*, *Mesorhizobium*, *Microbacterium*, *Micrococcus*, *Veillonela*, *Rhizobium*, *Stenotrophomonas*, and *Lactococcus* present mostly in healthy individual cohort. The relative abundance of *Proteobacteria* is increased in asthmatic children. *Pseudomonas aeruginosa*, *Staphylococcus aureus*, and *Burkholderia cepacia* are found most often in cystic fibrosis patients.

High-throughput sequencing and the whole genome sequencing approaches will provide the further information about the complexity and physiological implication of commensal bacteria in the lower respiratory tract.

Oral Microbiology

Oral microbiology is the study of the microorganisms (microbiota) of the oral cavity and their interactions between oral microorganisms or with the host. The environment present in the human mouth allows the growth of characteristic microorganisms found there. It provides a source of water and nutrients, as well as a moderate temperature. Resident microbes of the mouth adhere to the teeth and gums to resist mechanical flushing from the mouth to stomach where acid-sensitive microbes are destroyed by hydrochloric acid.

Anaerobic bacteria in the oral cavity include: *Actinomyces*, *Arachnia*, *Bacteroides*, *Bifidobacterium*, *Eubacterium*, *Fusobacterium*, *Lactobacillus*, *Leptotrichia*, *Peptococcus*, *Peptostreptococcus*, *Propionibacterium*, *Selenomonas*, *Treponema*, and *Veillonella*. Genera of fungi that are frequently found in the mouth include *Candida*, *Cladosporium*, *Aspergillus*, *Fusarium*, *Glomus*, *Alternaria*, *Penicillium*, and *Cryptococcus*, among others. Bacteria accumulate on both the hard and soft oral tissues in biofilms. Bacterial adhesion is particularly important for oral bacteria.

Oral bacteria have evolved mechanisms to sense their environment and evade or modify the host. Bacteria occupy the ecological niche provided by both the tooth surface and gingival epithelium. However, a highly efficient innate host defense system constantly monitors the bacterial colonization and prevents bacterial invasion of local tissues. A dynamic equilibrium exists between dental plaque bacteria and the innate host defense system. Of particular interest is the role of oral microorganisms in the two major dental diseases: dental caries and periodontal disease. Additionally, research has correlated poor oral heath and the resulting ability of the oral microbiota to invade the body to affect cardiac health as well as cognitive function.

Oral Bacteria

Putative Periodontal Pathogens Presumptive Identification	% Cultivable Microbiota	ANTIBIOTIC RESISTANCE TESTING S = 100% in vitro inhibition at threshold value. R = resistant			
		Doxycycline 4 µg/ml	Amoxicillin 8 µg/ml	Metronidazole 16 µg/ml	Clindamycin 4 µg/ml
Actinobacillus actinomycetemcomitans	0.0				
Porphyromonas gingivalis	12.9	S	S	S	S
Prevotella intermedia group species	3.4	S	R	S	R
Peptostreptococcus micros	2.6	S	S	S	S
Streptococcus constellatus	0.0				
Streptococcus intermedius-anginosus	0.0				
Campylobacter (Wolinella) rectus	0.0				
Fusobacterium nucleatum	11.2	S	S	S	S
Tannerella (Bacteroides) forsythia	0.3	S	S	S	S
Enteric gram negative rods	13.8	R	R	R	R
Enterococcus faecalis	0.0				
Staphylococcus aureus	0.0				
Candida species (yeast)	0.0				

Microbial Morphotypes (% direct microscopic wet-mount count)		
Spirochetes	Non-motile rods	Other:
Motile rods	Cocci	

Oral Microbiology Lab Analysis Report.

The environment present in the human mouth allows the growth of characteristic microorganisms found there. It provides a source of water and nutrients, as well as a moderate temperature. Resident microbes of the mouth adhere to the teeth and gums to resist mechanical flushing from the mouth to stomach where acid-sensitive microbes are destroyed by hydrochloric acid.

Anaerobic bacteria in the oral cavity include: *Actinomyces*, *Arachnia*, *Bacteroides*, *Bifidobacterium*, *Eubacterium*, *Fusobacterium*, *Lactobacillus*, *Leptotrichia*, *Peptococcus*, *Peptostreptococcus*, *Propionibacterium*, *Selenomonas*, *Treponema*, and *Veillonella*.

The oral cavity of the new-born baby does not contain bacteria but rapidly becomes colonized with bacteria such as *Streptococcus salivarius*. With the appearance of the teeth during the first year colonization by *Streptococcus mutans* and *Streptococcus sanguinis* occurs as these organisms colonise the dental surface and gingiva. Other strains of streptococci adhere strongly to the gums and cheeks but not to the teeth. The gingival crevice area (supporting structures of the teeth) provides a habitat for a variety of anaerobic species. Bacteroides and spirochetes colonize the mouth around puberty. Of particular interest is the role of oral microorganisms in the two major dental diseases: dental caries and periodontal disease.

Fusospirochetes

Spirochetes and fusi-form bacilli live as normal flora in the mouth, but in the case of bleeding in the oral cavity, the bacteria can cause infection and diseases to oral cavity:

- Acute necrotizing ulcerative gingivitis (ANUG)
- Vincent angina with a membrane covering the throat area

Veillonella

Veillonella are gram-negative anaerobic cocci. It is thought that this species thrives in the acidic environment of caries and is thought to slow the development of dental caries. It converts the acidic products of other species to less acidic products.

Actinobacillus actinomycetemcomitans

Actinobacillus actinomycetemcomitans is considered an oral pathogen due to its virulence factors, its association with localized aggressive periodontitis in young adolescents, and studies indicating that it can cause bone loss.

Lactobacillus

Some *Lactobacillus* species have been associated with dental cavities although these bacteria are normally symbiotic in humans and are found in the gut flora.

Dental Plaque

Dental plaque is the material that adheres to the teeth and consists of bacterial cells (mainly *S. mutans* and *S. sanguis*), salivary polymers and bacterial extracellular products. Plaque is a biofilm on the surfaces of the teeth. This accumulation of microorganisms subject the teeth and gingival tissues to high concentrations of bacterial metabolites which results in dental disease. If not taken care of, via brushing or flossing, the plaque can turn into tartar (its hardened form) and lead to gingivitis or periodontal disease.

Cell-cell Communication

Most of the bacterial species found in the mouth belong to microbial communities, called biofilms, a feature of which is inter-bacterial communication. Cell-cell contact is mediated by specific protein adhesins and often, as in the case of inter-species aggregation, by complementary polysaccharide receptors. Another method of communication involves cell-cell signalling molecules, which are of two classes: those used for intra-species and those used for inter-species signalling. An example of intra-species communication is quorum sensing. Oral bacteria have been shown to produce small peptides, such as competence stimulating peptides, which can help promote single-species biofilm formation. A common form of inter-species signalling is mediated by 4, 5-dihydroxy-2, 3-pentanedione (DPD), also known as autoinducer-2 (Al-2).

Vaccination Against Oral Infections

In the case of dental caries, proteins involved in colonization of teeth by *Streptococcus mutans* can produce antibodies that inhibit the cariogenic process.

Other Microbiota

Bacteria species typically associated with oral flora have been found to be present in women with bacterial vaginosis.

Genera of fungi that are frequently found in the mouth include *Candida*, *Cladosporium*, *Aspergillus*, *Fusarium*, *Glomus*, *Alternaria*, *Penicillium*, and *Cryptococcus*, among others.

Role in Non-oral Disease

Additionally, research has correlated poor oral heath and the resulting ability of the oral microbiota to invade the body to affect cardiac health as well as cognitive function.

REFERENCES

1. Origin: • Endogenous • Microbial
2. Consortium of Scientists Map the Human Body›s Bacterial Ecosystem. ucsf.edu.
3. Mouth bacteria can change its diet, supercomputers reveal. medicalxpress.com.
4. NIH Human Microbiome Project defines normal bacterial makeup of the body. NIH News. 13 June 2012.
5. Abeles, Shira R.; Robles-Sikisaka, Refugio; Ly, Melissa; Lum, Andrew G.; Salzman, Julia; Boehm, Tobias K.; Pride, David T. (2014-09-01). Human oral viruses are personal, persistent and gender-consistent. The ISME Journal. 8 (9): 1753–1767. doi:10.1038/ismej.2014.31. ISSN 1751-7362. PMC 4139723 . PMID 24646696.
6. Alison Abbott for Nature News. Jan 8 2016 Scientists bust myth that our bodies have more bacteria than human cells
7. American Academy of Microbiology FAQ: Human Microbiome January 2014
8. Antonio, M. A. D.; Hawes, S. E.; Hillier, S. L. (1999). The Identification of VaginalLactobacillusSpecies and the Demographic and Microbiologic Characteristics of Women Colonized by These Species. The Journal of Infectious Diseases. 180 (6): 1950–1956. doi:10.1086/315109. PMID 10558952.
9. Erdogan A, Rao SS (April 2015). Small intestinal fungal overgrowth. Curr Gastroenterol Rep. 17 (4): 16. doi:10.1007/s11894-015-0436-2. PMID 25786900.
10. NIH Human Microbiome Working Group (2009). The NIH Human Microbiome Project. Genome Res. 19 (12): 2317–2323. doi:10.1101/gr.096651.109. PMC 2792171. PMID 19819907.
11. Cavicchioli R, Curmi P, Saunders N, Thomas T (2003). Pathogenic archaea: do they exist?. BioEssays. 25 (11): 1119–28. doi:10.1002/bies.10354. PMID 14579252.
12. Chyan YJ, Poeggeler B, Omar RA, Chain DG, Frangione B, Ghiso J, Pappolla MA (1999).

13. Cui L, Morris A, Ghedin E (July 2013). The human mycobiome in health and disease. Genome Med. 5 (7): 63. doi:10.1186/gm467. PMC 3978422. PMID 23899327. Figure 2: Distribution of fungal genera in different body sites

14. Duncan SH, Louis P, Flint HJ (2007). Cultivable bacterial diversity from the human colon. Lett. Appl. Microbiol. 44 (4): 343–50. doi:10.1111/j.1472-765X.2007.02129.x. PMID 17397470.

15. Eckburg P, Lepp P, Relman D (2003). Archaea and their potential role in human disease. Infection and Immunity. 71 (2): 591–6. doi:10.1128/IAI.71.2.591-596.2003. PMC 145348. PMID 12540534.

16. Eckburg PB, Bik EM, Bernstein CN, et al. (2005). Diversity of the human intestinal microbial flora. Science. 308 (5728): 1635–8. Bibcode:2005Sci...308.1635E. doi:10.1126/science.1110591. PMC 1395357. PMID 15831718.

17. Faderl, M; et al. (Apr 2015). Keeping bugs in check: The mucus layer as a critical component in maintaining intestinal homeostasis. IUBMB Life. 67 (4): 275–85. doi:10.1002/iub.1374. PMID 25914114.

18. Falony G, Vieira-Silva S, Raes J (2015). Microbiology Meets Big Data: The Case of Gut Microbiota-Derived Trimethylamine. Annu. Rev. Microbiol. 69: 305–321. doi:10.1146/annurev-micro-091014-104422. PMID 26274026. we review literature on trimethylamine (TMA), a microbiota-generated metabolite linked to atherosclerosis development.

19. Florin TH, Zhu G, Kirk KM, Martin NG (2000). Shared and unique environmental factors determine the ecology of methanogens in humans and rats. Am. J. Gastroenterol. 95 (10): 2872–9. doi:10.1111/j.1572-0241.2000.02319.x. PMID 11051362.

20. Fox, Chelsea; Eichelberger, Kacey (2015). Maternal microbiome and pregnancy outcomes. Fertility and Sterility. 104 (6): 1358–1363. doi:10.1016/j.fertnstert.2015.09.037. ISSN 0015-0282. PMID 26493119.

21. Franasiak, Jason M.; Scott, Richard T. (2015). Reproductive tract microbiome in assisted reproductive technologies. Fertility and Sterility. 104 (6): 1364–1371. doi:10.1016/j.fertnstert.2015.10.012. ISSN 0015-0282. PMID 26597628.

22. g Quigley, EM (2013). Gut bacteria in health and disease. Gastroenterol Hepatol (N Y). 9 (9): 560–9. PMC 3983973. PMID 24729765.

23. Gaci N, Borrel G, Tottey W, O›Toole PW, Brugère JF (November 2014). Archaea and the human gut: new beginning of an old story. World J. Gastroenterol. 20 (43): 16062–16078. doi:10.3748/wjg.v20.i43.16062. PMC 4239492. PMID 25473158. Trimethylamine is exclusively a microbiota-derived product of nutrients (lecithin, choline, TMAO, L-carnitine) from normal diet, from which seems originate two diseases, trimethylaminuria (or Fish-Odor Syndrome) and cardiovascular disease through the proatherogenic property of its oxidized liver-derived form.

24. Grice, Elizabeth A.; Kong, HH; Conlan, S; Deming, CB; Davis, J; Young, AC; NISC Comparative Sequencing Program; Bouffard, GG; et al. (2006). Topographical and Temporal Diversity of the Human Skin Microbiome. Science. 324 (5931): 1190–2. Bibcode:2009Sci...324.1190G. doi:10.1126/science.1171700. PMC 2805064. PMID 19478181.

25. Hamady, M.; Knight, R. (2009). Microbial community profiling for human microbiome projects: Tools, techniques, and challenges. Genome Research. 19 (7): 1141–1152. doi:10.1101/gr.085464.108. PMID 19383763.

26. Hannigan, Geoffrey D.; Meisel, Jacquelyn S.; Tyldsley, Amanda S.; Zheng, Qi; Hodkinson, Brendan P.; SanMiguel, Adam J.; Minot, Samuel; Bushman, Frederic D.; Grice, Elizabeth

A. (2015-10-30). The Human Skin Double-Stranded DNA Virome: Topographical and Temporal Diversity, Genetic Enrichment, and Dynamic Associations with the Host Microbiome. MBio. 6 (5): e01578–15. doi:10.1128/mBio.01578-15. ISSN 2150-7511. PMC 4620475. PMID 26489866.

27. Human Microbiome Project Consortium (2012). A framework for human microbiome research. Nature. 486 (7402): 215–221. Bibcode:2012Natur.486..215T. doi:10.1038/nature11209. PMC 3377744. PMID 22699610.

28. Judah L. Rosner for Microbe Magazine, Feb 2014. Ten Times More Microbial Cells than Body Cells in Humans?

29. Katherine Harmon (16 December 2009). Bugs Inside: What Happens When the Microbes That Keep Us Healthy Disappear?. Scientific American. Retrieved 27 December 2008.

30. Kuczynski, J.; et al. (2011). Experimental and analytical tools for studying the human microbiome. Nature Reviews Genetics. 13 (1): 47–58. doi:10.1038/nrg3129. PMID 22179717.

31. Lavigne, Jean-Philippe; Sotto, Albert; Dunyach-Remy, Catherine; Lipsky, Benjamin A. (2015). New Molecular Techniques to Study the Skin Microbiota of Diabetic Foot Ulcers. Advances in Wound Care. 4 (1): 38–49. doi:10.1089/wound.2014.0532. ISSN 2162-1918. PMC 4281861. PMID 25566413.

32. Lepp P, Brinig M, Ouverney C, Palm K, Armitage G, Relman D (2004). Methanogenic Archaea and human periodontal disease. Proc. Natl. Acad. Sci. U.S.A. 101 (16): 6176–81. Bibcode:2004PNAS..101.6176L. doi:10.1073/pnas.0308766101. PMC 395942. PMID 15067114.

33. Ly, Melissa; Abeles, Shira R.; Boehm, Tobias K.; Robles-Sikisaka, Refugio; Naidu, Mayuri; Santiago-Rodriguez, Tasha; Pride, David T. (2014-07-01). Altered Oral Viral Ecology in Association with Periodontal Disease. MBio. 5 (3): e01133–14. doi:10.1128/mBio.01133-14. ISSN 2150-7511. PMC 4030452. PMID 24846382.

34. Marcon MJ, Powell DA (1 April 1992). Human infections due to Malassezia spp. Clin. Microbiol. Rev. 5 (2): 101–19. PMC 358230. PMID 1576583.

35. Minot, Samuel; Sinha, Rohini; Chen, Jun; Li, Hongzhe; Keilbaugh, Sue A.; Wu, Gary D.; Lewis, James D.; Bushman, Frederic D. (2011-10-01). The human gut virome: inter-individual variation and dynamic response to diet. Genome Research. 21 (10): 1616–1625. doi:10.1101/gr.122705.111. ISSN 1549-5469. PMC 3202279. PMID 21880779.

36. Monaco, Cynthia L.; Gootenberg, David B.; Zhao, Guoyan; Handley, Scott A.; Ghebremichael, Musie S.; Lim, Efrem S.; Lankowski, Alex; Baldridge, Megan T.; Wilen, Craig B. (2016-03-09). Altered Virome and Bacterial Microbiome in Human Immunodeficiency Virus-Associated Acquired Immunodeficiency Syndrome. Cell Host & Microbe. 19 (3): 311–322. doi:10.1016/j.chom.2016.02.011. ISSN 1934-6069. PMC 4821831. PMID 26962942.

37. Noble JM, Scarmeas N, Papapanou PN (2013). Poor oral health as a chronic, potentially modifiable dementia risk factor: review of the literature.. Curr Neurol Neurosci Rep. 13 (10): 384. doi:10.1007/s11910-013-0384-x. PMID 23963608.

38. Norman, Jason M.; Handley, Scott A.; Baldridge, Megan T.; Droit, Lindsay; Liu, Catherine Y.; Keller, Brian C.; Kambal, Amal; Monaco, Cynthia L.; Zhao, Guoyan (2015-01-29). Disease-specific alterations in the enteric virome in inflammatory bowel disease. Cell. 160 (3): 447–460. doi:10.1016/j.cell.2015.01.002. ISSN 1097-4172. PMC 4312520. PMID 25619688.

39. Onderdonk, A. B.; Zamarchi, G. R.; Walsh, J. A.; Mellor, R. D.; Muñoz, A.; Kass, E. H. (1986). Methods for quantitative and qualitative evaluation of vaginal microflora during menstruation. Applied and Environmental Microbiology. 51 (2): 333–339. PMC 238869. PMID 3954346.
40. PLoS Human Microbiome Project Collection Manuscript Summaries June 13, 2012
41. Roth RR, James WD (1988). Microbial ecology of the skin. Annu. Rev. Microbiol. 42 (1): 441–64. doi:10.1146/annurev.mi.42.100188.002301. PMID 3144238.
42. Schwiertz, Andreas (2016). Microbiota of the human body : implications in health and disease. Switzerland: Springer. p. 1. ISBN 978-3-319-31248-4.
43. Sender, R; Fuchs, S; Milo, R (Jan 2016). Are We Really Vastly Outnumbered? Revisiting the Ratio of Bacterial to Host Cells in Humans. Cell. 164 (3): 337–40. doi:10.1016/j.cell.2016.01.013. PMID 26824647.
44. Sherwood, Linda; Willey, Joanne; Woolverton, Christopher (2013). Prescott›s Microbiology(9th ed.). New York: McGraw Hill. pp. 713–721. ISBN 9780073402406. OCLC 886600661.
45. Sutter, V. L. (1984). Anaerobes as normal oral flora. Reviews of infectious diseases. 6 Suppl 1: S62–S66. doi:10.1093/clinids/6.Supplement_1.S62. PMID 6372039.
46. Tap, Julien; Mondot; et al. (2009). Towards the human intestinal microbiota phylogenetic core. Environmental Microbiology. 11 (102): 2574–2584. doi:10.1111/j.1462-2920.2009.01982.x. PMID 19601958.
47. The Human Microbiome Project Consortium (2012). Structure, function and diversity of the healthy human microbiome. Nature. 486 (7402): 207–214. Bibcode:2012Natur.486..207T. doi:10.1038/nature11234. PMC 3564958. PMID 22699609.
48. The Normal Bacterial Flora of Humans. textbookofbacteriology.net.
49. Beringer, P M; M D Appleman (November 2000). Unusual respiratory bacterial flora in cystic fibrosis: microbiologic and clinical features (PDF). Current Opinion in Pulmonary Medicine. 6 (6): 545–550. doi:10.1097/00063198-200011000-00015. ISSN 1070-5287. PMID 11100967.
50. Clarke, G; et al. (Aug 2014). Minireview: Gut microbiota: the neglected endocrine organ. Mol Endocrinol. 28 (8): 1221–38. doi:10.1210/me.2014-1108. PMID 24892638.
51. Garrett, Wendy S. (3 April 2015). Cancer and the microbiota. Science Magazine. doi:10.1126/science.aaa4972. Retrieved 2015-06-29.
52. Zhang LS, Davies SS (April 2016). Microbial metabolism of dietary components to bioactive metabolites: opportunities for new therapeutic interventions. Genome Med. 8 (1): 46. doi:10.1186/s13073-016-0296-x. PMC 4840492. PMID 27102537. Lactobacillus spp. convert tryptophan to indole-3-aldehyde (I3A) through unidentified enzymes . Clostridium sporogenes convert tryptophan to IPA , likely via a tryptophan deaminase. ... IPA also potently scavenges hydroxyl radicals
53. Table 2: Microbial metabolites: their synthesis, mechanisms of action, and effects on health and disease
54. Figure 1: Molecular mechanisms of action of indole and its metabolites on host physiology and disease
55. Witkin, S. S.; Linhares, I. M.; Giraldo, P. (2007). Bacterial flora of the female genital tract: Function and immune regulation. Best Practice & Research Clinical Obstetrics & Gynaecology. 21 (3): 347–354. doi:10.1016/j.bpobgyn.2006.12.004. PMID 17215167.

56. Martins N, Ferreira IC, Barros L, Silva S, Henriques M (June 2014). Candidiasis: predisposing factors, prevention, diagnosis and alternative treatment. Mycopathologia. 177 (5–6): 223–240. doi:10.1007/s11046-014-9749-1. PMID 24789109. Candida species and other microorganisms are involved in this complicated fungal infection, but Candida albicans continues to be the most prevalent. In the past two decades, it has been observed an abnormal overgrowth in the gastrointestinal, urinary and respiratory tracts, not only in immunocompromised patients, but also related to nosocomial infections and even in healthy individuals. There is a widely variety of causal factors that contribute to yeast infection which means that candidiasis is a good example of a multifactorial syndrome.

57. Petrova, Mariya I.; Lievens, Elke; Malik, Shweta; Imholz, Nicole; Lebeer, Sarah (2015). Lactobacillus species as biomarkers and agents that can promote various aspects of vaginal health. Frontiers in Physiology. 6. doi:10.3389/fphys.2015.00081. ISSN 1664-042X.

58. Rogers A H (editor). (2008). Molecular Oral Microbiology. Caister Academic Press. ISBN 978-1-904455-24-0.

59. to:a b Shen S, Wong CH. Bugging inflammation: role of the gut microbiota. Clin Transl Immunology. 2016 Apr;5(4):e72. Review. doi:10.1038/cti.2016.12 PMID 27195115 PDF

60. Sommer, F; Bäckhed, F (Apr 2013). The gut microbiota--masters of host development and physiology. Nat Rev Microbiol. 11 (4): 227–38. doi:10.1038/nrmicro2974. PMID 23435359.

61. Todar, Kenneth (2012). The Normal Bacterial Flora of Humans. Todar›s Online Textbook of Bacteriology. Madison, WI: Kenneth Todar. Retrieved 2012-04-06.

62. Vestheim, H.; Jarman, S. N. (2008). Blocking primers to enhance PCR amplification of rare sequences in mixed samples – a case study on prey DNA in Antarctic krill stomachs. Frontiers in Zoology. 5: 12. doi:10.1186/1742-9994-5-12. PMC 2517594. PMID 18638418.

63. Wang H, Lee IS, Braun C, Enck P (July 2016). Effect of probiotics on central nervous system functions in animals and humans - a systematic review. J. Neurogastroenterol Motil. doi:10.5056/jnm16018. PMID 27413138.

64. Wang ZK, Yang YS, Stefka AT, Sun G, Peng LH (April 2014). Review article: fungal microbiota and digestive diseases. Aliment. Pharmacol. Ther. 39 (8): 751–766. doi:10.1111/apt.12665. PMID 24612332.

65. Wassenaar, T.M.; Panigrahi, P. (2014). Is a foetus developing in a sterile environment?. Letters in Applied Microbiology. 59 (6): 572–579. doi:10.1111/lam.12334. ISSN 0266-8254. PMID 25273890.

66. Wikoff WR, Anfora AT, Liu J, Schultz PG, Lesley SA, Peters EC, Siuzdak G (2009). Metabolomics analysis reveals large effects of gut microflora on mammalian blood metabolites. Proc. Natl. Acad. Sci. U.S.A. 106 (10): 3698–703. doi:10.1073/pnas.0812874106. PMC 2656143. PMID 19234110. Production of IPA was shown to be completely dependent on the presence of gut microflora and could be established by colonization with the bacterium Clostridium sporogenes.

67. IPA metabolism diagram

68. Young, J. C.; Chehoud, C.; Bittinger, K.; Bailey, A.; Diamond, J. M.; Cantu, E.; Haas, A. R.; Abbas, A.; Frye, L. (2015-01-01). Viral metagenomics reveal blooms of anelloviruses in the respiratory tract of lung transplant recipients. American Journal of Transplantation: Official Journal of the American Society of Transplantation and the American Society of Transplant Surgeons. 15 (1): 200–209. doi:10.1111/ajt.13031. ISSN 1600-6143. PMC 4276431. PMID 25403800.

CHAPTER 9

Human Virome

Chapter Contents

Low-cost DNA sequencing has greatly democratized genomics, especially for the typically very small genomes of viruses. The recent acceleration in human virus discovery by metagenomics indicates that many viruses escaped prior detection due to limitations of preexisting technologies. It is now conceivable that all viral species commonly infecting human (i.e., the human virome) will soon be determined.

INTRODUCTION

Human virome is the collection of viruses in and on the human body. Defining the virome is thought to provide an understanding of microbes and how they affect human health and disease. Viruses in the human body infect both human cells as well as other microbes such as bacteria. For instance, many viruses (the bacteriophages) actually infect bacteria. Some viruses cause infections, while others may be asymptomatic. Certain viruses are integrated in the human genome. Viruses evolve rapidly and hence the human virome changes constantly. Every human being has a unique virome with a unique balance of species.Lifestyle, age, geographic location, and even the season of the year affects an individual›s exposure to viruses; while their susceptibility to disease is effected by preexisting immunity and both viral and human genetics. The human virome is far from being completely explored and new viruses are discovered frequently.

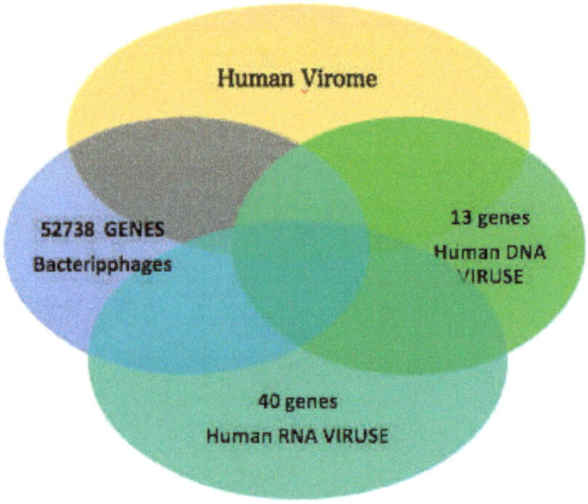

Figure 1: Diversity of human virus genomes sequences in NCBI /Gene (as of date 11-14-2016)

DIVERSITIES OF VIROME

Methods and Tools

Multiple methods are available for the isolation and study of human viruses. Deep sequencing: Deep sequencing is a rapid DNA sequencing technique that is useful for characterizing virome richness, stability, gene function and the association with disease phenotypes. This technology creates large amounts of sequence information and is capable of detecting rare components of a microbial community. Current methods combining the removal of human and bacterial DNA from samples, large scale sequencing, and bioinformatics are very efficient in the identification of unknown viruses. Unlike other discovery methods, viruses do not need to be grown in cell cultures. Without any prior knowledge of genome sequence or growth methods, novel viruses can be discovered. Therefore deep sequencing is well suited for rapid identification of an unknown or unexpected viruses involved in a disease outbreak or associated with conditions not thought to be caused by viruses. Deep sequencing also allows for large scale screenings with minimal hands on effort. A systematic exploration of the viruses that infect humans (the human virome) is important and feasible with these methods.

Polymerase chain reaction: Polymerase chain reaction is a tool to amplify and detect specific DNA sequences. It can be used to help characterize the virome, but it is limited by the need for at least partial DNA sequence information. The Human Metagenome: The Human Metagenome includes all organisms that live on or in us. Viruses contribute to the metagenome and establish chronic infection that infest chromosomes; this method will formulate new estimate of the number of genes that confer susceptibility to a given virus and specify alleles for some viruses.

ELISA: Large scale antibody studies with ELISA using donated blood could help to determine human exposure to particular viruses in different geographic regions.

Diversity of human viruses

The human virome is not stable and may change over time. In fact, new viruses are discovered constantly. With an increasing number of known viruses, diagnosis and treatment of novel viral-associated conditions will become easier as well. Lastly, studying the virome could help improve drug development and limit antibiotic usage.

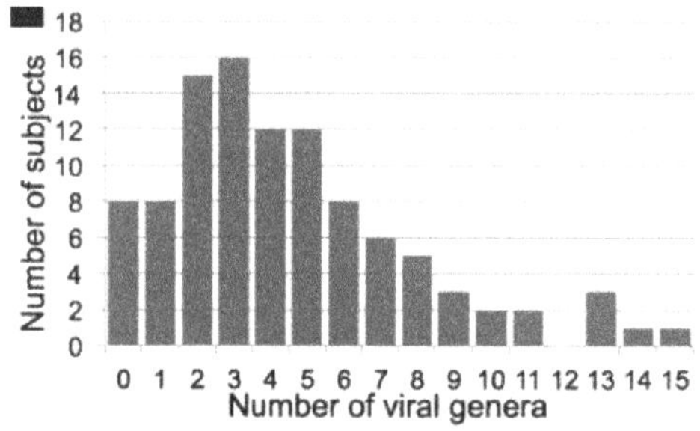

Figure 2:The human virome in healthy, asymptomatic adults. The histogram shows the number of individuals (x-axis) who were positive for a given number of different viral genera (y-axis).

One of the first studies that used high-throughput DNA sequencing to describe the diversity of eukaryotic dsDNA viruses in normal individuals included 706 samples from 102 subjects. This study detected an average of 5.5 viral genera in each individual and these viruses included herpesviruses, papillomaviruses,polyomaviruses, adenoviruses, anelloviruses, parvoviruses, and circoviruses. Each individual had a distinct viral profile, demonstrating the high interpersonal diversity of the virome. One to 15 viral genera (average 5.5) were detected in 92% of the 102 individuals sampled (Figure 2). Figure 3 illustrates the viromes of the 102 individuals defined by sampling up to five major body habitats, showing that a broad range of viruses was detected in healthy people (Figure 3).

The 102 individuals carried seven distinct families of human DNA viruses (Figure 4A). Sequences were detected predominantly in the nose and skin, similarity to 17 papillomavirus genera.Roseoloviruses, predominantly HHV-7 and to a lesser extent HHV-6, were present among 98% of the individuals who provided mouth samples.

In addition, the same viruses were prevalent in multiple body habitats within individuals. For instance, the beta- and gamma-papillomaviruses were the viruses most commonly found in the skin and the nose (anterior nares; Figure 4A,B), which may reflect proximity and similarities in microenvironments that support infection with these viruses.

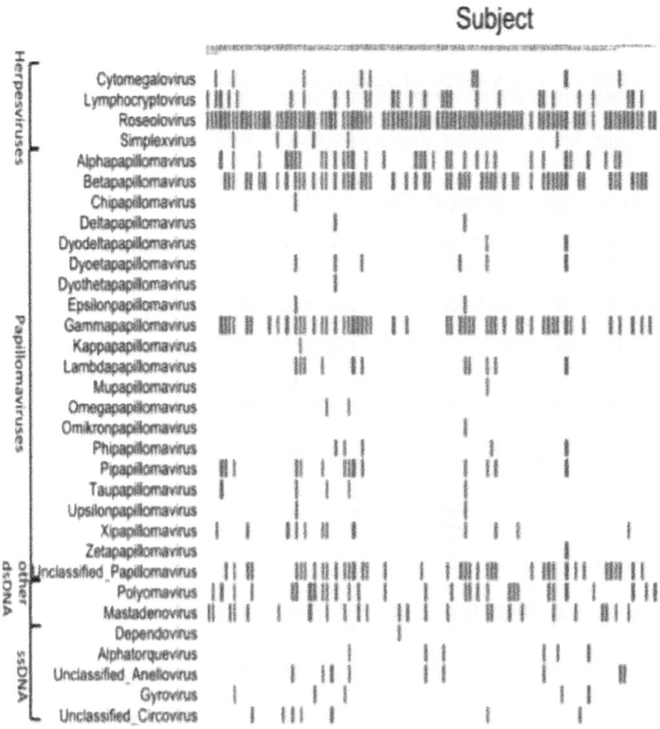

Figure 3: The human virome in healthy, asymptomatic adults.The viral genera (x-axis) detected in each subject (y-axis) are represented by black bars. The virome of each individual is viewed by looking at the black bars in a given row.

Impact the Human Health

The human virome is a part of our bodies and will not always cause harm. Many latent and asymptomatic viruses are present in the human body all the time. Viruses infect all life forms; therefore the bacterial, plant, and animal cells and material in our gut also carry viruses. When viruses cause harm by infecting the cells in the body, a symptomatic disease may develop. Contrary to common belief, harmful viruses may be in the minority compared to benign viruses in the human body. It is much harder to identify viruses than it is to identify bacteria, therefore our understanding of benign viruses in the human body is very rudimentary.

The health effects of viruses on an individual are dependent on the individual›s immune system.

The hygiene hypothesis

Recent research has linked the emerging idea of the hygiene hypothesis to viruses. This hypothesis attempts to explain and justify some of the high incidences of diseases such as asthma and eczema in the Western world to Western society's overuse of antibiotic and antiviral agents. This overuse potentially disrupts not only the bacteria of the gut but also the viruses that have long lived in harmony with the human body and now play a role in regulation of human health. This hypothesis generally refers to microorganisms but is now being extended to include airborne viruses and common viral infections of childhood that are becoming increasingly less common.

Effect of skin location

Diverse viruses colonize the human skin and differ by skin site. These skin virome includes human viruses (i.e. Human Papillomavirus) and bacteriophages (bacterial viruses) that infect commensal skin bacteria such as Staphylococci. Virus communities differ by moisture levels and degree of protection from the external environment.

Effect of diet

Many studies have demonstrated that the bacteria and viruses in the human gut (the gut microbiome) can be altered by changes in diet. One study that focused on bacterial viruses, called bacteriophages, in the gut found a significant relationship between diet and the type of bacteriophages present. This was done by comparing the distance between bacteriophage gut communities in individuals both before and after they started a controlled diet. The results were that the distance between the bacteriophage gut communities of individuals on the same diet was significantly smaller at the end of their dietary treatment than it was at the start, while there was no increase in community similarity for individuals on different diets over time.

REFERENCES

1. "bacteriophage - Gene - NCBI". www.ncbi.nlm.nih.gov. Retrieved 2016-11-15.
2. "Human AND RNA Virus - Gene - NCBI". www.ncbi.nlm.nih.gov. Retrieved 2016-11-15.
3. Wylie, Kristine M.; Mihindukulasuriya, Kathie A.; Zhou, Yanjiao; Sodergren, Erica; Storch, Gregory A.; Weinstock, George M. (2014-01-01). "Metagenomic analysis of double-stranded DNA viruses in healthy adults". BMC Biology. 12: 71.doi:10.1186/s12915-014-0071-7. ISSN 1741-7007. PMC 4177058 . PMID 25212266.
4. Williams, S. C. P. (6 February 2013). "The other microbiome". Proceedings of the National Academy of Sciences. 110 (8): 2682–2684. doi:10.1073/pnas.1300923110.
5. Wylie, Kristine M.; Weinstock, George M.; Storch, Gregory A. (1 October 2012). "Emerging view of the human virome". Translational Research. 160 (4): 283–290.doi:10.1016/j.trsl.2012.03.006.
6. Delwart, Eric; Racaniello, Vincent (14 February 2013). "A Roadmap to the Human Virome". PLoS Pathogens. 9 (2): e1003146. doi:10.1371/journal.ppat.1003146.
7. Dalke, Kate. "The Human Virome". Genome News Network. Retrieved 2 April

2013.

8. Fontana, Judith M.; Alexander, Elizabeth; Salvatore, Mirella. “Translational research in infectious disease: current paradigms and challenges ahead”. Translational Research. 159(6): 430–453. doi:10.1016/j.trsl.2011.12.009.
9. Foxman, Ellen F.; Iwasaki, Akiko (1 April 2011). “Genome–virome interactions: examining the role of common viral infections in complex disease”. Nature Reviews Microbiology. 9 (4): 254–264. doi:10.1038/nrmicro2541.
10. Hannigan, Geoffrey D.; Meisel, Jacquelyn S.; Tyldsley, Amanda S.; Zheng, Qi; Hodkinson, Brendan P.; SanMiguel, Adam J.; Minot, Samuel; Bushman, Frederic D.; Grice, Elizabeth A. (2015-10-30). “The Human Skin Double-Stranded DNA Virome: Topographical and Temporal Diversity, Genetic Enrichment, and Dynamic Associations with the Host Microbiome”. mBio. 6 (5): e01578–15. doi:10.1128/mBio.01578-15.ISSN 2150-7511. PMC 4620475 . PMID 26489866.
11. Zimmer, Carl. “Your Inner Lions: Get to Know Your Virome”. National Geographic. Retrieved 29 April 2013.
12. Allander, T. (6 September 2005). “From The Cover: Cloning of a human parvovirus by molecular screening of respiratory tract samples”. Proceedings of the National Academy of Sciences. 102 (36): 12891–12896. doi:10.1073/pnas.0504666102. PMC 1200281 .PMID 16118271.
13. Anderson, Norman G.; Gerin, John L.; Anderson, N. Leigh (1 July 2003). “Global Screening for Human Viral Pathogens”. Emerging Infectious Diseases. 9 (7): 768–773.doi:10.3201/eid0907.030004.
14. Butler, Christopher C (September 2013). “Asthma prevalence and humoral immune response in Somali immigrants in the US: implications for the hygiene hypothesis.”.Primary Care Respiratory Journal: Journal of the General Practice Airways Group. 22 (3): 262–264. doi:10.4104/pcrj.2013.00081.
15. Daley, D (October 2014). “The evolution of the hygiene hypothesis: the role of early-life exposures to viruses and microbes and their relationship to asthma and allergic diseases.”.Current opinion in allergy and clinical immunology. 14 (5): 390–396.doi:10.1097/ACI.0000000000000101.
16. Focà, Alfredo; Liberto, Maria Carla; Quirino, Angela; Marascio, Nadia; Zicca, Emilia; Pavia, Grazia (2015-01-01). “Gut Inflammation and Immunity: What Is the Role of the Human Gut Virome?”. Mediators of Inflammation. 2015. doi:10.1155/2015/326032.ISSN 0962-9351. PMC 4405218 . PMID 25944980.
17. Grice, Elizabeth A.; Kong, Heidi H.; Conlan, Sean; Deming, Clayton B.; Davis, Joie; Young, Alice C.; Program, NISC Comparative Sequencing; Bouffard, Gerard G.; Blakesley, Robert W. (2009-05-29). “Topographical and Temporal Diversity of the Human Skin Microbiome”. Science. 324 (5931): 1190–1192. doi:10.1126/science.1171700.ISSN 0036-8075. PMC 2805064 . PMID 19478181.
18. Handley, SA, Thackray, LB, Zhao, G, Presti, R, Miller, AD, Droit, L, Abbink, P, Maxfield, LF, Kambal, A, Duan, E, Stanley, K, Kramer, J, Macri, SC, Permar, SR, Schmitz, JE, Mansfield, K, Brenchley, JM, Veazey, RS, Stappenbeck, TS, Wang, D, Barouch, DH, Virgin, HW (Oct 12, 2012). “Pathogenic simian

immunodeficiency virus infection is associated with expansion of the enteric virome.". Cell. 151 (2): 253–66.doi:10.1016/j.cell.2012.09.024. PMID 23063120.

19. Kristensen, David M.; Mushegian, Arcady R.; Dolja, Valerian V.; Koonin, Eugene V."New dimensions of the virus world discovered through metagenomics". Trends in Microbiology. 18 (1): 11–19. doi:10.1016/j.tim.2009.11.003. PMC 3293453 .PMID 19942437.

20. Minot, S.; Sinha, R.; Chen, J.; Li, H.; Keilbaugh, S. A.; Wu, G. D.; Lewis, J. D.; Bushman, F. D. (31 August 2011). "The human gut virome: Inter-individual variation and dynamic response to diet". Genome Research. 21 (10): 1616–1625. doi:10.1101/gr.122705.111.

21. Pennisi, E. (24 March 2011). "Going Viral: Exploring the Role Of Viruses in Our Bodies".Science. 331 (6024): 1513–1513. doi:10.1126/science.331.6024.1513. PMID 21436418.

22. Pride, David T; Salzman, Julia; Haynes, Matthew; Rohwer, Forest; Davis-Long, Clara; White, Richard A; Loomer, Peter; Armitage, Gary C; Relman, David A (8 December 2011). "Evidence of a robust resident bacteriophage population revealed through analysis of the human salivary virome". The ISME Journal. 6 (5): 915–926. doi:10.1038/ismej.2011.169.

23. Strachan, David P (June 10, 2014). "Siblings, Asthma, Rhinoconjunctivitis And Eczema: A Worldwide Perspective From The International Study Of Asthma And Allergies In Childhood.". Clinical and Experimental Allergy. 45: 126–136. doi:10.1111/cea.12349.

24. Thurber, Rebecca V; Haynes, Matthew; Breitbart, Mya; Wegley, Linda; Rohwer, Forest."Laboratory procedures to generate viral metagenomes". Nature Protocols. 4 (4): 470–483. doi:10.1038/nprot.2009.10.

25. Virgin, Herbert W.; Wherry, E. John; Ahmed, Rafi (1 July 2009). "Redefining Chronic Viral Infection". Cell. 138 (1): 30–50. doi:10.1016/j.cell.2009.06.036.

26. Woolhouse, M.; Scott, F.; Hudson, Z.; Howey, R.; Chase-Topping, M. (10 September 2012). "Human viruses: discovery and emergence". Philosophical Transactions of the Royal Society B: Biological Sciences. 367 (1604): 2864–2871. doi:10.1098/rstb.2011.0354.

Index